Health Education

Foundations for the Future

Health Education
Foundations for the Future

Laurna Rubinson, Ph.D.

Associate Professor, Department of Health and Safety,
University of Illinois, Urbana-Champaign,
Champaign, Illinois

Wesley F. Alles, Ph.D.

Associate Professor, Health Education Department,
The Pennsylvania State University,
University Park, Pennsylvania

with 44 illustrations

TIMES MIRROR/MOSBY College Publishing

St. Louis • Toronto • Santa Clara   1984

Editor: Nancy K. Roberson
Assistant editor: Michelle A. Turenne
Manuscript editor: Mark Spann
Design: Diane Beasley
Production: Carolyn Biby, Teresa Breckwoldt, Judith England

Library of Congress Cataloging in Publication Data

Main entry under title:

Health education.

    Bibliography: p.
    Includes index.
    1. Health education. I. Rubinson, Laurna.
II. Alles, W.F. [DNLM: 1. Health education. 2. Health
promotion. WA 590 H4345]
RA440.H365 1984   613'.07'1   83-17357
ISBN 0-8016-4233-7

GW/VH/VH 9 8 7 6 5 4 3 2 1   01/C/075

Contributors

William H. Creswell, Jr., Ed.D.

Professor,
Department of Health and Safety,
University of Illinois,
Champaign, Illinois

Lawrence W. Green, Dr. P.H.

Director, Center for Health Promotion, Research and Development;
Professor, Medical School and School of Public Health,
University of Texas, Health Science Center,
Houston, Texas

Donald C. Iverson, Ph.D.

Director, Health Promotion/Disease Prevention Programs,
Mercy Medical Center,
Denver, Colorado

Richard Lussier, Dr. P.H.

Professor of Health Education,
University of California at Long Beach,
Long Beach, California

Samuel Monismith, D.Ed.

Assistant Professor of Health Education,
Pennsylvania State University,
University Park, Pennsylvania

James J. Neutens, Ph.D.

Associate Professor,
Department of Health Sciences,
Western Illinois University,
Macomb, Illinois

Richard W. St. Pierre, Ed.D.

Chairman and Associate Professor of Health Education,
Pennsylvania State University,
University Park, Pennsylvania

v

Janet A. Shirreffs, Ph.D.
Associate Professor,
Health Science Department,
Arizona State University,
Tempe, Arizona

Robert Shute, D.Ed.
Associate Professor of Health Education,
Pennsylvania State University,
University Park, Pennsylvania

To

My parents, Fred and Sylvia Goldberg

L.R.

To

My family, whose encouragement
and love enabled me to contribute
to this project.

W.A.

Preface

This book is designed to provide a generic introduction for students enrolled in programs of professional preparation in health education. From the beginning of the project we had three major purposes. First, we wanted to spark an appreciation for the heritage of past efforts and for the challenges that remain ahead of us. Second, we wanted to provide a text that students would find helpful as they embark on a career in health education. Finally, we wanted to engender a feeling on the part of the reader that there is an underlying philosophy and set of competencies unique to health education that are shared by many others who have chosen a career in this emerging profession.

Regardless of a person's areas of specialization, there are commonalities shared by all of us because we are health educators. Throughout our presentation we explore the various health settings: the community, the school, the hospital, and the worksite. As offspring of more established professions, notably education, medicine, and the behavioral sciences, it is not always easy to envision the specific qualities of our own field. Nor is it easy to feel a part of a profession when there are so many career paths available to those who share the title of health educator. But a sense of identity is important because it is the collective abilities of those who are now studying health education that will shape the future of the profession. They should be proud of their title and be prepared to assume positions of leadership in order to advance the profession. It is hoped that this textbook presents something of the nature of health education by considering its history, philosophy, current and future issues, and competencies related to program planning, teaching, research, evaluation, and advocacy.

Major Features

There have been other books whose purposes were similar to ours. However, this book contains several important pedagogical features that will enhance the teaching-learning process. The most significant feature is that the book is composed of chapters that were written by leading health educators from across the country. Each person contributed in an area of personal interest and each is considered to be an expert in that particular aspect of health education. This contributing author concept brings greater breadth of perspective than could have been presented by any one author.

Several helpful *learning aids* included throughout the text will enhance students' understanding of the content. Each chapter contains an *introduction* to help focus the reader's attention on important ideas. The *chapter summary* helps to clarify these concepts through a brief reiteration. To add perspective, the editors provide *end-of-chapter analysis* of issues considered to be of prime importance to the practitioner. *Discussion questions* are presented at the end of each chapter to facilitate dialogue among students. The questions encourage students to consider the personal meaning of each chapter, and as such make interesting out-of-class assignments for in-class discussion. Additional *suggested readings* from the current literature have been selected by the editors. The readings will add even more perspective to the concepts presented in this textbook. A *glossary* of key terms is provided to assist students in interpreting major concepts. Numerous *appendixes* supplement the content by providing useful and detailed information. The appendixes include:

Promoting health-preventing disease: objectives for the nation
Government-sponsored health promotion programs
Protection, prevention, and health promotion
Federal health information clearinghouses
Sample worksite health promotion programs
Employee health promotion resource lists
Educational materials available from three voluntary health agencies

This work will be appreciated by students and teachers who prefer a textbook that stimulates learning through introspection, discussion, and reflection rather than by trying to convey the impression that, having read the book, the student has nothing left to do but take the test and pass the course. Learning is not limited to the words contained on the pages between the covers. A good textbook can never replace a good teacher. A college course should never be recalled in the student's mind by the textbook that was used in the course. The purposes of a textbook are to stimulate thinking and to facilitate an exchange of ideas. We think *Health Education: Foundation for the Future* will achieve these purposes.

Acknowledgments

Many people have enabled us to develop this textbook from its conception to its completion. Our first debt of gratitude is to Chuck Hirsch, who believed in the concept and encouraged us with the project. Nancy Roberson, our editor, who ably completed the project, has provided both insight and forethought. Nancy's assistant, Michelle Turenne, has kept the text moving on schedule and has graciously dealt with the many details of publication. Mark Spann did an excellent job of editing the manuscript.

This text would never have been possible without the contributors. They all are provocative writers, excellent scholars, and humanitarians. We do appreciate their patience and understanding in the arduous process of manuscript preparation.

For their thoughtful suggestions and constructive criticisms, we would also like to thank the reviewers who received the many drafts of the manuscript: Marian V. Hamburg, Ed.D., New York University; Altha M. Crouch, Ed.D., and Linda Sue King, Ph.D., both of the University of New Mexico; James H. Dotson, Jr., University of Maryland; Stuart W. Fors, Ph.D., University of Georgia; Debra L. Sutton, University of Northern Colorado; Mal Goldsmith, Ph.D., Southern Illinois University at Edwardsville; and Alice Ennis, State University of New York College at Brockport.

Finally, we would like to note our appreciation to our students and colleagues, for without their influence on our careers this text would never have been possible.

Laurna Rubinson
Wesley F. Alles

Contents

Health Education
Foundations for the Future

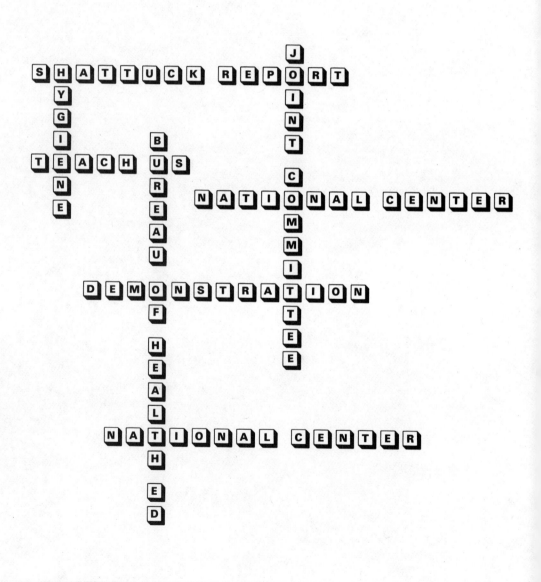

1 History of Health Education

Introduction

This textbook appropriately begins with a look through history at the people and events that have helped shape our profession. It has been a long, winding road from ancient superstitions and formal codes of health to the contemporary role of health education in the 1980s. Professor Lussier describes how our profession emerged from the European traditions of education and physical education, the public health movement at the turn of this century, and the development of twentieth century medicine. Gradually the "blood and bones" study of hygiene gave way to a more exciting, relevant, and educationally prudent approach to the study of individual health behavior. The struggle for professional identity that has persisted for decades (also discussed in Chapter 4) is nearly over, and health education stands on the threshold of a great future. As health educators of the future you are about to make your own contributions to the profession. This chapter is a tribute to those pioneering health educators who have created the opportunity that lies ahead.

Professor Lussier offers a chronology of important events in the evolution of health education. The following is a brief calender of events to help guide your reading of this chapter.

1837	The first of Horace Mann's *Annual Reports* campaigned for mandatory programs of hygiene.
1850	*Report of the Sanitary Commission of Massachusetts*, better known as the Shattuck Report, called for public health reforms and mandatory hygiene education.
1850-1900	The creation of voluntary agencies and professional associations to promote health, education, and professional preparation.
1901	Thomas D. Wood, M.D., who has been called the father of health education, established a program of professional preparation in hygiene at Columbia University.
1901	The first of many White House conferences on the health of children.
1911	Creation of the Joint Committee on Health Problems in Education (NEA and AMA), a forum for the study of innovative ideas.
1918	Establishment of the American Child Health Association to protect and improve the health of children.
1921	The Summerville and Malden Studies were conducted by Clair Turner to clarify the status and role of health education.
1931	The Cattagaugus Study, directed by Ruth Grout, studied the impact of health education and the competency of health teachers.
1934	Mary Spencer, the first student to complete all three degree programs in health education, was awarded a Ph.D. by Columbia University.
1936	The Astoria Study was directed by Dorothy Nyswander. Although the focus was on school health services it had an impact on all aspects of the school health program.

1943	The School Community Health Project in Michigan demonstrated the effectiveness of a comprehensive school-community health program.
1944	The School Community Health Project in California demonstrated the effectiveness of a comprehensive school-community health program.
1945	The Denver Interest Study, a needs assessment for the development of curriculum, was conducted.
1948	National Conference on Undergraduate Professional Preparation in Health, Physical Education and Recreation identified competencies needed by the health educator.
1949	The first U.S. Office of Education Conference on Undergraduate Professional Preparation of Students majoring in health education was directed by H.F. Kilander.
1950	The National Conference on Graduate Study in Health, Physical Education and Recreation established guidelines for graduate education.
1950	The official beginning of the Society of Public Health Educators (SOPHE).
1950	Mid-Century White House Conference on Children and Youth recommended greater emphasis of health education in the school curriculum and quality instruction achieved through adequately prepared teachers.
1953	Creation of the U.S. Department of Health, Education, and Welfare.
1954	The School Health Education Evaluation Study in Los Angeles examined the effects of comprehensive school health education.
1956	Two College Health conferences were chaired by Edward B. Johns; the first one analyzed health content and methodology and the second one studied the professional preparation of school health educators.
1958	The Inter-Agency Conference on School Health Education recommended effective communication among the various elements involved in health education.
1959	The Highland Park Conference established commissions to study specific issues; committee Chairs included Delbert Oberterffer on philosophy, Sarah Louise Smith and Edward B. Johns on health instruction, Fred Hein on research, Charlotte Leach on intergroup relationships, and William Creswell on accreditation.
1961	The School Health Education Study (SHES) surveyed nearly 1 million students nationwide and initiated the writing of a K-12 curriculum guide.
1966	The Committee on Graduate Curriculum in Health Education offered recommendations for a core curriculum that included health science, behavioral science, education, and research.
1969	Teach Us What We Want to Know, a needs and interest survey of 5000 Connecticut students, was directed by Ruth Byler.
1971	Coalition of National Health Organizations was formed to mobilize the resources of the profession.
1971	President's Committee on Health Education was established.
1974	Bureau of Health Education within the Centers for Disease Control.
1976	Office of Health Information, Health Promotion, Physical Fitness and Sports Medicine created by PL 94-317.
1978	National Center for Health Education facilitated the Role Delineation Project.
1978	Office of Comprehensive School Health within the Department of Education created by PL 95-561.
1978	Conference on the Commonalities and Differences in the Preparation and Practice of Health Educators held in Bethesda, Md.; it led to the National Task Force on the Preparation and Practice of Health Educators.
1980	The *Initial Role Delineation for Health Education, Final Report* published.

| 1980-1982 | Further national efforts halted as a result of cutbacks in federal funding. |
| 1981 | National Conference for Institutions Preparing Health Educators Role Delineation Conference held in Birmingham, Alabama. |

The Beginnings

Health education has an ancient and complex history. Its beginnings can be located within the very foundation of civilization. Much of the early history of the profession closely parallels that of medicine and its associated sciences. In later times, particularly since 1800, the history of health education has taken on a richness and character uniquely its own.

Let us go back to the distant past, to that time when history begins to fade into speculation, and examine the genesis of health education. When the earliest societies emerged from independent families into gatherer-hunter communities people began to examine the forces that were shaping their lives. Two forces that they were able to identify were illness and death. Although unable to identify the specific cause and effect relationship that led to illness and death, they were nevertheless able to determine that disease had some relationship to illness and death and therefore should be avoided. They also recognized that some members of the community lived longer than others. It was believed that people with great longevity must have had some special knowledge that enabled them to remain healthy and alive. This belief is still reflected in the fact that people who survive into their 80s and beyond are frequently asked to reveal their secret of longevity. In primitive civilizations the survivors were respected and revered. Eventually the status of such survivors evolved to that of headmen or shamans whose role was to define and enforce the taboos of the culture. Compliance with taboos was believed to result in a longer and healthier life.

Superstition evolved through taboos and mores to become laws that shaped public policy. The headmen gradually emerged as leaders who ultimately became the institutional heads. The evolution of superstition into scientific fact and the role of shamans into what we call teachers, doctors, and other health specialists comprises the history of health education. Although much of this history lies outside the purview of this book, it is nevertheless important for the sake of continuity to identify some of the people and events that constitute landmarks in this long and eventful history.

The earliest traces of the history of health are found among paleontologic relics. They are composed of wall paintings, artifacts, and trephined skulls. The oldest written documents related to health are the Smith Papyri dating from 1600 BC, which describe various surgical techniques.

It described forty-eight cases in clinical surgery, from cranial fractures to injuries of the spine. Each case is treated in logical order, under the heads of provisional diagnosis, examination, semeiology, diagnosis, prognosis, treatment, and glosses on the term used.[1]

This modest document is followed by The Code of Hammurabi, which contains the earliest medical fee schedule and serves as proof of the existence of an organized system of medicine 4000 years ago.

Ancient writings, particularly those of Homer, credit the god Asclepius with superior knowledge and ability in medicine. Legend slowly developed around the great healer. The cult of Asclepius gradually spread throughout Greece until more than 200 temples, or Asclepia, were known. Visitors to the Asclepia included the sick of course but also perhaps even greater numbers of healthy persons who came to worship in order to ensure their good health.[1] Members of the cult of Asclepius believed in maintaining health as well as in curing illness. Fom the Asclepia the great healers began to emerge: Susruta (the first of many great Indian physicians), Hippocrates (the father of modern medicine), Galen (the first great anatomist), Rhazes (the first to write about diseases of children), Vesalius (the father of modern anatomy), and Roger of Salerno (the father of hygiene), who laid down his *Gemimen Sanitas,* or rules of healthful living, which served as the beginnings of the science of hygiene. The temples and cult of Asclepius (500 BC to 500 AD) have left their symbol as a permanent reminder of the past—the staff and serpent of the physician known as the caduceus.

The Dark Ages were replaced with the vitality and dynamism of the Renaissance. The Renaissance, having gradually lost its vitality was replaced by an era of religious reformation. As the Reformation ended medical science and health care began an age of discovery and innovation. More than anything else this era after 1650 was characterized by the dominance of science and the replacement of superstition with the analysis of cause and effect. The latter half of the seventeenth century also saw the emergence of leaders in medicine. Anton van Leeuwenhoek (developer of the microscope) was a man whose single-minded dedication to discovery opened a window, albeit a window as tiny as the eyepiece of a microscope, through which others like Morgagni (father of pathology) and Malpighi (discoverer of the function of capillaries) would see.

During the eighteenth century John Hunter (father of modern surgery) initiated a more orderly exploration of the workings of the human body. His work eventually resulted in a systematic assault on chronic disease. Phillippe Pinel (an early supporter of the humane treatment of the emotionally disturbed) fostered the recognition that abnormal behavior is an illness that can be cured. During the mid-nineteenth century philosophers were reexamining the essays of eighteenth century European philosophers such as

Diderot, Locke, Rousseau, and Voltaire, all of whom promoted the worth of each human life and the importance of individual health for the well-being of society. People such as Pasteur, Lister, and Koch are associated with the germ theory of disease. Their scientific studies helped to change the nature of morbidity, mortality, and medical technique. Thus medicine and philosophy combined to improve the health of society and plant the seeds of a new profession known as health education.

Health Education in the United States

From the time of the earliest permanent settlements in North America (1607) issues of health were of major concern. In colonial America physicians were struggling against disease. Scholars were seeking "the good life," for themselves and for their fellow citizens. In 1760 New York state passed a law requiring the licensing of all physicians. This was one of the earliest official documents relating to health in America. In the last third of the eighteenth century additional laws were passed that had a significant impact on health. One such law, promulgated in 1770 by the Continental Congress, required physical education for all men found to be unfit to bear arms. This law was created as a result of the French and Indian Wars and established in the same year as the Boston Massacre; obviously the Continental Congress recognized the approaching need for healthy citizens to defend their freedom. From such beginnings came the early relationship between health education and physical education.

Germany was well ahead of the United States in the study of exercise and human movement. The Turnverein (German fitness organizations) and other physical activity–oriented programs were enjoying great popularity. It is not surprising to discover that in 1792 the first course related to the study of hygiene came from this culture and that an instructional guide that gained popularity throughout Europe was translated into English. Copies brought to the United States from England quickly became popular; by 1798 copies were being printed in New York. Thus hygiene, the earliest form of health education in the United States, owed its initial popularity to a text from Europe. As the nineteenth century began health instruction was present in the public schools as part of the physical education curriculum.

During the first half of the nineteenth century education established itself as a profession. There were an increasing number of colleges, known as normal schools, that specialized in the training of teachers. This formal training in pedagogy demonstrated that classroom instructors were in need of special skills not found among the general population, even among the learned within the population. Soon the specialized training in teacher preparation became even more specialized as programs evolved according to content areas. People were not only studying to become teachers but also to become science teachers, English teachers, history teachers, and health and physical education teachers. This professionalization was important because it helped enhance the role of the teacher and demonstrate the value of instruction by specialists in each area of study.

A great spokesman for education appeared in the person of Horace Mann, whose writings and speeches helped to promote the importance of education and the role of the educator in the learning process. Mann, who had become a member of the Massachusetts legislature in 1827 and Secretary of the State Board of Education in 1837, would ultimately be recognized as one of the great educational reformers in history. He directly contributed to improvements in school construction, instructional materials and equipment, classroom instruction, and teacher training. Beginning in 1837 with the publication of his *First Annual Report* and continuing through the publication of the *Sixth Annual Report* in 1843, Mann campaigned for mandatory programs of hygiene that would result in all students having an understanding of their bodies and the relationship between their conduct and health.

Health education began to grow because of leaders who were able to envision the positive outcomes for society. These were people who popularized their ideas through personal contact and the written word. William Alcott was such a person. Alcott, who was born in 1798, the same year the Marine Hospital Service was established, was an educational reformer who first became interested in providing a healthful school environment. This initial interest gradually broadened so that eventually he was concerned about the total health of the school-aged child. Alcott popularized his ideas through a series of essays and books published between 1829 and 1850. Samuel Hall wrote the first text on professional preparation for hygiene in 1823. The publication of the *Report of the Sanitary Commission of Massachusetts,* commonly referred to as the Shattuck Report,[2] had a significant impact on health education. This report was written by Lemuel Shattuck and had as a part of its text a bold call for mandatory instruction in hygiene. It also promoted the idea that hygiene was absolutely necessary for achieving "the good life." It further described a strategy for implementing education for healthful living.

Consolidation and Growth (1850-1900)

From 1850 to 1900 the growth of public health was marked by a number of significant events. In 1859 the American Dental Association was founded; in 1861 the United States Sanitary Commission was established; in 1864 the International Red Cross was created; in 1869 the first State Board of Health was established in Massachusetts; in 1872 the American Public Health As-

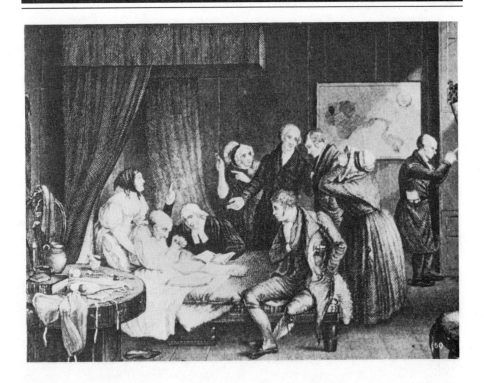

Fig. 1-1. Changing patterns of disease in America have created the need for a shift in the nature of health education. (From Eddy, J.M., and Alles, W.F.: Death education, St. Louis, 1983, The C.V. Mosby Co.)

sociation was founded and the first City Board of Health was created in Boston; and in 1881 the American Red Cross was founded. Against this backdrop of progress the potential for health education began to be recognized.

From 1850 to approximately 1880 education in hygiene could best be described as going through a period of consolidation. The growth of hygiene-related instruction in secondary and elementary schools had slowed. A number of diverse views were emerging as to what instruction in hygiene should include and what its focus should be. At the college and university level, however, hygiene was continuing to experience steady growth in the number of institutions that offered instruction. Health education was for the most part limited to the college curriculum. Public health education and public school curricula were strictly confined to principles of personal hygiene.

Another indicator of the consolidation occurring in hygiene at this time was the emergence of professional organizations that included within their membership many persons who were actively engaged in teaching hygiene.

The American Public Health Association (APHA) began in 1872. The National Teacher's Association was founded in 1857. This organization, which had among its early members many teachers of hygiene and physical education, changed its name in 1907 to the National Education Association (NEA). Because of the close association between hygiene and physical education another organization, known as the American Association for Health, Physical Education and Recreation (AAHPER), came into existence in 1885. Not only was hygiene taught in more colleges and universities than ever before but also those who taught the subject now had professional meetings they could attend. These meetings provided a forum for discussion and for the exchange of ideas regarding the teaching of hygiene.

In 1874 an increased public concern with the use of drugs, particularly alcohol and tobacco, resulted in the creation of the Women's Christian Temperance Union. Mary H. Hunt, one of the leaders of the organization, had been a teacher and believed the schools provided a perfect forum to teach an impressionable audience. The Women's Christian Temperance Union directed a great deal of its efforts to the passage of laws that would require health instruction on the "evils" of alcohol, tobacco, and drugs in the nation's schools. Their efforts were so successful that by 1890 all states had established requirements that the effects of alcohol, tobacco, and drugs be taught in public schools. The impact on health education was threefold. First, the number of hygiene classes being taught throughout the country increased dramatically. Second, the content of hygiene classes began a process of diversification. And last, these requirements set the precedent for tying instruction to contemporary health problems of public concern. This phenomenon would occur repeatedly in the history of health education, as with such topical concerns as venereal disease, human sexuality, teenage pregnancy, and mental health.

In the 1890s another major event affected school health education. The Medical Inspection Program brought illness care specialists (doctors, nurses, and dentists) into the schools to conduct examinations of schoolchildren. This practice had a profound effect on the concept of health education. Health education was not only a matter of instruction by the classroom teacher; its overall goal of child health could be enhanced through school health services and a healthful school environment.

From Hygiene to Health Education (1900-1920)

Although the teaching of hygiene in the early 1900s was enjoying more widespread influence than in the past, there was disenchantment with the term itself, largely as a result of the teaching methods used by many hygiene teachers and the "blood and bones" nature of its curriculum. Hygiene was

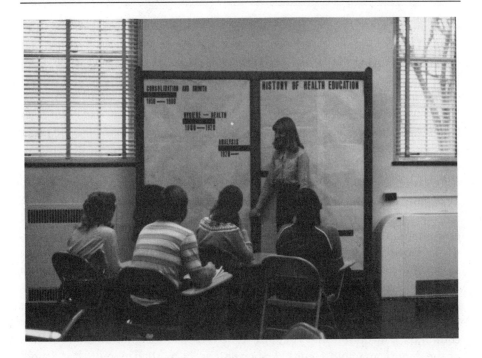

Fig. 1-2. Health education has experienced significant growth since 1850. Historical perspective enhances one's appreciation of the profession.

coming under increasing attack for its sterility and proscriptiveness. The very word *hygiene* was beginning to take on an undesirable connotation. Ideas for change came from three sources: (1) related educational disciplines such as physical education and the life sciences, (2) professional conferences, and (3) the increased pool of teachers who had been prepared to teach hygiene.

From physical education came the message that hygiene was a crucial part of its educational responsibility and a subject that should be included in all school programs. The life sciences, including medicine, gave strong and consistent support for hygiene education. The primary concern voiced by these professionals was that accurate information needed to be transferred to people who were learning to make important life decisions. The American School Hygiene Association held 12 meetings between its founding date in 1906 and the year 1920. The focus of these meetings was on the improvement of school hygiene wherever it was being taught.

In 1909 the first of many White House Conferences on the Health of Children was held. These meetings, held at roughly 10-year intervals, provided a forum for significant changes in health education. The Joint Committee on Health Problems in Education, composed of representatives of the American Medical Association (AMA) and the NEA, was assembled in 1911. This committee was crucial to the changes occurring in hygiene, not only because it focused attention on the role of public education in fostering health nor because it represented a marriage between two major forces (education and medicine) but also because it provided a highly respected forum for the publication of new and innovative ideas in the field. The Joint Committee helped demonstrate that public schools had an obligation to provide students with health instruction, health services, and a healthy environment. The information and experiences received as a child would inspire good health practices as an adult.

In 1901 Thomas D. Wood, M.D., formerly a faculty member at Sanford University, arrived at Columbia university to establish a program in physical education and hygiene. He remained at the university for 30 years and his work helped to establish health education as a discipline. Wood played a significant role in almost all of the events in health education from 1900 to 1940 and has been called the father of health education. His accomplishments were many. He served as chairman of the previously mentioned Joint Committee of the AMA and NEA. He held this chairmanship from the committee's inception in 1911 until 1938. He also was one of the founders of the American Child Health Association and was chairman of the "School and the Child" committee at the 1930 White House Conference on Child Health. Wood's greatest contribution, however, was the development of programs of professional preparation for school teachers in health education. His work at Columbia University resulted in the development of the finest undergraduate and graduate programs in hygiene (and eventually in health education) in the country. At that time, Wood prepared students who were to become the new leaders in school health education. Professional preparation programs such as those at Columbia University and Georgia State College for Women, which established the first undergraduate major in hygiene, resulted in a vast improvement in the professional preparation of hygiene teachers.

In 1918 the American Child Health Association (ACHA) was established. This body was committed to protecting and improving the health of children. Although this organization was health oriented, it had a somewhat different view of how individual health could be improved. Rather than didactic teaching of basic hygiene its membership believed that people should be taught to make decisions about their health behavior, an extremely different approach from memorization of facts. This reorientation away from rigid content and a curriculum that proscribed specific behaviors to one that emphasized the interrelationship between knowledge and decision making was significant. Whereas the hygiene group had tried to teach "correct" behavior, the ACHA wanted to help people become health educated so they could make appropriate decisions to enhance the quality of their lives.

The idea of health education had been maturing since the late 1800s, but it was through the ACHA that it became a reality. In 1918 this new orientation away from hygiene instruction and toward instruction for health was termed *health education* by Sally Lucas Jean, director of the association. As with most transitions it would take years before health education replaced hygiene in many schools and universities. Health education had reached a new plateau in its progress, and hygiene/health education had achieved new popularity in public schools. Professional programs were being developed in colleges and universities, and professionals were emerging in the field who would accelerate the growth of the profession and serve as models for young people who would be the leaders of the future.

Earlier in this chapter it was mentioned that during the late 1800s medical inspection programs became popular in schools. These programs gradually evolved into what were called demonstration projects. A demonstration project is an experiment that attempts to demonstrate the viability of a concept or idea. If the demonstration is successful, the hope is that other programs will use the pilot test as evidence that the project is worthwhile. The first demonstration project in health education is believed to have occurred in 1914. Additional demonstrations were to occur at increasingly frequent intervals as they became more popular through the mid-1930s. The importance of these demonstrations to health education was that they provided a visible activity to popularize and spread the concept of health education.

Analysis and Synthesis (1920-1935)

The period from 1920 to 1935 is best described as one of analysis and synthesis. Research studies and demonstration projects conducted in these years played an important part in clarifying the role of health education. An ambitious project was begun in Malden, Massachusetts, as the result of a 1921 pilot study conducted in Sumerville, Massachusetts, by Clair Turner. This research, known as the Malden Study, was an attempt to analyze the practicability and effectiveness of health instruction and the relative merits of various teaching strategies. In a report on the study issued in 1928 Turner stated "the health education program proved to be a sound, practicable, and acceptable public school procedure. Definite improvement in health habits was shown."[3]

Responding to the continued public concern about the poor health of many who had applied for service in the armed forces in World War I, President Warren G. Harding appointed the Committee of Fifty on College

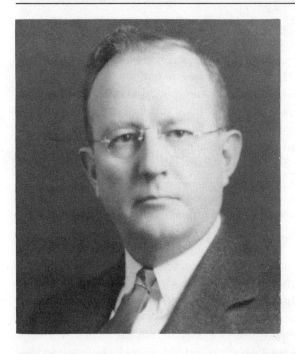

Fig. 1-3. Clair Turner served as the first president of SOPHE in 1950. Earlier he had directed the Malden Study, which began in 1921. (Courtesy Association for the Advancement of Health Education.)

Hygiene. This committee was composed primarily of university and college presidents and had as its goal the development of health education in normal schools, colleges, and universities. In 1927, in an effort to clarify the situation, Thomas Storey, M.D., Director of Hygiene and Physical Education at Stanford University, wrote *The Status of Hygiene Programs in Institutions of Higher Education in the United States.*[4] The report described as deplorable the minor role being given health education in the curriculum of colleges and universities. Another study sponsored by the National Tuberculosis Association in 1924 reported that there was a lack of sufficient training of health educators in teacher preparation institutions.[5]

The Cattaraugus Study took place in New York under the auspices of the Milbank Memorial Fund.[6] It was directed by Dr. Ruth Grout, who was later known for her leadership in health education programs at the University of Minnesota. The Cattaraugus Study began in 1931 and was completed in 1936. Its objectives were to evaluate the influence of health education on student behavior, the effects of a health program on a school environment, and the competency of health teachers. The study found that in the area of behavior change among students

The difference in the results of health knowledge tests to both groups was small but moderately significant statistically. The Cattaraugus County group made slightly better scores than did the control group for nearly every field of subject matter. The older pupils, under the influence of the school for a longer period, showed greater changes in certain habits over the four-year period than the younger pupils who were closer to the influences of the home.[7]

The effects of the health education program on the school environment were found to be positive. As for teacher performance in health education, it was determined that there was a correlation between the amount and quality of training the teacher had received and the teacher's performance as a health education teacher.

Apparently the education of teachers was especially effective in creating an awareness of the more desirable types of incentives to healthful living. In every respect, however, the experimental group was rated somewhat higher by judges who did not know the group to which the individual records belonged.[8]

This study and others conducted during this era provided an increasingly sophisticated data base that health educators could use for program evaluation and as evidence that health education can have a positive influence on the knowledge and health behavior of young people exposed to school health education.

Health demonstration projects, which had come into vogue in the early 1900s, continued to be valuable devices for popularizing health education. Their basic goal was to demonstrate the effectiveness of properly designed health programs. During the 1920s and 1930s there were a number of such demonstrations. Those of particular significance were in Fargo, North Dakota; Salem, Oregon; Clark County and Athens, Georgia; Rutherford County, Tennessee; and Mansfield and Richland Counties in Ohio. Of particular note were the demonstration projects held in Ohio and Oregon because Walter H. Brown, M.D., was the director of both projects.

Brown, a former "horse and buggy" doctor and health officer who became a dynamic teacher, was the inspiration for health education programs on the West Coast. He directed the Mansfield, Ohio, and Salem, Oregon, Child Health Demonstrations that offered health services for children and showed the importance of these services to parents. From Salem Dr. Brown went on to establish the first complete health education professional preparation program at Stanford University. After his retirement from Stanford he designed and developed the School of Public Health at Berkeley, California. It was his positive influence that led to the development of the University of California Department of Public Health and Health Education at UCLA. This department later became the School of Public Health. Through the programs he developed, the professional standards he established, and the many professional health education students he inspired and prepared Brown continues to be a force in health education.

To leave this period of time without mentioning two additional events would be irresponsible. The first was the publication in 1924 of a book titled *Health Education, A Program For Public Schools And Teacher Training Institutions* issued by the Joint Committee of the NEA and AMA.[9] This book, a report of research on the school health program and its major curricular issues, was a milestone. It is probably the most important document written on the subject of school health education to date and served as a set of guidelines for the development of many of the programs that were established after its publication.

The second event was the emergence of safety education in the early 1920s as an identifiable teaching area. Beginning in 1913 with the founding of the National Safety Council, a number of events occurred that emphasized an increasing awareness of the importance of safety and the realization that it deserved a place in the school curriculum. Some of these events were (1) the beginning of safety instruction in the schools of San Antonio, Texas, in 1913 and in Philadelphia and Detroit in 1916; (2) the organization of a safety education section of the National Safety Council in 1919; and (3) the presentation "Safety Education in Public Schools" given by Albert Whitney at the NEA Convention in Milwaukee in 1919. The growth of safety education, with its many health-related issues, would parallel that of health education, and in some instances elements of the two fields would merge to form academic departments of health and safety education.

Consolidation and Diversification (1935-1950)

From 1935 to 1950 health education was shaped by the continued use of surveys and other studies. It was also affected by the impact of World War II, the continuation of demonstration projects to assess the feasibility of health education in a variety of settings, the fine tuning of professional preparation, and the emergence of health education in community settings.

In 1942 Dorothy Nyswander published a report on research conducted on school health services in Astoria, New York (the Astoria Study), entitled *Solving School Health Problems.*[10] This report described the results of research conducted between 1936 and 1940 and also drew from a number of other studies related to school health services that had been published as early as 1925. Although the focus of the study was on school health services, its findings affected all aspects of the school health program. The Astoria Study resulted in improvements in instruction, administration, and school health services. Perhaps its greatest impact was on the team approach for nurses, teachers, and parents working together for the health of the child. Health appraisal forms developed by the study are still in use today.

Another study of significance to the field was the New York City Evaluation Study.[11] Designed to evaluate health education in the public schools of New York, the study began in 1944 and isued its report in 1949. The recommendations that resulted from this research were important to health education. They included suggestions for a minimum amount of instructional time, strategies for teaching, content areas to be emphasized, and the recommendation that education in health be conducted under the title of health instruction. It emphasized the importance of the school's cooperation with community health agencies and organizations:

> The School Health Education program cannot operate effectively in a vacuum. The wise school administrator should tap the resources of the community, and bring community health and welfare agencies into cooperative relationship with the school to the end that a more dynamic and vastly enriched health program should result . . . Upon the caliber of these relationships depends the success or failure of the Health Education program.[11]

Demonstration projects carried on during this time also popularized the role of health education. In 1936 the U.S. Office of Education issued a pamphlet entitled *Training of Elementary Teachers For School Health Work.*[12] This pamphlet placed responsibility for the health education of children squarely on the shoulders of the classroom teacher. It called for elementary teachers to be well trained not only in the content to be taught in health education classes but also in the methods and procedures of effective health instruction:

> Elementary teachers should be sufficiently informed not only concerning the facts of physiology and hygiene but have adequate schooling in planning and presenting lessons to children of various grades. The subject certainly deserves to be taken as seriously as any other of the curriculum.[12]

In 1943 a series of demonstration projects was sponsored by the W.K. Kellogg Foundation. The first of these was conducted in Michigan and was called the Community Health Service Project (later the School Community Health Project). This project, which began as a training program for nurses, evolved into a major demonstration of the effectiveness of a comprehensive school-community health program. Eventually 24 states participated in this project, which had three significant effects on health education. First, it helped establish the foundation of public confidence in both school and community health education, which would facilitate a postwar growth in the program. Second, the findings of the study validated the need for health instruction as a joint effort of the home, school, and community:

> 1. Effective health education is best accomplished through the cooperative services of the professional personnel of the schools and health agencies.
> 2. This essential cooperation at all levels can be most effectively and agreeable secured through a health council.
> 3. The superiority of the functional approach . . . was outstanding in the attainment of results directly affecting health conduct and attitudes.
> 4. An effective health education program is directly dependent upon community understanding and support.[13]

The third positive outcome of the Community Health Service Project was that it set the stage for the California School Community Health Project. One of the outcomes of the latter project was the establishment of health education courses within the curriculum of the state colleges in California. Like the Michigan project, the California project was funded by the Kellogg Foundation and directed by the California State Department of Education. The California project began in 1944 and was first implemented at Fresno State College under the leadership of Cecil Havelin of the State Department of Education. This program was so successful that it was quickly expanded to San Diego State, San Francisco State, and Chico State colleges. All of these programs continued to function after the project ended because the Kellogg grant required the institutions at which the programs had been implemented to assume financial responsibility after the original funds were terminated. This effort represents an example of the best type of cooperative effort between private enterprise and higher education at the state level.

Another major study during this era was the Denver Interest Study, which began in 1945 and was concluded in 1954. Its goals, as stated in *Health Interests of Children*, were "to discover interests and needs of pupils as a basis for providing the most meaningful health experience for boys and girls at the same time to find out at what grade level, or levels, those experiences should be provided."[14] On completion of the study a number of conclusions were evident. Among these were three that particularly related to health education:

1. From percentage enrollments and time allowed it would appear that health instruction too frequently is playing second fiddle not only to traditional school subjects but also to the closely related fields of physical education and competitive sports.
2. As a major goal of education, health deserves a more prominent place in the school program.
3. More school systems of all sizes should give careful consideration to the merits of the school health council.[14]

These conclusions brought forth the following recommendations:

1. That all teachers become increasingly aware of the health interests and needs of the children with whom they work and of the contribution that teachers can make to the health of those children.
2. That teachers discover through abundant experimentation increasingly effective techniques for health instruction.
3. That to facilitate these important understandings and skills of teachers, a teacher-education program in the field of health should be developed.
4. That a parent education program in the field of health be developed in order that parents may have a greater understanding of the part

that environment plays in the health of children and knowledge of their responsibility in modifying it.[14]
The Denver Interest Study is generally regarded as one of the first large-scale needs and interest assessments in health education.

Between 1948 and 1950 three conferences took place that were important to the continued growth of the field. The first of these conferences was held at Jackson's Mill, Weston, West Virginia, in 1948. Entitled The National Conference on Undergraduate Professional Preparation In Health Education, Physical Education and Recreation, the conference resulted in the development of a list of personal qualifications for successful leadership in health education and identified a list of general competencies of the health educator.[15] This was the forerunner of competency-based health education programs that are described more fully in Chapter 4. The work of this conference was a prelude to the School Health Education Study of the 1960s and the Role Delineation Project of the 1980s.

The second conference also dealt with undergraduate professional preparation in health education. It was called The First U.S. Office of Education Conference on Undergraduate Professional Preparation of Students Majoring in Health Education.[16] The conference was held in Washington, D.C. in 1949 under the direction of H.F. Kilander. The major outcome of the conference was the familiarization of professionals in the field with the state of the art in health education as reflected in the programs being taught in colleges and universities all over the country. It also provided a greater understanding of the needs of health education undergraduate students and a description of the status of graduate programs in health education. This conference was so successful that a second one took place in 1953.

The third and most significant of these three conferences was the National Conference on Graduate Study in Health Education, Physical Education and Recreation held at Pere Marquette State Park in Illinois in 1950. This conference was a milestone in the history of health education. It was held with the conviction that the preparation of personnel is the key to favorably affecting the health of people, and it resulted in the establishment of guidelines for the professional preparation of health educators at the graduate level. The core areas of the graduate program included:

1. Scientific foundations of health education (knowledge of scientific facts and principles relating to personal, family, and community health, including national and international implications)
2. History, philosophy, and principles
3. Administration and supervision
4. Curriculum and teaching
5. Evaluation and research[17]

In addition, the doctoral-level student was expected to develop a high level

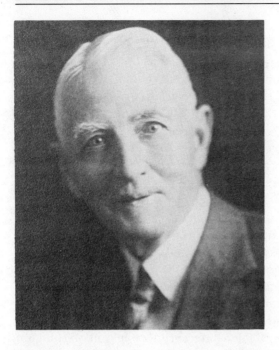

Fig. 1-4. William Howe, M.D., one of the founders of the American School Health Association (ASHA). ASHAs highest award is named after Dr. Howe. (Courtesy American School Health Association.)

of competence in an area of health education such as teaching, administration, or research. Experiences should be included in the cultural foundations in health education, the literature of the field, and in research through seminars, individual study, and an acceptable dissertation. A supervised school-community field work experience was also recommended. The impact of this conference and its resulting guidelines are still affecting graduate programs.[18]

Professional preparation of health educators during the period from 1935 to 1950 enjoyed a golden age. The number of undergraduate programs increased from 8 in 1942 to 38 in 1950. The number of graduate programs grew to 25.

During this era a number of new agencies and organizations relating to health or health education were created. Prominent among these was the establishment of the School Health section of the American Public Health Association (APHA) in 1936, the Health Education section of the American Association of Health, Physical Education and Recreation in 1937, and the creation of the Society of Public Health Education (SOPHE) in 1950.

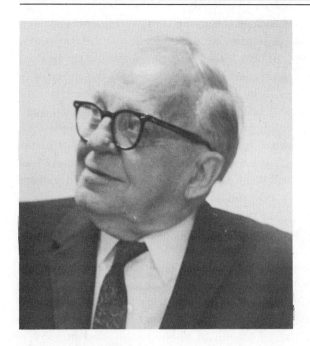

Fig. 1-5. Dr. A. O. DeWeese, first Executive Director of ASHA and one of the founders of the organization who served 25 years. (Courtesy American School Health Association.)

By 1948, when the Third Annual Working Conference for Health Education Alumni was held by the School of Public Health of the University of North Carolina at Chapel Hill, there had developed a strong desire among many health educators who worked in community settings for a professional organization that would be uniquely their own. This desire had been growing since the establishment of the first health education programs in schools of public health during the 1920s. Prominent among those who were interested in establishing a professional organization for community health educators were Lucy Morgan, Eunice Tyler, Mayhew Derryberry, Sally Lucas Jean, Clair Turner, and Dorothy Nyswander. Thus it was at the Chapel Hill conference that the 56 people who attended dedicated their efforts to establishing a new professional organization for public health educators. Specifically, they decided to canvas other health educators to determine if there was sufficient support for their idea and to meet in New Orleans later that year (1948) for further discussion. At the meeting in New Orleans it was decided to continue the sampling of opinion of health educators on the establishment of a new professional organization and to meet again at the annual APHA meeting in Boston in 1948.

Two informal meetings took place at the APHA convention. These meetings resulted in the idea of holding an open meeting at the convention to get a sense of the sentiment of health educators on the idea of establishing a new organization. They also decided to create a steering committee of 33 people to guide their efforts in creating a new professional society and discussed what the objectives of this new organization should be. In 1949, just before the APHA convention in New York, the steering committee met as the Society of Public Health Educators, Interim Commission. This was the real beginning of SOPHE. The official beginning of the society took place on October 27 and 28, 1950. Thus SOPHE, with a membership of less than 100, had become a reality. It would be several years before the organization would become a major force in health education.

The era of 1935 through 1950 had been one of unparalleled professional growth in health education. The growth had been provided by demonstration projects, by the impetus of war, and through research and conferences. All these occurrences had strengthened the field and given it new vitality. In addition, the APHA began to accredit schools of public health in 1945. Between 1945 and 1949 there were only 18 master of health education degrees conferred among the 10 schools of public health, and in 1949-50 there were only 430 students enrolled in all Master in Public Health degree programs. Altogether in that year there were only slightly over 1000 members in the APHA. Recruitment of new members was identified as the most pressing need.

The Conceptual Approach (1950-1970)

The period from 1950 to 1970 was a time of refined professional preparation, increased research, and clarification of professional purpose. This era opened in 1950 with the Mid-Century White House Conference on Children and Youth sponsored by the National Committee on Children and Youth.[19] This conference, which featured substantial public participation, had among its recommendations:
1. That health instruction should be given more time in the curriculum
2. That those entrusted with teaching health should be well prepared
3. That school districts and counties should have health coordinators to facilitate the implementation and coordination of health-related programs

The conference identified the concerns of the time as being the quality of health instruction regardless of the setting, the competency of the health educator, and the administrative framework in which health education operated.

The year following the While House Conference on Children and

Youth saw the establishment of the President's Commission on the Health Needs of the Nation. This Commission had been charged to conduct a wide-ranging study of the organizational and administrative problems of health-related systems in the United States. It issued its findings in a 5-volume report.[20] One of the outcomes of this work was the creation of the U.S. Department of Health, Education and Welfare in 1953. In this same year the Second Conference on the Professional Preparation of Students Majoring in Health Education was held in Washington, D.C.[21] It concerned itself with recruitment, placement, research, accreditation, admissions, student teaching, and field experiences. The conference found that

> We are making slow, but sure progress toward identifying and developing health education as a unique field of professional study at both the undergraduate and graduate levels. Health education is being established as a profession open to both men and women who wish to follow a life time career of humanitarian service.[21]

In 1954 the School Health Education Evaluation Study was launched in Los Angeles. This study was funded by the Tuberculosis and Health Association of Los Angeles County and sponsored by the Health Education Unit of UCLA and the Los Angeles County schools. This project was designed to evaluate health education programs in schools and colleges. Conducted between 1954 and 1959, the project was specifically designed to consider the effectiveness of the school health program, "including administrative organization, school health services, health instruction, and healthful school living; the health behavior of pupils including knowledge, attitudes and practices; and the process of evaluation."[22]

In 1956 two college health conferences were sponsored by the Health Education Division of the American Association for Health, Physical Education and Recreation. This association and its health education division had become an increasingly important force in health education since the inception of the division in 1937. These conferences were just two of the many important contributions of this association.

The first conference was chaired by Edward B. Johns of UCLA, who had also played a significant role in the 1954 School Health Education Evaluative Study. The conference dealt with a wide range of topics, particularly those of health content and methodology, that were of concern to college health educators.[23] One week later those who had participated in this conference became delegates to the Second National Conference on College Health Education sponsored by the American Association of Colleges for Teacher Preparation, the National Commission on Teacher Education and Professional Standards, and the Association for Higher Education. Whereas the first conference considered health education at the college level, this second conference was convened to examine the preparation in health education that would best meet the needs of elementary and secondary school teachers.[24] This unique "back-to-back" conference format allowed a body of professionals to examine a wide range of issues affecting health education, such as objectives, content, organization and administration, resources, and evaluation, and to formulate guidelines or position statements regarding each.

In 1958 the Inter-Agency Conference on School Health Education was held at West Point, New York. This conference resulted from the growing awareness of the need for cooperation between organizations with a common interest in providing improved health education. The result of the conference was the identification of a number of needs for the improvement of health education, including the need for greater and more effective communication between entities, improved and expanded teacher preparation, improved health education in schools, and better cooperation between all those involved in health education.

In 1959 the Highland Park Conference (Health Education Planning Conference)[25] in Illinois made additional contributions to the growth of health education. The conference established commissions to study specific health education issues that resulted from discussion. For example, Delbert Oberteuffer's Commission on Philosophy presented *A point of view for health education;* the Curriculum Commission, first chaired by Sara Louise Smith and later by Edward B. Johns, produced a publication entitled *Health concepts: an approach to health instruction;* Fred Hein's Commission on Research held a successful conference on health education research; Charlotte Leach's Relationships Group developed a directory of health education organizations; and William Creswell's Commission on Teacher Education and Accreditation produced an *Appraisal guide for professional preparation in health education* in 1967. Cumulatively, these commission reports helped to establish long-range goals and strategies in health education, thereby giving the profession a sense of direction for the future.

In 1966 the Committee on Graduate Curriculum in Health Education of the American Academy of Physical Education delivered the report of its findings.[26] These findings represented a careful analysis of the graduate curricula in health education. They helped to identify more closely the core of the graduate program and the role of each of its elements. The core of graduate study in health education comprised four broad content areas:

1. Health science
2. Behavioral science
3. Education, the school, and society
4. Evaluation and research

The report indicated that the master's degree was designed to prepare teachers, supervisors, and coordinators for elementary and secondary schools as well as teachers for the junior colleges and for the first 2 years of a 4-year college program. In addition, the master's degree should provide basic graduate education for those who want to proceed to the doctorate degree. It further stated that the doctorate program in health education was designed to prepare university and college teachers, research workers, and leaders at higher levels of responsibility in schools, colleges, universities, and in the community setting.[26]

In 1969 one of the last major studies of the decade was reported in a volume entitled *Teach Us What We Want To Know*.[27] This "needs and interest" study, which involved 5000 students from kindergarten through high school in the state of Connecticut, was sponsored by the Connecticut Department of Education and the U.S. Office of Education. Like the one previously conducted in Denver in 1954, this study was a large-scale attempt to identify the health education needs and interests of students. The uniqueness of this effort was the care taken to report student responses with as much detail as possible. A description of the interrelated nature of student needs from grade level to grade level presented in Section III of the report and the professional analysis available in Section IV made this document extremely valuable to the school health educator and to those establishing curricula in health education.

Spanning the time from 1960 to 1970 was a single project that may have surpassed all others in importance. This was the School Health Education Study. Through the efforts of First Deputy Commissioner Granville Larimore, M.D., and Commissioner Herman E. Hilleboe, M.D., of the New York State Department of Health and through the generosity of the Samuel Bronfman Foundation, the School Health Education Study was established in 1961 with offices in Washington, D.C. Dr. Elena Sliepcevich, Professor of Health Education at Ohio State University, was selected as the director of the study. The first major activity of this study was to conduct a survey of the status of health education in the United States. This survey involved 135 school systems, 1460 schools, and 840,832 students in 38 states and was the largest and most comprehensive survey in the history of health education.

The results of the research, published in 1964, showed the overall performance of school health education programs to be lacking. The study also demonstrated that the general level of health education among students was poor. The situation was judged to be so crucial that significant and fundamental changes in school education were desperately needed.[28]

After the Bronfman Foundation was no longer able to support the study, the Minnesota Mining and Manufacturing Company (3M) agreed to finance its further efforts. This relationship continued until 1972. With new support and the clear recognition of the need to carry out a comprehensive curriculum development task, the study began the process that would revolutionize curriculum development in health education. First, after exhaustive research it was decided to implement a conceptual approach to the formulation of curriculum materials. This resulted in a format that linked content together conceptually and in four progressive stages of sophistication. In 1964, members of the writing team and their consultants began the ambitious task of producing a comprehensive curriculum for students from kindergarten through the twelfth grade. This project was immensely successful. Thus when it ended in 1972, not only had the School Health Education Study produced and popularized its instructional materials but also it had established a new perspective on health education. The study provided a sophisticated conceptual approach with a unique way to structure and organize knowledge; a learning process including long-range goals, behavioral objectives, learning experiences, a wealth of useful resources, and evaluation procedures; a model describing the discipline of health education; a *Directory of Institutions Offering Programs of Specialization in Health Education;* and through all of its activities and relationships, greater status to health education both within and outside the profession.

In 1972 the Joint Committee on Terminology in Health Education, chaired by Edward B. Johns, examined and amended the common terminology used in the field. Because words are the tools of the health educator, the importance of this project to define old terms and to forge new ones should not be underestimated. The committee's efforts resulted in more exact communication between health educators, between health educators and their students, and between health educators and educators in other fields.

Today: Tomorrow's History (1970-Present)

There have been a number of events since 1970 that are potentially historic, although there has been insufficient time to evaluate their impact or significance. Some of these events are described briefly below. They include (1) the creation of the Coalition of National Health Education Organizations, (2) the work of the President's Committee on Health Education, (3) the establishment of the Office of Health Information, Health Promotion, Physical Fitness and Sports Medicine, and (4) the creation of the Office of Comprehensive School Health within the Department of Education.

The Coalition of National Health Organizations was founded in 1971 after receiving its initial impetus from the Executive Committee of the School Health Division of the American Association for Health, Physical Education and Recreation in the form of a unanimously approved motion to study the feasibility of a federation of national health education organizations.[29] The coalition comprises organizations that have members who are professional health educators or who have a major commitment to health education. There are eight health education units representing seven national organizations:

1. American College Health Association (Health Education Section)
2. American Public Health Association (Public Health Education Section)
3. Amerian Public Health Association (School Health Education and Services Section)
4. American School Health Association
5. Association for the Advancement of Health Education (American Alliance for Health, Physical Education, Recreation and Dance)
6. Conference of State and Territorial Directors of Public Health Education
7. Society for Public Health Education
8. Society of State Directors for Health, Physical Education and Recreation.

The primary goal of the coalition as stated in the *Eta Sigma Gamman*, is to "mobilize the resources of the health education profession in order to expand and improve health education—be it community based or occupational, or whether it involves patient education or school health education."[29] The major purposes of the coalition include the following:

1. To facilitate national-level communication, collaboration and coordination among the member organizations.
2. To provide a forum for the identification and discussion of health education issues.
3. To formulate recommendations and take appropriate action on issues affecting the member interests.
4. To serve as a communication and advisory resource for agencies, organizations and persons in the public and private sectors on health education issues.
5. To serve as a focus for the exploration and resolution of issues pertinent to professional health educators.[29]

Another important event that took place in the early 1970s was the creation by President Richard M. Nixon of the President's Committee on Health Education. The committee held nationwide hearings in eight regions to determine what should be recommended tó develop in the general public a sense of health consumer citizenship.[30] The major finding was that there was a need for community health programs that could foster a healthy citizenry. To help meet this need it was recommended that two agencies for the promotion of health be created, one a federal agency and one a private organization.

The Bureau of Health Education (now the Center for Health Promotion and Education) within the Centers for Disease Control was created as a federal agency in 1974. Its mission is "to provide for the prevention of disease, disability, premature death, and undesirable and unnecessary health problems."[31] Although the title of the bureau has now changed as noted above, its primary goal remains the same.

The private sector has as its representative for health concerns the National Center for Health Education. The center is a nonprofit organization that has been awarded several contracts and grants to improve the health of Americans. One of its most noteworthy contributions to the progress of health education was the Role Delineation Project for Health Education. This project began in 1978 and ended in 1982 because of federal cutbacks in funding such projects.

The first phase of the project began with the Conference on the Commonalities and Differences in the Preparation and Practice of Health Educators, held in February 1978 in Bethesda, Maryland. This meeting resulted in the foundation of the National Task Force on the Preparation and Practice of Health Educators. A contract between the Bureau of Health Manpower and the National Center for Health Education began the first phase of the Role Delineation Project: to identify roles and competencies of health educators as perceived by professionals working in school, community, or other health care settings (role specification). In January 1980 this phase was completed and the findings were published as the *Initial Role Delineation for Health Education, Final Report.*

Phase II of the project, Role Verification and Refinement, began in May, 1980. In this phase professionals in the field and those in training institutions tried to verify the roles and competencies identified in the first phase of the project. This involved a review of materials by selected health educators and a conference at which virtually all health education training programs were represented. The conference, held in Birmingham, Alabama, was called the National Conference for Institutions Preparing Health Educators. Initially, there were five phases to the project; however, only the first two phases were completed, again because of federal funding cutbacks.

In 1976 the Office of Health Information and Health Promotion (OHP) (later to include physical fitness and sports medicine) was created because PL 94-317, Title I, was signed by President Gerald R. Ford on June 23, 1976. Section 1706 of the law directed the Secretary of Health, Education and Welfare (now Health and Human Services) to establish, within the office of the Assistant Secretary for Health, an office (1) to coordinate all activities within the Department of Health, Education and Welfare that related to health information and promotion; (2) to coordinate its activities with similar activities of organizations in the private sector, and (3) to establish a national information clearinghouse to facilitate the exchange of information on matters relating to health information and promotion, preventive health services, and education in the appropriate use of health care.

The OHP has published many documents and reports and has assisted in the development of the surgeon general's reports on the nation's health. The OHP became extremely active under the direction of Dr. Lawrence Green, with the assistance of Dr. Donald Iverson, During 1980 alone the OHP contacted 600 people who became part of a network that the office used to carry out its activities. The OHP remains a vital part of federal activities concerned with health education.

In 1978, PL 95-561, the Health Education Act, was passed. This act helped to create an Office of Comprehensive School Health within the Department of Education. The primary purpose of that office was to serve as a link for policy development in the Department of Education for health education issues that affect children and youth. Although the office was never fully funded, a director (Dr. Peter Cortese) was appointed in 1980. However, the office was deactivated with the advent of the Reagan administration's budget cuts.

The future of health education holds great promise, as can be witnessed by:

> increased emphasis and recognition that has been given to disease prevention and health education in the form of officially published statements as represented in the series of reports, *A Forward Plan for Health*, FY 77-81, FY 78-82, and FY 79-83. Also, Congress has rewritten the missions of the two institutes, NHLBI and NCI, in order that they might encourage and support research on disease prevention and health education in addition to their traditional support of biomedical research.[32]

Which of these events will be the focus of historians is unknown. But certainly these are dramatic times, full of possibility and hope. As health educators we have an obligation to our rich past, and to all those who preceded us, to make these historic times.

Editors' Remarks

It may seem strange for a chapter on history to begin in the year 1850. But the chapter presents a historical perspective of a discipline that has yet to fully emerge. Although many health-related events that occurred before 1850 could be cited, they had little to do with the development of health education. The fact that bubonic plague killed nearly half the earth's population during the Middle Ages is an interesting historical fact but is not important as an event that contributed to the foundations of health education.

The current state of the art in health education has been shaped by and actually grew from several other professions, notably medicine and education. The purpose of this section is to provide the reader with some insight into how our historical roots have led us to where we are today.

First, let us consider medicine. Before 1850 little was known about the cause, diagnosis, and treatment of disease. Remember that the American Civil War had not yet begun. The exciting wild west portaryed in "western" movies and books occurred a little more than 100 years ago, between 1865 and 1875. Many physicians were self-proclaimed. Treatment consisted of elixirs concocted from roots and spices, septic surgery, and a good deal of misinformation. Whiskey served as anesthesia, surgery was performed with a hunting knife "sterilized" over the flame of a candle, and the operating room was a doctor's office above a saloon. Hanlon states that it was not until 1910 that a patient in the United States had a 50/50 chance of being accurately diagnosed.[33] It is safe to say that the accumulated knowledge of medical science grew at an exponential rate during each year of the twentieth century.

By examining some of the historical theories of disease it is possible to demonstrate that health education could not have emerged earlier than it did. The religious theory of disease, popular well into the nineteenth century, states that people get sick as punishment for sins. The demonic theory states that people become ill because the devil inhabits the body or mind. If one accepts these beliefs about sickness, then health education (if you want to call it that) must be conducted by religious clerics who tell people how to avoid sin and calamity. Sickness would not be treated by a physician but instead by a minister. Prevention would not be an educational task but instead a religious one.

The miasmatic theory of disease states that sickness results from bad air or vapors that emanate from the bodies of those who are diseased or dead. The way to prevent sickness therefore is to bury or burn the dead and to isolate the sick so that sickness cannot spread. Even today this is a healthy and practiced technique, although it offers no potential for health education. Public health activities conducted ex post facto were fairly effective at preventing the further spread of disease.

The microscope was developed around 1650. Because most of the diseases prevalent then, and until the middle of the twentieth century, were caused by microorganisms, scientists believed that if they could find a deterrent, then people would be able to live a long life. In 1796 Edward Jenner discovered vaccination as a means of preventing smallpox. Here was an opportunity for health education. If disease could be prevented through immunization, then people needed to be informed. At the time the belief was popularly held that if the public was made aware of the facts, they would "do the proper thing" to protect their health. Other than some basic knowledge of the issue, the information given required none of the special skills that are currently required of an effective health educator. Keep in mind that the health belief model, which helps to explain why people choose to act on information, was not created until the mid-twentieth century.

The ecologic theory of disease also evolved in the mid-twentieth century. Books such as *Mirage of Health* by René Dubos helped us to understand that health and disease result from pluricausal factors. We learned that health is a positive quality and that in addition to heredity and environment, life-style is a definite factor in our overall health status. In a complex way these factors interact to produce a health potential. However, the research to support this concept is a recent development. The Framingham Study, which identified the risk factors for heart disease, was not begun until 1950. The first report from the surgeon general of the United States to use epidemiologic data to link cigarette smoking to lung cancer was not published until 1964. Even now there are individuals who do not accept these data as being valid.

All of this demonstrates the fact that health education has been shaped by factors related to the nature of disease and beliefs about causation that placed disease causation outside the realm of individual control. Only recently were superstition and taboo replaced by knowledge based on objective evidence. Can you imagine a health educator in nineteenth century America? What would the instructional content be? How would this health educator hope to convince a school board, a corporation, or a hospital that health education had merit? Assuming that colleges could find someone interested in becoming a health educator, what would be the nature of their professional preparation?

At the same time consider the working environment at the turn of the century. With the continent finally united, interests turned to industrialization. Workers were struggling to make a living in the factory and on the farm. Their concern was for survival rather than a recently popular concept called "quality of living." Children didn't stay in school through graduation. In 1890 fewer than 10% of children aged 14 to 17 years were enrolled in secondary schools. Factories were not interested in paying decent wages to employees, let alone providing release time for educational programs. Public health officials were so busy dealing with epidemics they did not have time to develop creative classroom strategies. And hospitals were places where people went to die, so health education seemed a little out of place there too.

Another area that had to emerge before health education could stand by itself was social science and appropriate techniques for research. The development of the social science discipline is a recent occurrence. The only way to demonstrate accountability is to prove a point through controlled study. Before 1950 the social sciences were not that sophisticated. Consequently it was difficult if not impossible to justify the existence of health education in a school curriculum or a public health department budget. Although some people were willing to accept health education on faith, most were not. In retrospect it is curious that health educators would have expected anything other than skepticism from the general public. To decision makers all those conferences, committees, and commissions that addressed health education were only so much rhetoric. Without supporting evidence, the final reports were insufficient to convince legislators, policymakers, and financial supporters that health education had merit.

Return to the chronology of events presented in the introduction of this chapter. The first professional preparation program, the White House Conference, the Joint Committee, and the American Child Health Association were all established before the Cattaraugus Study in 1931 that evaluated the impact of health education and the competency of health teachers. From then until the present there have been sporadic studies to demonstrate that health education can affect personal and community health. However, the chronology of events lists many conferences to discuss the role of professional preparation and the curriculum appropriate for public schools. We cannot help but think that health education would have progressed further had more efforts such as the School Community Health Project been conducted before the 1948 National Conference on Undergraduate Professional Preparation and the 1950 National Conference on Graduate Study.

This is not intended to second guess or criticize the pioneers who nurtured health education in the early days. The events must have occurred in what seemed to be a logical sequence in the best interest of the profession. Remember also that research in the social sciences did not come of age until after World War II. Statistical analysis appropriate for behavioral research came even later, and computers were not widely available until about 1960. So even if the pioneers had wanted to demonstrate the potential of an emerging profession, the tools were not yet available to do so. Furthermore, the professional associations that promote health education by encouraging research and publication were established fairly recently (APHA in 1872 and School Health Section in 1936, AAHPER in 1885 and Health Education Section in 1937, ASHA in 1927, and SOPHE in 1950).

Health education has evolved from the efforts of a few dedicated individuals such as Thomas D. Wood, Sally Lucas Jean, Clair Turner, Ruth Grout, and Walter H. Brown. It grew from demonstration projects and from eight professional preparation programs in existence before 1942. It began as public health education and gradually moved into the public schools. Only after 1960 did it also become prominent in community settings (other than as a public health activity), hospitals, and worksites. Its foundations are still being built. Some of those who are now providing leadership to the profession will be referred to in the future as "pioneers."

One of the necessary ingredients in the composition of a discipline's foundation is the creation of a philosophy. As health education developed, a philosophy also began to form. Although we could point to statements of philosophy reported by individual authors or professional organizations, it would be wrong to believe that on a particular date the philosophy suddenly appeared. The next chapter describes some of the philosophical tenets of our profession that have slowly evolved as our history unfolded. In order to appreciate the philosophy it is necessary to understand the events that have helped to fashion a current set of beliefs.

Summary

We hope that this brief historical orientation has stimulated your professional appetite and that this chapter enables you to appreciate the important events that have led to the current state of the health education profession. Just as the past has shaped our current situation, it is the present that will shape our future. A clear picture of the past can be useful in helping to make decisions about that future. Philosophy, issues, trends, and occurrences take on added significance when viewed in a historical perspective.

A review of these conferences, studies, and reports demonstrates the key areas of concern with which health education has had to deal. They seem to fall into three major categories: (1) professional preparation of health educators, including clarification of competencies, (2) curriculum development based on the needs and interests of schoolchildren, and (3) evaluation of the effectiveness of comprehensive school health education. The Role Delineation Project mentioned in this chapter, is described more fully in Chapters 4 and 8.

Questions for Review

1. What single historical event do you think has made the greatest contribution to the development of health education? Why?
2. In what ways does our current status reflect the fact that health education emerged from the disciplines of medicine and education?
3. In what ways has health education begun to take on an identity all its own?
4. How do you think the early pioneers of health education, such as William A. Alcott, Thomas D. Wood, and Sally Lucas Jean, would react to the current state of the profession?
5. How would you characterize the differences between hygiene education and the modern concepts of health education?
6. Speculate on the differences one would find between the 1969 survey entitled *Teach Us What We Want to Know*, conducted by Ruth Byler, and a contemporary needs and interest survey of students.

References

1. Durant, W.: Our oriental heritage, New York, 1963, Simon and Schuster.
2. Shattuck, L.: Report of the sanitary commission of Massachusetts, fasc. ed., Boston, 1850, Dutton & Wentworth.
3. Turner, C.E.: Malden studies on health education and growth, Am. J. Public Health **18:**1217-1230, 1928.
4. Storey, T.A.: The status of hygiene programs in institutions of higher education in the United States Report: of the President's Committee of Fifty on College Hygiene, Stanford, 1927, Stanford University Press.
5. Strachan, M.L.: Fifteen years of child health education, New York, 1932, National Tuberculosis Association.
6. Education of a rural school health education project, New York, 1939, Milbank Memorial Fund.
7. Grout, R.E.: and Pickup, E.G.: A study of pupil health practices, Milbank Mem. Fund Q. **16:**1-21, 1938.
8. Strang, R.M., Grout, R.E., and Wiehl, D.G.: Evaluation of teachers work in health education, Milbank Mem. Fund Q. **15:**355-370, 1937.
9. Wood, T.D.: Health education—a program for public schools and teacher training institutions, Joint Committee on Health Problems in Education of the National Education Association and the American Medical Association, with the cooperation of the Technical Committee of Twenty-Seven, New York, 1924, National Education Association.
10. Nyswander, D.B.: Solving School Health Problems: the Astoria demonstration study, New York, 1942, Commonwealth Fund.
11. Evaluation study of health education in the public schools of the city of New York, Brooklyn, 1949, Board of Education of the City of New York.
12. Rogers, J.F.: Training of elementary teachers for school health work, U.S. Department of the Interior, Office of Education, Pamphlet No. 67, Washington, D.C., 1936, U.S. Government Printing Office.
13. An experience in health education, Battle Creek, Mich., 1950, W.K. Kellogg Foundation.
14. Report of a research study of health interest and needs of children as a basis for health instruction. In Health interests of children, rev. ed., Denver, 1954, Board of Education, Denver Public Schools.
15. Report of the National Conference on Undergraduate Professional Preparation in Health Education, Physical Education and Recreation (Jackson's Mill, Weston, West Virginia, May 16-27, 1948, Chicago, 1948, The Athletic Institute.
16. Conference Report on the Undergraduate Professional Preparation of Students Majoring in Health Education November 28-December 2, 1949, Washington, D.C., 1950, U.S. Office of Education.
17. Graduate Study in Health Education, Physical Education and Recreation, Chicago, 1950, The Athletic Institute.
18. Johns, E.B.: Graduate health education: past, present, and future, Paper presented before Eta Sigma Gamma (National Health Science Honorary) Annual Meeting, Atlanta, October 14, 1977.
19. Richards, E.A., editor: Proceedings of the Mid-century White House Conference on Children and Youth, Raleigh, N.C., 1951, Health Publications Institute, Inc.
20. President's Commission on the Health Needs of the Nation. Vol. I, Building America's health; vol II, America's health status, needs and resources; vol. III, Statistical appendix; vol. IV, Financing a health program for America; vol. V, The people speak, Washington, D.C., 1953, U.S. Government Printing Office.
21. Second Conference on the Professional Preparation of Students Majoring in Health Education (January 5-9, 1953), Washington, D.C., 1953, U.S. Office of Education.
22. Report of an evaluation research study: School health education evaluative study—Los Angeles area, 1954-1959, Berkeley, 1960, University of California Press.

23. Report of the National Conference on College Health Education: A Forward Look in College Health Education, Washington, D.C., 1956, American Association for Health, Physical Education and Recreation.
24. Report of the National Conference on College Health Education: Health education for prospective teachers, Washington, D.C., 1956, American Association for Health, Physical Education and Recreation.
25. Health Education Planning Conference Report: Guidelines for health education: a suggested plan of action (Highland Park, Illinois, October 10-12, 1959), Washington, D.C., 1959, American Association for Health, Education, Physical Education and Recreation.
26. Creswell, W.H., Jr.: Research relationships and relevancy, School Health Review **2**:2-11, 1971.
27. Byler, R., editor: Teach Us What We Want To Know. Published for Connecticut State Board of Education, New York, 1969, Mental Health Materials Center, Inc.
28. School health education study, a summary report, New York, 1964, The Samuel Bronfman Foundation.
29. Coalition of National Health Organizations: Facts about the coalition of national health organizations, Eta Sigma Gamman **13**(2):12-13, 1981.
30. Means, R.K.: Historical perspectives on school health, Thorofare, N.J., 1975, Charles B. Slack, Inc.
31. Bureau of Health Education: Facts, Atlanta, 1975, U.S. Department of Health, Education and Welfare.
32. Creswell, W.H., Jr.: Health education: the state of the art, Paper presented at the American Heart Association Meeting, 1980.
33. Hanlon, J.J., and Pickett, G.E.: Public health administration and practice, ed. 8, St. Louis, 1984, The C.V. Mosby Co.

Additional Readings

Hahn, D.B.: The Malden Studies: the first experimental research project in school health education, *Health Education*, **13**(4):8-9, 1982.

Hanlon, J.J., and Pickett, G.E.: Public health administration and practice, ed. 8, St. Louis, 1984, The C.V. Mosby Co.

Healthy people: the surgeon general's report on health promotion and disease prevention, United States Department of Health Education and Welfare, Public Health Service, Office of the Assistant Secretary for Health and Surgeon General, DHEW (PHS) Publication No. 79-55071 A, Washington, D.C., 1979, U.S. Government Printing Office.

Initial role delineation for health education, final report, United States Department of Health and Human Services, Public Health Service, Health Resources Administration. Washington, D.C., 1980, U.S. Government Printing Office.

National Conference for Institutions Preparing Health Educators: Proceedings, United States Department of Health and Human Services, Office of Disease Prevention and Health Promotion, and Physical Fitness and Sports Medicine, Washington, D.C., 1981, U.S. Government Printing Office.

Preparation and practice of community, patient, and school health educators, Proceedings of the Workshop on Commonalities and Differences, Washington, D.C., 1978, United States Department of Health, Education, Welfare and Public Health Science, Health Service Administration.

Promoting health and preventing disease, objectives for the nation, United States Department of Health and Human Services, Office of the Assistant Secretary for Health, Washington, D.C., 1980, U.S. Government Printing Office.

Reagan, P.A.: In search of health history—Margaret Sanger: health educator, Health Education **13**(4):5-7, 1982.

Andringa, R.C.: Recommendations for school health education, a handbook for state policy makers: report No. 130, Denver, Colorado, 1981, Education Programs Division, Education Commission of the States.

Weber, N.B.: Historical research as it applies to groups and institutions, Health Education **13**(4):10-11, 1982.

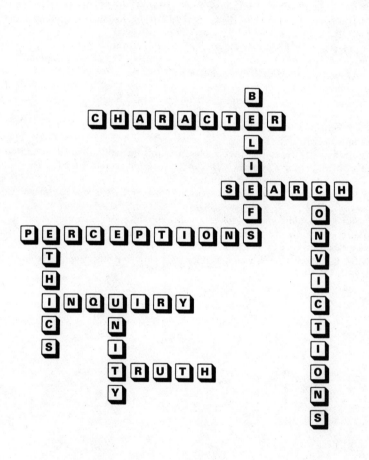

2 The Nature and Meaning of Health Education

Introduction

After a brief introduction on the nature of philosophy this chapter considers some important issues facing health education. There is a pressing need to define the values, significance, and purposes of the profession. We need to establish a theoretical and conceptual basis for our activity. The substantive boundaries of the discipline have yet to be defined. There does seem to be ample evidence that health education is moving toward the establishment of a uniform philosophy. When this process is completed members of the profession will be able to describe clearly the purposes, values, and significance (indeed, the fundamental character) of health education. In the broad field of study known as the social sciences it is becoming ever more imperative that a niche for health education be established.

Dr. Shirreffs seeks to blend fragmented thoughts, beliefs, and ideas into a cohesive philosophy on which theoretical precepts can operate. She seeks to identify common understandings and convictions by integrating them into a unified statement of purpose, acknowledging that before we can communicate our position to others we must first reach agreement on that position among ourselves.

Dr. Shirreffs cautions us to be open-minded in the search for professional values. She defines philosophy as a humanistic discipline that pursues an informed understanding of reality. The purpose of philosophy is to seek truth, to test one's convictions and beliefs. This can only take place when examination is not hindered by preconceived bias. Without a willingness to consider a variety of possibilities we become slaves to existing ideas at the expense of horizons that never expand and challenges that remain unexplored. In seeking truth pursue all pathways, not just the one that is worn bare by frequent traffic.

The Nature of Philosophy

What is philosophy? Is it a formal subject in academia? Is it a process in which people such as Plato and Aristotle engaged? Is it an individual's hierarchy of beliefs about life and living? Indeed, philosophy is all these things and more.

Philosophy is a humanistic discipline that attempts to obtain an informed understanding of reality. It is in effect the most general form of human understanding by which we understand and live our lives. The philosopher within each of us seeks answers to such profound yet basic questions as Who am I? Where am I? Why am I living?

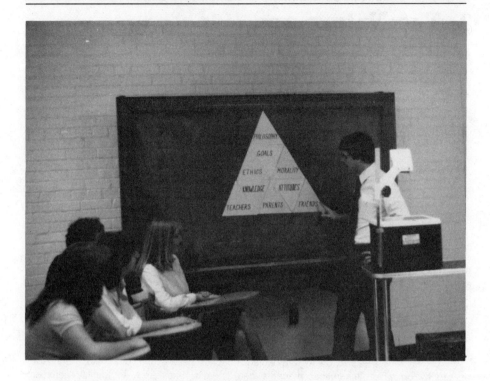

Fig. 2-1. Many factors lead to the establishment of a philosophy. By considering these factors separately we are able to integrate them into a unified set of beliefs.

Philosophy is concerned mainly with the process of pursuing philosophic truths and speculating about this process. It seeks to recognize the underlying relationship between all things in life, however varied they may be and however unrelated they may seem. It tries to establish an essential unity of reality that accounts for the many varied aspects of that reality, not as fragmented bits and pieces but as participants in unity—a cohesive whole.[1] Yet it is not so much concerned with answers or solutions as it is with exploring, examining, and identifying elements of a situation in order to reveal a special type of truth.

Philosophy requires that we look beyond the obvious and the known, beyond what appears to be fact or final truth. It begs us to speculate, to question assumptions, to break habits or "talking from ignorance" or "lack of preciseness" or "overclaiming" an inconsequential point. This so-called reflective attitude involves a desire coupled with persistence to constantly strive to increase our understanding and to identify justifiable bases of our convictions and beliefs. Such things as loose thinking, closed-door attitudes and biased minds have no place in philosophic inquiry because they are obstacles to straight thinking that cause trouble when people want to be certain of the validity of their beliefs.

It should be apparent at this point that philosophic inquiry is not for those who favor expediency over deliberate efforts, not for those who prefer to remain in their secure and familiar "comfort zones." It is also not for those who are afraid to make errors, for the possibility is good that errors in reasoning and generalization may crop up in the philosophic process. It is in this spirit this chapter is written.

Philosophy of Health Education

This chapter on the philosophy of health education entails a philosophic examination of the discipline itself, a systematic investigation into the whole of the discipline—its concepts, its nature, its fundamental character, and its goals. The chapter will examine

The essential nature or fundamental character of health education.

The value, significance, and purpose of health education.

The relationship of health education and the human condition.

The phrase *philosophy of* has come alive in many fields in the past decade, and health education is one of those fields. If you were to conduct a review of literature today you would find many more articles in our professional journals devoted to philosophic topics than ever before. Professional associations are sponsoring workshops and other sessions as part of their programs at national meetings on various aspects of philosophy and health education, and increasing numbers of graduate students are selecting philosophic topics for study. Given all this, it seems reasonable to say that health educators are recognizing the need to acquire the ability to understand their discipline more accurately and be able to explain it more clearly to others.

Why a Philosophy is Needed

There are a number of questions today that indicate the need for health educators to develop their acumen in philosophic inquiry. The most outstanding question perhaps is Do health educators now have the abilities to produce a reasoning about and an explanation and interpretation of their field? Think about this question.

Why is health education still not considered a viable and legitimate academic discipline on many campuses in the United States? For example, the fine arts have managed to gain acceptance as legitimate academic disciplines. Is it because those in the fine arts have demonstrated their abilities in thinking, discussing, and writing about things such as the theory of art, the philosophy of art, and art as a department of knowledge?[2]

Health education is considered by some (outside the field) as a prime component of health and medical systems, yet many remain skeptical about the relative impact of health education on the prevention of health problems and the promotion of health. Why is this? Could it be that health educators lack the ability to communicate with those in other fields? In reality all fields have a common language that includes such things as values, purposes, relationships, and outcomes. This common language also includes the abilities to think, discuss, and write about each field.[2] Can health educators speak this common language?

Another factor present in health education that indicates the need for more intensive philosophic inquiry is related to something I shall call professional "self-centeredness." Does health education identify with society's needs? Does it respond to the predominant societal values? Or do we as health educators conduct our day-to-day business the way "we know" it should be done? Davis and Miller have this to say:

> For a profession's interest to continue chiefly to spin inwardly upon itself is not a sign of a healthy professional personality, if such an analogy is acceptable. Such inward-looking-upon-itself forces the field to begin to lose touch with the life of the people and their way of life.[2]

In this regard, Sliepcevich has said:

> We must stay attuned to cultural, economic, legal, political, social and technological forces and to the myriad of social movements—for these will affect the human condition—and in turn our professional roles. Activists movements related to human rights, ecological issues, the changing role of women, protection of the abused and the battered, rights of consumers, demands for cultural identity, futurism, bioethics, transitions in values and family patterns, global issues, government interventions, interplanetary space stations—these cannot be ignored as if they had no meaning . . . It may seem paradoxical to say that, while striving for standards for our specialized professional field, we must also be generalists—interested in making connections, identifying relationships, recognizing the interdependence of all forces and trends—in essence, not just learning more and more about less and less.[3]
>
> Are health educators even in the remotest way guilty of professional self-centeredness? Do we spend enough of our professional time and energy attempting to identify and understand the values and culture of the people with whom we work? Do the values of our field parallel the values of our society? Have we moved in directions beyond self-concerns?

Philosophic inquiry will be needed to move us closer to "our rightful place as a major instrument for improving health of the nation and its people." Yet is is clear that the challenge is far too great for philosophy alone to meet. Indeed, just as health education is not a panacea for all the ills in society, philosophy is not a panacea for the problems affecting health education. It does, however, present us with a significant opportunity to at the very least begin to understand our discipline more clearly. And although we may not find tacit answers and solutions to our problems, at least we will have begun to examine the elements of the discipline, be they good or bad.

Essential Nature or Fundamental Character of Health Education

Underlying professional thought and work are certain assumptions, hypotheses, and beliefs about the meaning of ideas. These form the philosophic base of any profession. The questions are these: What is health education? What is its substance and nature? How is health education included by or distinguished from disciplines such as nursing, patient education, hospital administration, medicine, physical education, psychology, physiology, and sociology?

To attempt to answer these questions it is essential that we first seek an appreciation and understanding of the idea of *health*. In simple terms, what do you believe about health? What does the term really mean?

Etymologically *health* is derived from the Anglo-Saxon word *haelth*, meaning safe, sound, or whole. In a number of languages *health* and *wholeness* as well as *health* and *holiness* are etymologically linked.[4]

Over the years health has had a variety of meanings, including freedom from disease and quality of life. Traditionally, health was viewed as physical well-being and as a static state. Contemporary views of health define it as a process instead of a condition and as a concept with physical, social, emotional, and spiritual dimensions.

The first attempt to rectify the limitations of defining health in the physical sense alone was made by the World Health Organization (WHO), which redefined health as a "state of complete physical, mental, and social well-being and not merely the absence of disease or infirmity."[5] Jesse Feiring Williams, a progressive thinker in the 1930s, observed that "health as freedom from disease is a standard of mediocrity; health as the quality of life is a standard of inspiration and increasing achievement."[6]

Relating health to quality of life was a dramatic departure from traditional thought. The enlightened thinking of scholars such as Dubos, Hoyman, and Dunn has resulted in more comprehensive philosophic interpretations of the meaning of health. The contemporary view of health is perhaps best expressed by Hoyman:

> A (person) wants health as a means of living the kind of life and striving toward the kinds of goals that he sets for life. Only the health crank or hypochondriac values health as an end in itself. A truly healthful person will sacrifice his physical health and if need be his life, for values he considers greater than himself.[7]

In line with this thinking is the general agreement among health educators that emphasizing increased life span as an indicator of health is insufficient and that the quality of life a person experiences is far more important than longevity. Health is now considered *one* means of achieving a full life.

According to Webster, a definition is "A word or phrase expressing the essential nature of a person or thing." It sounds simple enough, but capturing in a word or phrase the essential nature of what we call *health* is a very difficult, and perhaps not very useful, task. So explained Carlyon when describing his concept of health. He continued: "For these reasons, I'd sooner describe health as I see it, rather than define it."[8]

Before stepping off into that realm of speculation, social science, and sentiment wherein we customarily grope for meaning for the world *health* it might be useful to separate the health territory from two adjacent territories with which it is frequently confused.

Disease. Disease is largely a scientific, medical, and technical territory that encompasses what is known about biologic impairment. It has been explored with diligence and its many variations weighed and measured, and their labels are considered more or less universal.

Illness. Illness is the territory in which social judgment defines that deviance for which the physician and other health practitioners are considered the official remedial agents. It includes biologic deviance but encompasses a wide range of human behavior also judged to be deviant. Illness is culturally defined.

Health. Health is entirely a philosophic territory. It begins beyond disease and illness. Health can no more be defined as the absence of illness or disease than New York City can be defined as the absence of Chicago or Los Angeles. Health is a territory by itself. It is erroneous to imagine that people spend their lives sliding up and down a continuum marked by levels of illness and wellness, with death at one end and some sort of superhealth at the other. Health and illness are separate territories. They can coexist. It is possible to be ill and still be healthy.

The outstanding feature of health is that it is a quality and therefore cannot be weighed and measured. Health is not a single entity or condition. There are levels of health that can be distinguished one from the other, but it is easier to observe the differences than to define health itself. That it exists seems certain, but getting a firm hold on it is virtually impossible. In fact, the health territory has no independent existence at all. It is a state of mind, a projection of our beliefs about the nature and perfectibility of humans and our value judgments about what constitutes a good person in a good society.[8]

In concluding this section it should be pointed out that in a national survey of health educators on the meaning of health and the scope and nature of health education no consensus was reached on the definition of health.[9] These results prompt the question, Does it then seem reasonable to assume that Carlyon's belief that capturing the essential nature of what we call 'health' is a very difficult, and perhaps not very useful, task? What then is health education?

Over the years health education has been defined and conceived of in various ways. It has been called a "quasi-academic area," "an emerging discipline which has grown from infancy to adolescence," and "a vital component of health and medical programs which utilizes educational processes to achieve disease-preventive, curative, rehabilitative and health-promotive ends."

In 1977 a *Report on Current Status and Needs for Health Education* was prepared with the support of the Bureau of Health Education. The rationale for this report was as follows:

> Health Education as a profession and as a field of endeavor is fragmented among a variety of organizations and disciplines. This fragmentation is accompanied by a panorama of notions about what health education is and about what competencies are needed for its adequate performance. This fragmentation and lack of definition often results in a lack of recognition and priority for the professional health educator.[10]

Let us focus on what health educators themselves consider to be the nature of health education.

In 1976 a Conference on Professional Preparation was held in Towson, Maryland. One focus of this conference was a discussion of the question What is health education? It was not the purpose of the Towson conference to redefine health education, but participants accepted the following statements concerning health education:

1. Health education is a professional field and an academic discipline, and eclectic in nature for its scientific base.
2. Health education strategies provide needed approaches to bridging the gap between scientific discovery and its application for everyday healthful purposes.
3. Health education is an integral part of the school curriculum at all levels and an integral component of community-based health programs.
4. Health education contributes to the total education of the individual by providing meaningful experiences that can positively influence health behavior.
5. Health education principles and strategies are based on and improved through basic and applied research.
6. Health education is most appropriately engaged in by the professionally prepared health educator.
7. Health education facilitates the primary prevention of health problems.[11]

Mico and Ross have stated the beliefs of many professionals in the field:

> (1) Health education is an educationally-oriented process; (2) its target is the individual, even when conducted in community or mass-media settings; (3) it focuses on closing the gap between that which is known to be good for health and that which is actually being practiced by the individual; and (4) it is concerned with the behavior of the individual and the forces of needs, values, motivations and perceptions that influence those behaviors.[12]

Health education was defined by the working group on The Role Delineation Project as a "process, based upon scientific principles, which employs planned learning opportunities to enable individuals, acting separately or collectively, to make and act upon informed decisions about things affecting their health."[14] Encompassed in this definition are efforts directed toward assisting people to achieve an optimal level of health, to prevent disease and debilitating conditions from occurring, and to minimize the impact of such diseases and conditions on individuals who have been afflicted. The focal points for health education activities are individuals and individuals acting collectively in groups and organizations. Through education, health education specialists work to enhance those factors that predispose, enable, and reinforce healthy behavior.[13]

As such, is health education a unique and distinct discipline, different from nursing or medicine through its purpose and its methods?

Recently two fields have emerged that bear close resemblance to health education as it has been defined and described. One of these new multidisciplinary fields is called behavioral medicine. The field is defined as being concerned with "the development of behavioral science knowledge and techniques relevant to the understanding of physical health and illness and the application of this knowledge and these techniques to prevention, diagnosis, treatment and rehabilitation."[14]

Dwore and Matarazzo discuss in a scholarly paper another development germane to health education—the emergence of "behavioral health." This is an interdisciplinary field dedicated to promoting a philosophy of health that stresses individual responsibility in the application of behavioral and biomedical science knowledge and techniques to the maintenance of health and the prevention of illness and dysfunction by a variety of self-initiated individual or shared activities.[15] The purpose of behavioral health is promoting health among currently healthy people.

The behavioral sciences are generally considered to include such areas as psychology, sociology, anthropology, economics, political science, and geography. These disciplines are concerned with individual and collective behavior of people in various situations. The extent to which they focus on health varies from discipline to discipline. Obviously health education is rather significantly involved in health-related individual and collective behavior. But so are behavioral health and behavioral medicine.

What then are the ramifications of these recently developed fields for health education? Dwore and Matarazzo suggest

> The behavioral sciences and health education have many common means and ends, strengths and weaknesses. Both are oriented toward studying human behavior and improving the quality of life for the individual, family and society through teaching, research

and service . . . Both are seeking to increase their scientific knowledge base and hence improve the potential of the services they provide . . . Neither area, nor any area, has a monopoly over the study of human behavior, including the factors and processes involved in health promotion (i.e., decision making, learning theory, behavior modification, human values or personal growth and development). Instead, differences largely are based on degrees of emphasis and issues of content. Traditionally the behavioral sciences have been more academic than applied. Health education developed somewhat untraditionally, with problem solving and application preceding theory.[16]

Dwore and Matarazzo suggest three ways in which the behavioral sciences and health education may relate to one another, including (1) to continue as at present with little formal articulation, (2) to compete with each other for larger resource allocations through claiming primacy in common areas, and (3) to interact with each other for multidisciplinary collaboration in which cross-fertilization of ideas is stimulated.

What are the implications of three fields so closely related? What is the best way for these fields to relate to one another? How should "best way" be defined, both to the professions and to society? Is health education a unique and distinct discipline?

Settings for Health Education

At the 1978 Bethesda Conference entitled Commonalities and Differences in the Preparation and Practice of Health Educators, Helen Cleary[17] suggested three possible classifications for health educators. The first of these was by function. Cleary suggested that although most health educators perform both teaching and planning functions, each has major responsibility for one of two functions: (1) those who teach in schools, colleges, medical care institutions, or community settings or (2) those who plan, organize, coordinate, and evaluate health education programs in schools, colleges, medical care settings, or community settings.

The second classification offered was by the type of institution in which the health educator works. The classification of nonmedical care institution versus medical care institution is an example of this scheme. Cleary suggests that by and large health educators in medical institutions perform disease education and health educators in nonmedical institutions perform primarily health education.

A third classification proposed by Cleary was by professional identity. In this regard, SOPHEs Committee on Professional Preparation and Practice identified three types of health educators: (1) those who teach health education in the schools, (2) those who plan, coordinate, and evaluate health education programs in schools and other settings, and (3) those with a professional identity other than health educator who perform health education.

Cleary suggests that the distinction by professional identity may be the most useful. Thus when we talk about health educators we are referring to professionals who identify health or disease education as their major responsibility.

In discussing the community, patient, and school settings in which health education takes place, Sliepcevich says, "If you examine the locus of each of these three elements, you will note that: 'community' is an *abstraction,* 'patient' refers to a *being,* 'school' is an identifiable *place.*" Further Sliepcevich observes that some health educators would view community as

> the territory of a designated kind of health educator, whereas my concept of "community" would include the school or university as a "community"; the workplace as a "community"; the home as a "community"; the neighborhood, the state, the nation, the world, the universe as "communities," as well as, the "community of solution." All of these settings would meet the criteria of community. Community as health has no boundaries. Perhaps we are talking about "community based health education." In that case, the parameters of the setting in which a health education program takes place delimits the community (e.g., hospital based, school based, home based).[3]

In referring to the sometimes subtle, sometimes resounding differences of opinion regarding health education, its substance and goals, between public health educators and school health educators, Sliepcevich warns, "We cannot let territorial imperatives implied in titles interfere with our common goal of education for health." Sliepcevich is hopeful that there will "emerge awareness that health education should be reinforcing as individuals move from one setting to another and interact with others in their environments, who also may have been health educated in other settings," and further that

> Role, Function and Setting are interrelated and interdependent. As any one of these change, so will the other two. In . . . reality that the orientation of the social structure and the setting determines the boundaries of the health educator's role and functions.[3]

Missions and Goals of Health Education

Perhaps the first and most basic questions in the philosophy of a profession are: What is this discipline for? What is its body of knowledge for? On this topic Burt says that "professionalism begins with a group of people bound together by common purpose or purposes and operating within recognizable boundaries—boundaries known to those within and those outside the group."[18] Has health education as a profession identified its basic mission? Are health educators bound together by common purpose(s)? Are we operating within clearly delineated boundaries? Some would respond affirmatively to all three of these questions. These health educators would say that our basic mission is health promotion—social, physical, and emotional— among population groups. They would also say that the use and value of health education is that it helps the individual and society in general to achieve, restore, and maintain health.

Other health educators would unequivocally say "no" in response to each question and ask

How many times will it take carefully selected groups to go to the well and return without water before someone discovers that a pitcher without a bottom, without a base should be replaced by one that has such an essential, if they expect to come back with the water.[2]

These health educators express frustration with what they call "the intrinsic superficiality" in health education as it now exists. Others suggest that although we do not have our act together yet as a profession, we are making some progress and that perhaps what we need to do is go back and explore the values of the field before we can identify goals.

At this point let us examine the efforts of health education that focus on identifying its goals and parameters. At the 1978 Bethesda Conference on Health Education participants were asked to respond to the question, "What do you perceive as the goals of health education?"

After an initial generation of goal statements, participants realized that the statements they had come up with were quite diverse in terms of scope and content. They decided therefore to identify an overall or "umbrella" goal separately and to place more specific goal statements into a subgoal or supporting goal category. These goals, as viewed by the workshop participants, in essence set the parameters of the field. The goal statements listed below represent a synthesis of views expressed in the various discussion groups.

Goal. The goal of health education is to maintain, promote, and improve individual and community health through educational processes.

Background: The discussants agreed that there are certain fundamental elements that should be incorporated into a general goal for the profession. The overall goal stated above sets forth the important link between health and education that is characteristic of the profession. It points out that the impact of health education is broader than that of disease prevention or therapeutic educational intervention. It covers educational activities relating to the maintenance, promotion, and improvement of health. This goal therefore suggests a wide continuum between health and disease, spanning both prevention and treatment. Moreover, it illustrates the dual concern for affecting health on both an individual and community level.

Subgoal I. To foster or facilitate individual and community responsibility for the prevention of disease and the management of optimum health status.

Background: One of the issues raised by the discussants was the question of responsibility for health. The discussants defined the difference between ultimate responsibility for disease prevention and health maintenance and the responsibility of the profession to facilitate individual and community acceptance of this ultimate responsibility. Although they concurred that health educators help define behaviors that are positive or negative to health status, their prime responsibility is to facilitate health behavioral change processes that have already begun within the society. In providing activities that motivate and stimulate people toward health-related behavior, health educators assist providers and advance wellness maintenance. In addition to defining responsibility for disease prevention and health maintenance, this subgoal also points out the continuum implied in the meaning of health, from disease to optimum health status.

Subgoal II. To facilitate opportunities among individuals and communities to make informed decisions or intelligent choices regarding health and health behavior.

Background: The general consensus of the participants was that health education should provide a milieu in which change is possible. It should make the range of choices and the consequences of each choice apparent to the target population. The participants indicated that health education as much as possible should involve facilitation rather than coercion or manipulation regarding health and health behavior.

Subgoal III. To effectively stimulate community interest in health resulting in the development of consumerism, participation, conservation, and prevention.

Background: The participants viewed health for any individual as being to a large extent a result of community decision. They agreed that health education therefore must be specifically concerned with the role of the community in the maintenance, promotion, and improvement of health. Reflecting the central importance of this issue, they concluded that community interest leads to or depends on informed decisions and increased acceptance of responsibility for health.[18]

This compilation of goals represents the work of various health education professionals who came together for a 3-day period to consider the discipline of which they were members. This is indeed one useful way to identify the goals of a profession. Philosophers have always emphasized the need for bringing together or synthesizing experiences, ideas, and beliefs. This workship provided a type of synthesizing experience for participants. It brought together those who identified themselves as public health educators, school health educators, and patient educators. It offered participants an opportunity to explore centers of belief and promoted the recognition of relationships between and within the experiences of health educators who function in various settings.

However, the viewpoint of the participants is of equal importance in attempting to identify the goals or values of a field. What do participants in health education encounters get out of the experience? What do participants want to get out of health education encounters? Answers to these questions will partially provide us with the information we need to decide if health education has a place in schools, community health agencies, worksites, and health care institutions; for that matter, if health education even has a place in American life. These are crucial questions when determining goals.

Before you discount this last statement as pure heresy remember that the philosophic process is impossible when emotional involvement is strong or when a closed-door attitude exists. As Davis and Miller stated: "Personal interest can be so emphasized and insisted upon that almost everything else seems unimportant. Perspective is lost. Sound thinking becomes difficult, even impossible."[2] You must be careful not to become a slave to an idea; rather control and modify ideas and beliefs as you gather truth. In a similar way, by side-stepping the difficult and searching for security, the philosophic process is thwarted. As health educators we need to guard against being satisfied with lists of words that represent values that reflect credit on the profession and its members.

In order to clarify these thoughts on the value derived and perceived by the participants in health education let us go back and analyze the goals identified earlier in this chapter.

Subgoal I. To foster or facilitate individual or community responsibility for the prevention of disease and management of optimum health status.

Do individuals want responsibility for their own health promotion? If so, why is it that 80% of patients treated by physicians have self-limiting illnesses that they could have managed themselves?

What causes people to behave in unhealthy ways? Why is 60% of the adult population in the United States overweight? Why does 33% of the population smoke cigarettes? Why do only about 33% of Americans exercise regularly?

Is it possible that people just want to be left alone and live health-destructive lifes in hopes that someone else can "fix them up" if they become ill and not be bothered about "taking responsibility for their own health?"

Is it possible that some people just value things more than health and that moneymaking or lovemaking is more important, or that comfort, convenience, and immediate gratification are more important than the long-term concern of good health?

Should we be trying to make individuals assume ultimate responsibility for their health? If as professionals we truly believe in freedom, would not we also believe in "informed refusal?" The question is not can we but rather should we be providing activities that motivate people toward adopting health behaviors? Is this what participants want?

Subgoal II. To facilitate opportunities among individuals and communities to make informed decisions or intelligent choices regarding health and health behavior.

Do participants want to know about the importance to good health of eating breakfast each day, or exercising three times a week, or practicing self-hypnosis daily? Or do participants want to know how to start and maintain a regimen of exercise, self-hypnosis, and eating breakfast?

Is it knowledge the participants want and value? Do they merely want information they feel they can use? Or do they want more? Do participants want to be able to make informed choices about health and health behavior?

Subgoal III. To effectively stimulate community interest in health, resulting in the development of consumerism, participation, conservation, and prevention.

Of what benefit to the individual is community interest in health? Do individuals believe that they want a profession like health education to help them participate as active health consumers? Do all people, or even most people, value conservation?

John Burt emphasizes the necessity of a profession identifying with and understanding the "wants" of its constituency. He explains it this way:

> To develop a successful enterprise it is necessary to market a product or service for which there is a consumer. To become a legitimate enterprise the product or service must be reliable and worthwhile. To become both successful and legitimate, an enterprise must acquaint the consumer with a product or service that is worthwhile and, in turn, the consumer must "try it and like it." Health education could become a very successful and legitimate enterprise. The market is right. In fact, "Our time has come" is an echo often heard. But somehow the price of our stock has failed to exhibit a spurt—a condition exacerbated by the rapid growth of related stocks. Someone ought to research both the market and the service. Indeed, maybe all health educators ought to research the matter.[19]

Approaches of Health Education

At the present time there is considerable agreement among health educators that the ultimate goal of the profession is health behavior. That is, most would concur that the critical outcome of a health education intervention is that the individual possess the understanding, skills, and experience needed to make and implement informed health decisions. However, there continues to be disagreement among health educators as to the method by which this outcome is best achieved.

Until recently, both the public and school health education branches of the discipline concentrated on the information-giving aspect of health education. Most believed that what people do about health is more important than what they know about health. However, the goal of many health education programs has been to increase knowledge or to change attitudes.

The theory that has predominated in health education for many years is simple: An increase in knowledge plus a more favorable attitude will lead to a behavior change that is health-generating.

Dwore and Matarazzo, among others, express concern about health knowledge being the main goal of health education. They suggest that

> health education's concentration on merely providing information has resulted in consistent liabilities throughout its history. The major issue has revolved around demonstration of results: namely, what good has this information done for the recipients?[16]

Green and associates[20] believe that

> No matter where, how, and by whom it is offered, health education is a process related to health decisions and practices. Knowledge, values, perceptions and motivation are, of course, causes of behavior, but the linkages between them is a matter of probability.[20]

In summary, the criticisms leveled against health education's focus on increasing knowledge of participants is related to several key points:

1. The assumption that the more health-related knowledge a person possesses the greater the likelihood of that person adopting health-generating behaviors is ill-founded.
2. The knowledge equals behavior approach has not been effective in the past and its effectiveness in the future is unlikely because it is based on an ill-founded assumption.
3. As professionals we must be able to document that we provide our society with a valuable service and the knowledge equals behavior approach has failed to accomplish this.

Another school of thought that is growing in popularity in health education holds that the emphasis of health education programs should be on altering behavior, not knowledge. The PRECEDE model developed by Green and associates recognizes the complexity of behavior change and uses a diagnostic approach for health education program planning based on the theory and techniques of four disciplines, including the behavioral sciences. The emphasis in this approach is placed on demonstrating an impact on behavior. The overriding principle in this approach to health education is that health behavior must be voluntary and that health behavior should be compelled only in cases in which the health of others is threatened.

The proponents of the approach suggest that "in the final analysis, health education programs are effective only to the extent that they influence the health practices which in research are found to be causally related to desired health outcomes."[20] Consequently this apporach emphasizes a behavioral diagnosis in which it is necessary to establish a cause-and-effect relationship between behavior and health.

One method used in the behavior change approach is client-contract behavior modification. In this type of program a person voluntarily enters a program, is fully informed of the methods used, decides on and makes an open commitment to a degree of desired behavior change, and has full freedom to withdraw from the program at any time.

The behavior change approach also has been critized for reasons including the following:

1. The assumption that life-style behaviors are primary determinants of health status is ill-founded. Critics suggest that social and economic conditions in the United States directly determine some diseases and indirectly create or promote life-styles that contribute to other diseases.

2. The use of behavior change as the primary tool for health education raises ethical issues related primarily to freedom and power. A key is to influence behavior change in such a way as to increase the ability of people to control their own destiny. As Hochbaum has said, our charge is "to shape and free people" at the same time.

3. Although the behavior change approach has demonstrated success in changing the behavior of small groups of volunteers, there is no evidence that as a public health strategy it offers hope for reducing morbidity or mortality from the major health problems we face today.[21]

Another alternative method for health education that has been proposed is social change. This approach is based on the assumption that the primary determinant of health and disease is the social and economic structure of the United States. Freudenberg describes this approach:

> Health education for social change identifies the health-damaging elements in our society. Its goal is to involve people in collective action to create health-promoting environments and life-styles. . . . The following principles characterize health education for social change:
> 1. It recognizes the social and economic determinants of health and disease.
> 2. It combines education, services and political action. Each enhances the contribution of the other.
> 3. It emphasizes the need for collective action and mutual support.
> 4. Its starting point is the problems that people face in their daily lives.
> 5. Its primary allegiance is to the people it serves.[21]

The objections raised to a social change approach for health education revolve around three issues. First, some believe that the social change approach reflects a particular political philosophy and that health education should retain its objectivity outside of the political arena. Some argue that political action is ill-suited to professions and that this type of activity should remain the responsibility of private citizens. Some fear that if health education adopts a strategy that promotes social change, it runs the risk of alienating itself from the health care system in general and from physicians in particular, on whom health education depends for support. Finally, some believe that the assumptions underlying the social change approach to health education are both ill-founded and unrealistic.

Further Areas for Philosophic Inquiry
Limits and Organization of Knowledge

Clearly a key component of any profession is a body of knowledge that serves as a theoretical and practical base from which and within which the profession operates. Equally important is the generation and application of new knowledge by professionals. With this in mind I will now explore the subject of knowledge boundaries of health education and the conduct of research, seeking answers to such questions as, What are the substantive boundaries of health education? Does health education have theoretical and conceptual bases?

At the present time there is evidence to suggest that although health education does not yet have clearly defined boundaries nor a substantive body of knowledge, it is closer than ever before to achieving these. Green and associates, in the preface to a recently published health education text, have said:

> This book is the product of a period of growth and development in health education that was at times exhilarating but often painful in the recognition that the field has been without a clear articulation of its boundaries, its methods, its procedures. . . . Health education knowledge has been inadequately codified.[20]

In a recent study of the scope and nature of health education there was general agreement among health educators surveyed that if a discipline is unable to clearly define its boundaries, massive conceptual and methodologic problems may result.[22] These problems may involve areas such as professional preparation, continuing education, the conduct of research, protection of the public, and use to society.

However, as a profession we are closer to accumulating a body of knowledge to serve as the discipline's base, primarily through the development of paradigms. Paradigms and their underlying assumptions provide the context in which research is conducted and knowledge is accumulated. "Thus, paradigms not only comprise and define the body of knowledge that becomes a discipline, they also determine which problems or questions are to be addressed by research."[23]

Recently two paradigms have been proposed for health education— the Health Belief Model and the PRECEDE model. These models, according to Kolbe and associates have been designed to represent our understandings about the nature of, and relationships among, independent variables that influence health behaviors. The ultimate function of these paradigms is to describe how the component independent variables can be influenced to increase the probability that a given behavior will occur (or not occur as the case may be). The focus of these paradigms is on the question "What factors are important to understand and influence in order to elicit a desired decision about a specified behavior?"[23]

In discussing the factors that determine the development of health education, Green[26,27] conceives two overlapping cycles:

In the first cycle, professional decisions about theory influence policy, which influences practice, which influences research, which in turn influences theory. Decisions about policy also influence training, which influences research. In the second cycle, the public's understanding of health education theory and policy determine their demands and expectations of health education, which in turn influence health education policy and practice. These cycles illustrate the immense power of research paradigms to influence professional decisions and public expectations of health education.[23]

Ethics (the Common Good)

Ethics is a branch of philosophy that attempts to discover whether conduct is good or bad, right or wrong. It seeks to shed light on the relative rightness or wrongness of actions based on such moral principles as individual freedom, equality or justice, and beneficence or "doing goodness." What is an ethic? It is a value, a standard. It is what ought to be in a world of what is.

Health education, unlike most helping professions, lacks a code of ethics that is understood by its members and endorsed by all its professional organizations. The nature of health education is such that there is potential for ethical abuse that in turn may adversely affect both the profession and the society.

What are some of the ethical issues facing health education today? Here are some questions that in turn may generate discussion about professional ethics. Hochbaum[26] has raised the following questions relating to the ethical practice of health education:

1. Are we in a sense playing "big brother" when we decide what behaviors others should adopt and then influence for that behavior-change?
2. How far *can* and *should* we go to influence a skeptical public's attitudes and behaviors?
3. When are our means and methods so strong that they restrict the individual's ability to exercise a choice?

Other related questions about ethical conduct in health education that need to be addressed include, To what extent do health educators help people to fulfill themselves in their own unique ways? Are we as health educators consciously or unconsciously seeking power over people, expecting them to resemble ourselves in point of view and behavior? What constitutes professional integrity? What makes a health educator a dependable and reliable practitioner? What are the duties or responsibilities of a health educator to the public, to individual clients, and to colleagues and the profession?

Daniel Callahan, a noted ethicist, has developed moral propositions that are applicable to health educators and can serve as a guide to ethical conduct in our field:

1. We are responsible for the consequences of our voluntary and intentional actions, and unintended consequences resulting from negligence.
2. We are responsible for unforseeable consequences if the actions that caused them were capricious and irrational.
3. We must answer to those people affected by our actions when those actions violate their wishes and values and in particular when there are harmful consequences.[27]

Editors' Remarks

As previously noted, the philosophy of a profession does not just happen; it is shaped by history. It must be analyzed in the context of the society from which it grew. Dr. Shirreff has presented a philosophic statement that portrays current thinking toward health education. It is a statement that would not have accurately described the profession 10 years ago and may not describe the profession 10 years from now. Although some elements will remain the same, others undoubtedly will change in response to events as they unfold.

To understand how health education developed its current philosophy it will be useful to examine educational thought from a historical perspective. Over the centuries many philosophers have presented educational ideology, but by necessity it always reflected the circumstances of the larger society. A few examples will demonstrate the fact that one cannot separate educational philosophy from the times in which it is written. Philosophy must be interpreted as part of the milieu that influenced its creation.

The great Greek philosophers saw education from an idealistic point of view. Education was valuable to the extent that it enabled one to appreciate life and to take advantage of the aesthetic qualities not appreciated by the masses. Plato believed that education serves as a mechanism to redirect the entire personality toward goodness. He wrote that the most important state official should be the minister of education. Socrates observed that education had the potential to formulate attitudes and to shape behavior. Aristotle understood the relationship between the mental, physical, and spiritual aspects of human life. All three philosophers realized that education could enhance self-esteem, self-reliance, personal responsibility, and the attainment of individual goals.

Although these concepts are still appropriate, it must be recognized that the Greek educational system and the very idea of education is quite different from today's. The nature of Greek society encouraged such a philosophy. From among the elite, education was expected to produce leaders, thinkers, and doers. It was an opportunity available only to those of wealth and breeding. Education was intended not so much to benefit society directly as to provide the male nobility with the opportunity of attaining self-enhancement as well as the skills necessary to fulfill the responsibilities of their birthright. Indirectly, their knowledge and their benevolent decisions would benefit all of society.

The Roman civilization was more practical and less idealistic. Because of the complex and sophisticated nature of their society, schools were established by the State to train men for positions of responsibility and service to the state. Only gradually did a state-endorsed theory of education evolve. All schools were required to adopt the official curriculum. Originally Romans believed that education should take place in the home through family discussion. But as the empire spread and new territories were incorporated, it became necessary to reinforce the Roman way of life and the values that created the empire. Education in the state-run schools, using approved curricula and teachers, would not encourage self-actualization and independence, but it would effectively perpetuate the philosophy of the state.

The Middle Ages grew from the fall of the Roman Empire. Religion was important in nearly all aspects of medieval life. A new intellectual philosophy, known as Scholasticism, was popularized by St. Thomas Aquinas. Education centered on Latin, the classics, and religious philosophy. The Bible was the textbook and lessons came from the scriptures. Dramatic political and cultural changes during the Renaissance created a philosophy that glorified the individual. Consequently the writings of the humanists determined educational theroy and practice.

Health education in this country has been influenced by events taking place in the larger society. Consider the following examples. In 1874 the Women's Christian Temperance Union was established, and shortly thereafter every state required alcohol education in the public schools. When men were found to be physically unfit for military duty in World War II, schools received new impetus for encouraging personal fitness. When Russia launched its first Sputnik satellite in October of 1957, "frill" subjects such as health education were eliminated to make room for the basic sciences. In order to increase efficiency students were tested, labeled as college bound, and homogeneously grouped. Money was made available from the federal government to hire guidance counselors who could help to increase the proportion of graduating seniors who would attend college. The National Defense Education Act appropriated money to help pay tuition for students who would eventually contribute to the national security. Health education was temporarily stalled.

More specific examples can be identified in more recent history. In 1965 the Medicare and Medicaid bills were passed by Congress. Widely publicized abuses and the rising costs of health care led to consumer health education programs supported with government funds. Programs for the prevention of mental retardation were developed because President John F. Kennedy was vitally interested. President Lyndon B. Johnson promoted the "Great Society," and "humanistic" education became popular in schools and colleges. President Richard M. Nixon formed the President's Committee on Health Education in 1971 and from it came renewed interest in comprehensive school health education, creation of community health education centers, and a National Center for Health Education. President Jimmy Carter and his wife were interested in mental health, so many community health education programs were established. President Ronald Reagan's support of the "prolife" philosophy and of parental notification for minors who seek birth control will most definitely have an impact on the provision of women's health services.

Health education has been criticized for being a reactive profession. There are numerous examples of topical areas that burst onto the scene in response to contemporary events. To name a few: Earth Day 1972 produced interest in environmental health and ecology; the rise of a drug subculture, as typified by the Haight-Ashbury area of San Francisco in the 1960s, reestablished community interest in drug education; the increasing incidence of teenage pregnancy and sexually transmitted diseases demonstrated the need for family living and sex education; and increasing deaths on highways as a result of alcohol abuse brought forth public outrage that led to school and community programs intended to curb the fatalities. It is common to find similar shifts in priority even at the local level. Recently, in a Pennsylvania community three students were expelled from school for possession of illegal drugs. The community raised $5000 to bring in an "expert" for 2 days of intensive meetings with student and adult groups. Plans were made to reconsider the entire drug education curriculum, methodology, and time allotted for instruction.

In one respect health education deserves criticism for being reactionary, but on the other hand it has consistently attempted to meet the pressing health and social needs of the nation and the individual communities. Perhaps the time has come for health education to play an active role in society. From a variety of settings (school, worksite, community) health educators have assessed the nation's health concerns. It is possible to identify issues and predict trends in advance of the crisis stage (see Chapter 8). Effective program planning and intervention can reduce the consequences of transient but powerful social events.

There is another possibility that offers even more potential benefit. Comprehensive health education can coordinate the efforts of school and community health educators. The word *comprehensive* means not only offering diverse topical content, but also coordinating the efforts of diverse segments of society. An ongoing needs assessment for a planning guide enables school health educators to construct a meaningful K-12 curriculum. Public health educators can concentrate on specific community groups and prepare classroom activities appropriate for the audience. Community health educators can present the same topics to adult audiences as are being presented in the school classroom, with appropriate modifications in level of content and learning activities. School personnel can sit on the community health council and representatives from the community can belong to the school health council. The outcome of a coordinated community effort is likely to be greater than the sum of the parts. Messages received from and reinforced by different sources may effect better health behavior than single-source messages.

Regardless of the setting in which a health educator works, the basic objectives, activities, and skills necessary to perform those activities will be fairly similar. There may be differences in philosophy as they relate to the educational setting, the intended audience, or the individual educator (see Chapter 4), but we believe the similarities overshadow the differences. That is, health educators will share a good bit of ideology regardless of where they received their professional preparation or where they are employed. There should be a common core of beliefs that are shared throughout the health education profession.

In addition to health content and teaching methodology, health educators should understand the nature of the learner. Psychologists such as John Dewey, Carl Rogers, Jean Piaget, and Abraham Maslow have expressed their thoughts on human development and learning theory. All health educators should possess an understanding of human development and mental health because that understanding will most definitely influence decisions about the teaching-learning process.

Behavioral Foundations

In the space available for this section it is impossible to provide a thorough background in the behavioral sciences. The purpose of this brief discussion is to demonstrate the fact that health education depends heavily on the fields of psychology and sociology as foundations for program planning and implementation. Just as health education depends on the biologic sciences for much of its content and the educational discipline for much of its methodology, so too it depends on the behavioral sciences for the establishment of a philosophy about the teaching-learning process that is derived from social scientific research. If we accept the premise that the overall purpose of health education is the facilitation of healthful behavior, then we must also accept the fact that the behavioral sciences are indispensable foundations of our profession. It should be apparent that preparation as a health educator requires extensive course work in the behavioral sciences.

In a room full of people some will be cigarette smokers while others will not. Some individuals will regularly monitor their body for changes that may indicate the onset of disease, and others will not think twice about this kind of preventive activity. Still other people will buckle their seat belts during long trips on the interstate highway while others will choose to protect themselves even when they are close to home. What accounts for these differences of behavior when we know that factual information is equally available to each of these individuals? To understand we need to study the internal and external forces that guide a person's behavior. These two disciplines, psychology and sociology, are part of a broad field of study known as behavioral science.

For the most part, differences in health behavior are not attributable to differences in knowledge. In fact, studies have shown that smokers are more cognizant of the potential consequences of tobacco use than are nonsmokers. To understand why people behave as they do we need to understand the multitude of complex forces that motivate them. The concept of multiple forces is important because, returning to our examples, not all people smoke for the same set of reasons, not all people monitor their body for the same set of reasons, and not all people use their car's seat belts for the same set of reasons. Furthermore, some people who smoke cigarettes always use seat belts for safety, and some people who never use seat belts consider it a personal responsibility to regularly inspect themselves for the warning signs of cancer.

If all we had to do was dispense information to ensure proper behavior, then vending machines could certainly replace health educators. The purpose of health information is to effect positive health behavior. The challenge for health educators is to increase the likelihood that individuals in the intended audience will favorably respond to educational efforts. The opportunity for success is diminished when planning disregards the information available from the behavioral sciences.

Behavioral sciences are important to health educators regardless of the setting in which they work. Normally people in attendance in a community health program are already motivated; otherwise they would not take time from a busy schedule to attend. The issue of learner readiness is not a problem. On the other hand, the people most in need of education may be the ones who choose to watch television instead of coming to a community health education program. The community health educator needs to determine why the audience is present, and likewise the health educator needs to find alternative means of reaching the people who do not feel comfortable at a community forum. Good planning involves more than content. The health educator needs to consider all of the factors that may play a role in attendance and participation and the establishment of a personal action plan for better health.

The advantage of school health education is that we can reach young people at a time when their values are being formed and often before bad habits are established. The disadvantage is that they may not want to be in school, in health class, or studying a particular topic. Another disadvantage related to motivation is that most teenagers are healthy most of the time; discussions of disease seem irrelevant to present needs. Through the study of child development and adolescent psychology the teacher has a better understanding of what is important to students and their level of readiness to use the information. Peer acceptance, self-esteem, and the need for security are powerful forces in the life of a teenager. The health educator can use these forces to help them see the personal relevance of the educational message. To briefly demonstrate this point, a high school teacher once asked her pupils to raise their hands if they wanted to study dating, mental health, and family living. Not one student raised a hand. Several days later she asked them to raise their hands if they wanted to study interpersonal relationships, social psychology, and health aspects of spirituality. This time nearly all the hands went up. She was a teacher who understood psychology.

Obviously psychology is not quite that simple. For one thing, people develop a skill for selective perception. They filter out some stimuli and respond to others. Psychology enables the educator, like the advertising executive, to predict which stimuli will be attractive and which will not. Factors such as the appearance of the person giving the lesson, the type of learning activity selected, the size of the group, or the location of the program can be the difference between success and failure. This is why peer education is effective when dealing with people of low socioeconomic status who mistrust the establishment, why role playing works well with people who cannot read, why small groups are effective for value-laden issues, and why churches are better places than hospitals to hold community classes on death education.

The health educator must try to see the learning experience through the eyes of the student. For example, it may be easy for the health educator to talk freely about sex, but not everyone in attendance will have the same degree of comfort. A summer session graduate class is recalled in which the teacher wanted to break down the barriers related to terminology. Cards with proper terminology were turned upside down on each desk during the first class, with instructions not to turn over the card. A 64-year-old woman who was about to enter her final year of teaching took a front row seat in order to see the blackboard. The instructor told the students to write down and then read aloud as many slang names as they could think of that were synonymous with the word on the card. The older woman was so embarrassed that she dropped the class before the second meeting.

Just as health educators need to use their knowledge of psychology to improve their effectiveness, they also need to consider the sociologic dimensions of the educational process. Sociology is important to the field of education because the subject matter is often sensitive to one social group or another. Education planners benefit from understanding the social norms of their intended audiences in order to construct a program that is accepted by the group. For instance, it might be helpful to know that people who are well educated tend to trust scientists and respond favorably to presentations delivered by experts, whereas poorly educated individuals tend to mistrust scientists and instead believe respected members of their own social group. Regardless of content, believability is enhanced in the former case by using authorities and in the latter case by using peer opinion leaders or peer educators.

Health-related content often requires special consideration for the beliefs, customs, and traditions of the intended audience. This is true because so many health-related issues are also value-laden issues, with "right and wrong" strongly entrenched in the attitudes of the group. To illustrate the point, consider your approach to the following educational challenges.

1. Contraception in a Roman Catholic school in which religion teaches that artificial means of birth control are wrong
2. Health care delivery and medical technology to Christian Scientists, who believe that faith is the way to restore health
3. Prevention of childhood diseases to the Amish, who don't believe in vaccinations
4. Parenting in an alternative school for pregnant teenagers
5. Breast self-examination to Chicano women, who are taught modesty and are hesitant to touch body parts that pertain to sexuality
6. Blood donation and transfusions to Navajos, who believe that individual spirit resides in the body and the blood
7. Health promotion and well-baby care to poor mothers who do not have money to buy other necessities
8. Stress reduction to executives, who achieved success by virtue of their hard-driving, competitive, and aggressive personalities
9. Mental health to a patient undergoing renal dialysis
10. The effects of alcohol to a group of adults who were arrested for driving under the influence of alcohol and who must attend class by order of the courts

Each of these examples demonstrates that program planning and implementation must consider the educational effort in the social context of the intended audience and that the educational process must focus on people rather than information. What is important is that the health educator be aware of personal beliefs and social norms that may inhibit health behavior or interfere with acceptance of the educational message. Conversely, knowledge of personal beliefs and social norms can be helpful in constructing an educational package that meets the needs of the audience and therefore has a better chance of facilitating healthful behavior.

Health educators and other human service personnel often perform research studies to determine how people feel about or act toward some issue of concern. These studies may explore knowledge, attitudes, or behavior. Most studies of this type build into the design of the questionnaire a section that deals with demographic characteristics such as age, sex, religion, and socioeconomic status in order to determine whether any of these factors (or several in combination) can influence a response. Knowing that differences in knowledge, attitudes, or behavior can be associated with a given demographic characteristic provides useful information for program planning. If a public school teacher finds that students are knowledgeable about the harmful effects of tobacco, that they have appropriate attitudes toward its nonuse, and that they do not smoke cigarettes, then the curricular time might be better spent on another health opic. But if it is found that certain characteristics typify the smoker, then the educator would benefit from knowing that and would be able to better plan a program aimed specifically at the subgroup of students.

Whatever health educators can do to help the learner become interested in the topic, to see the personal relevance of the material, and to feel comfortable with the learning environment will contribute to the overall success of the program. It may be necessary to use materials printed in another language or to use illustrations that are culturally familiar. It may be wise to alter the vocabulary and presentation of ideas to accommodate the learner. It may be helpful to use examples that are appreciated by the social group. This kind of consideration will definitely lead to more successful health education because the teaching-learning process is focused on the learner instead of the teacher.

Summary

A central theme of this chapter is unification. To some extent we have been hampered in our efforts to gain status and recognition because of fragmented philosophy. This idea is reiterated in Chapters 4 and 5. Dr. Shirreffs presents a systematic investigation of the fundamental character of the profession. A common understanding is important not only for communicating with one another but for sharing our convictions with others outside the field.

The chapter begins with a definition of the word *health*. It is worth repeating that health is not 180° from disease—it is not the opposite of sickness. Instead it is a quality of life, a zest for living—and a manner of travel rather than the destination. Health is given greater importance when we examine the priorities of life and emphasize the fact that health makes all things possible.

Chapter 1 described some of the issues and events that helped elevate health education to its current status. This chapter on philosophy demonstrates that many important issues are still unresolved. Consider for instance (1) the Conference on Professional Preparation held at Towson, Maryland, in 1976; (2) the Report on the Current Status and Needs for Health Education, supported by the Bureau of Health Education in 1977; and (3) the 1978 Bethesda Conference on Commonalities and Differences in Preparation and Practice of Health Education. Although we have come a long way toward the development of a unifying philosophy, there are still many areas of disagreement. Health education not only is competing with other behavioral sciences but also is experiencing intraprofessional conflicts that limit its progress.

The traditional approach to health education, with its focus on knowledge, is challenged. Dr. Shirreffs recognizes that behavior is a complex event precipitated by a host of interacting variables. A behavioral diagnosis therefore should be an essential part of program planning. The Health Belief Model and the PRECEDE model (see Chapter 5) are offered as paradigms to represent our understanding of health behavior. The social change approach to health briefly presented in this chapter is discussed more fully in Chapter 3.

The final section of the chapter considers the subject of ethics. Health education has many unresolved issues that can be classified as ethical concerns. In fact there is no single code of ethics that is universally endorsed by the professional associations. Issues that need to be resolved include (1) the right or responsibility of health educators to influence a person's behavior, (2) responsibilities owed to clients, the public, and other professionals, and (3) the definition of professional integrity.

The chapter raises a lot of questions; you are encouraged to contemplate and discuss these questions and formulate initial impressions. Further study will either affirm those impressions or challenge you to reevaluate the evidence. Before a profession can attain collective unity the individual members must possess a cohesive philosophy that can be communicated to others.

Questions for Review

1. How would you respond to someone who asked you to describe your philosophy of health education?
2. What differences and similarities in philosophy do you think exist between school health education and community health education?
3. Are there differences between the way health educators see the profession and the way the general public sees the profession?
4. How does health education relate to larger social issues such as the changing role of women, ecology, human rights, family planning, religion, and bioethics?
5. Is a health educator created from years of study and guided practice or are certain personality prerequisites inherent in all successful health educators?
6. Of the dozens of articles written on the philosophy of health education, which one most appropriately describes your philosophy?
7. How does a person's definition of health influence his/her premises about health education?
8. Do you agree with the goal and subgoals that were expressed by the participants of the Bethesda Conference?
9. What cultural, economic, legal, political, social, and technologic forces do you see affecting our profession in the future?
10. Do you agree or disagree with the statement that the more knowledge a person possesses the greater the likelihood that healthful behavior will be adopted?
11. What did Hochbaum mean when he said, "Our charge is to shape and free people at the same time."?
12. Select a specific population group and a health topic. What implications are derived from the Health Belief Model and the PRECEDE Model?
13. What ideas would you incorporate into a code of ethics for health educators?

References

1. Osterhoudt, R.G.: An introduction to the philosophy of physical education and sport, Champaign, Ill., 1978, Stipes Publishing Co.
2. Davis, E.C., and Miller, D.M.: The philosophic process in physical education, Philadelphia, 1967, Lea & Febiger.
3. Sliepcevich, E.: Overviewer comments, Proceedings of the Workshop on Commonalities and Differences in the Preparation and Practice of Health Education, Bethesda, Md., Feb. 15-17, 1978.
4. Horrine, F.: Toward a philosophy of health education, International Journal of Health Education, **9**(3):106-112, 1966.
5. Constitution of the World Health Organization, Chronicle of the World Health Organization **1**:3, 1947.
6. Williams, J.F.: Personal hygiene applied, Philadelphia, 1934, W.B. Saunders Co.
7. Hoyman, H.S.: Rethinking an ecological system of man's health, disease, aging and death, Journal of School Health, **45**(9):509-518, 1975.
8. Carlyon, W.H.: Coming back from utopia, Health Education **9**(1):25-28, 1978.
9. Shirreffs, J.H.: Investigating the meaning of health and the scope and nature of health education, Health Education **9**(1):25-28, 1978.
10. Report on the current status and needs for health education: performance standards and recommendations for action, Washington, D.C., 1978, U.S. Department of Health, Education and Welfare.
11. Bruess, C.E., editor: Professional preparation of the health educator, J. of School Health **46**(7):418-421, 1976.
12. Mico, P.R., and Ross, H.S.: Health education and behavioral science, Oakland, Third Party Associates, Inc.
13. Initial role delineation for health education: final report, DHHS Pub. No. (HRA) 80-44, Washington, D.C., 1980, U.S. Government Printing Offce.
14. Simmonds, S.: Scholarship: building the knowledge base of health education, Eta Sigma Gamman **10**:4-9, 1978.
15. Matarazzo, J.D.: Behavioral health and behavioral medicine: Frontiers for a New Health Psychology, American Psychologist **35**:812-815, 1980.
16. Dwore, R.B., and Matarazzo, J.D.: The behavioral sciences and health education, Health Education **12**:4-8, 1981.
17. Cleary, H.: Health education, state-of-the-art, parameters of the profession, Proceedings of the Workshop on Commonalities and Differences in the Preparation and Practice of Health Education, Bethesda, Md., 1978.
18. Burt, J.J.: Proceedings of The Workshop on Commonalities and Differences in the Preparation and Practice of Health Education, Bethesda, Md., Feb. 15-17, 1978.
19. Burt, J.J.: Research and the health education enterprise: an editorial, School Health Review **3**(6):2, 1972.
20. Green, L.W., Kreuter, M.W., Deeds, S.G., and Partridge, K.B.: Health education planning: a diagnostic approach, Palo Alto, Cal., 1980, Mayfield Publishing Co.
21. Freudenberg, N.: Shaping the future of health education: from behavior change to social change, Health Education Monographs, **6**(4):372-377, 1928.
22. Shirreffs, J.H.: A survey of the health science discipline—its relationship to other academic disciplines, Journal of School Health **48**(6):330-336, 1978.
23. Kolbe, L.J., Iverson, D.C., Kreuter, M.W., and others: Propositions for an alternate and complementary health education paradigm, Health Education **12**:24-30, 1981.
24. Green, L.: National policy in the promotion of health, International Journal of Health Education **22**(3):164, 1979.
25. Green, L.: The changing state of science in health education practice, Focal Points **4**:19-21, 1980.
26. Hochbaum, G.: Is health education playing "big brother." Presented at the Third Annual Arizona Patient—Health Education Conference, Scottsdale, Az., March 27, 1980.

Additional Readings

Balog, J.: Conceptual questions in health education and philosophical inquiry, J. of School Health, **52**(4):201-204, 1982.

The behavioral sciences and health education, Health Education **12**(3):3-39, 1981.

Dwore, R.B.: Liberal education and health education: option for articulation in higher education, Health Values: Achieving High Level Wellness **6**(2):14-18, 1982.

Englehardt, T.H., and Callahan, D., editors: Knowing and valuing, Hastings-on-Hudson, New York, Institute for Society, Ethics, and the Life Sciences.

Englehardt, T.H., and Callahan, D., editors: The search for common routes, Hastings-on-Hudson, New York, Institute for Society, Ethics, and the Life Sciences.

Hochbaum, G.M.: Behavior change as the goal of health education, Eta Sigma Gamman **13**(2):3-6, 1981.

King, K.: Selected behavioral strategies for the health educator, Health Education, **13**(3):35-37, 1982.

Nolte, A.E., and Smith, B.J.: A philosophy of comprehensive school health: an enigma, Health Values: Achieving High Level Wellness **6**(1):21-24, 1982.

Oberteuffer, D.: Philosophy and principles of the school health program, Health Values: Achieving High Level Wellness **6**(1):8-13, 1982.

Purdy, C.O.: Must we wait for a crisis, Health Values: Achieving High Level Wellness **6**(1):41-43, 1982.

Reizen, M.S., Ruff, J., and Danielson, R.H.: Policy development and implementation issues for health education, Health Education Monographs, **6**(suppl. 1):74-90, 1978.

Simonds, S.K.: Health education: facing issues of policy, ethics, and social justice, Health Education Monographs, **6**(suppl. 1):18-27, 1978.

QUALITY OF LIFE

RESPONSIBILITY

LIFESTYLE

WELLNESS

PREVENTION

HEALTHY PEOPLE

RISK FACTORS

HUMAN SERVICES

3 Health Promotion

Introduction

Chapter 1 pointed out that health education emerged from the disciplines of education and medicine. In the early days health education was known as hygiene education. Before the midtwentieth century most of the sickness and deaths in this country were caused by infectious diseases, which had acute onset and occurred in apparently random fashion among the population; little could be done to prevent individual sickness. Hygiene education therefore focused on anatomy, physiology, and a few content areas such as contagion, alcohol education, and personal cleanliness. Pedagogy consisted of didactic lessons aimed at helping people understand the disease process.

In the past 50 years, however, the major causes of death have shifted toward the chronic diseases. These conditions develop over a prolonged period of time and result largely from the negative aspects of people's life-styles. It was during this era that health educators earned the colorful title of "Warriors against pleasure." It seemed as though anything that was fun and anything that tasted good was harmful to health. Therefore the primary word in the vocabulary of the midtwentieth century health educator was *don't*. "Don't eat sweets because they cause tooth decay." "Don't smoke cigarettes because you will get lung cancer." "Don't have sexual intercourse because you might get pregnant." Obviously, health education was not the most popular subject in the curriculum.

Between 1945 and 1980 a tremendous amount of money was spent on sophisticated medical technology and highly specialized providers of health care. During the 1970s it became apparent that although the health care delivery system could restore some level of health, it would not provide a zest for living and sense of vitality. Only the individual could do that. Merely treating the disease is a Band-Aid approach to our nation's health-related problems. What is needed is a strong sense of commitment to a life-style that promotes wellness.

During the 1970s the new buzzword became health promotion, and the educational approach adopted a whole new philosophy. The "don't do this because" theme (avoiding disease) shifted to a more positive orientation that focused on quality of life. This change required health educators to call on a broad area of study known as the behavioral sciences. If people were going to encourage others to make healthful life-style changes, it would be necessary to understand the principles of motivation, reinforcement, and behavior modification. After all, asking a person to sacrifice immediate gratification from nicotine, candy, and sex for an abstraction known as "high-level wellness" would require some fancy footwork.

Chapter 3 describes the concept of health promotion. It demonstrates that health needs vary from age group to age group because of the changing risks associated with each age group. The authors give examples of health promotion activities sponsored by the federal government, schools, voluntary agencies, corporate organizations, and professional associations. The federal government has taken a leadership role in programs of this type largely because it pays for about 40% of the nation's health care costs. Although longitudinal data that demonstrate effectiveness in reducing chronic disease have not yet become available, the short-term results of health promotion activities are definitely encouraging.

63

In the foreword to *Healthy people**, the surgeon general's report on health promotion and disease prevention, former Secretary of the Department of Health, Education and Welfare (now the Department of Health and Human Services) Joseph Califano expressed the hope that the document would encourage a second public health revolution. (The first having been the tremendous advances related to infectious diseases, which killed so many American citizens until the second half of this century.) The improvements in health since 1900 are not entirely a result of advances in medical science. Improvements in the key areas of sanitation, mass immunization, and good nutrition were so successful that today only 1% of Americans who die before the age of 75 are killed by infectious diseases. The impact of these improvements is staggering, and by way of illustration, consider these figures. In the year 1900 the death rate for influenza, pneumonia, diphtheria and gastrointestinal infections totaled 580/100,000. Today the rate is 30/100,000. If the rate that prevailed in the year 1900 were still accurate today, there would be 400,000 deaths from tuberculosis, 300,000 caused by gastroenteritis, 80,000 as a result of diphtheria, and 55,000 from polio. Instead, all four conditions combined account for less than 10,000 deaths each year.

The mortality pattern has shifted drastically since the turn of the century. In 1915, 100 of 1000 infants died during their first 12 months. By 1978 the infant mortality rate had dropped to 13.8/1000 live births. Conversely, the proportion of deaths caused by chronic afflictions, such as cardiovascular diseases and cancer, has increased by 250%, accounting for approximately 70% of the total deaths in 1978. Interestingly, the leading causes of mortality are related to several key risk factors, and some of these risk factors increase the probability of contracting more than one chronic disease. Whenever an individual combines two or more of the known risk factors (for example, hypertension and stress) the cumulative effect is greater than the sum of their parts. Controlling even a few of these factors greatly diminishes the potential for harm and greatly enhances the potential for health.

In the context of health, prevention requires action to reduce or eliminate specific risk factors. Promotion requires effort by those who are seemingly healthy to enhance their health status beyond its present level. Apparently the success of the second public health revolution will depend on our ability to promote the health of specific target populations; those who are not in immediate danger of acute illness but who, because of their life-style, are at risk of chronic disease. Encouragement of a positive social

---

*Unless otherwise noted, data reported in this chapter were taken from *Healthy People: The Surgeon General's Report on Health Promotion and Disease Prevention,* U.S. Public Health Service, DHHS Pub. No. 79-55071, Washington, D.C., 1979.

and personal ethic, which demands a high quality of life, can be achieved through personal action that eliminates or reduces specific risk factors for disease.

For instance, cigarette smoking is the single most important preventable cause of death. Alcohol has been cited as a factor in more than 10% of all deaths in the United States. Treatment for conditions associated with alcohol abuse represent $1 of every $5 spent on hospital care for adults.[1] The total economic cost of smoking and alcohol abuse in 1976 was estimated at nearly $60 billion, about one fourth of the total cost of illness in the United States.[2] Those who contribute to these figures have been candidates for sickness for many years. Because of the life-styles of these people certain diseases could have been predicted or prevented. With the exception of a major medical breakthrough, such as a cure for cancer, the health care delivery system can produce only marginal increases in the nation's health status. According to Joseph Califano:

> We are convinced that the road to better health in the nation's future cannot be paved only with the golden bricks of medication and expensive technology. The next dramatic breakthrough in the health of our people should be in prevention and health promotion.[3]

Health Promotion—A Concept

During the 1950s chronic diseases became the prominent cause of death. At this time little was known about the complex causes of heart disease, cancer, diabetes, and respiratory conditions. The 1960s witnessed a heavy investment in biomedical research, education of health professionals, and specialized therapeutic technology. This investment dramatically raised the cost of illness care and helped lead us to our present dependence on the medical model as the route to good health. The 1970s have been described as an era of fiscal restraint with regard to biomedical research, manpower development, and public financing of health care. During the 1960s and 1970s epidemiologic research began to unravel the intertwined and complicated causes of morbidity. Gradually it became apparent that many contemporary illnesses could be linked to a person's life-style. Health professionals, policymakers, economists, and (most importantly) average citizens began to consider the potential of disease prevention through personal activities that could actually raise one's level of health beyond its present state.

Health promotion is a broad subject. It takes place in a wide range of settings, including the home, school, worksite, and health care facility. A variety of techniques are employed to achieve the stated goals. Among them are health education, risk reduction programs, environmental controls, mass media presentations, and activities that promote a healthy life-style. These activities are sponsored by schools, colleges, professional associations, voluntary health agencies, government, business, labor unions, churches and synagogues, private clubs, and consumer and self-help groups. The target audience is the 220 million Americans who stand to benefit from these activities. The health education profession stands center stage in the theater of health promotion because health educators possess the knowledge of content, skills in facilitation of healthful behavior, and abilities to plan, organize, and evaluate the outcomes of these programs.

The concept of prevention has three distinct levels, each defined by the type of activity being conducted. Primary prevention, also known as health promotion, is represented by those activities designed to improve the well-being of an already healthy person or group. It is more than an attempt to prevent sickness. Primary prevention actually seeks to enhance well-being by reinforcing healthy behavior and discouraging life-styles that eventually lead to illness. Primary prevention recognizes that medicine, technology, and the entire medical (disease) care delivery system can do very little in this regard. Instead, it is the individual, and collectively the society, that can improve the overall level of health.

Using the major causes of death to illustrate primary prevention, consider the following:

1. Cardiovascular diseases—choosing not to smoke cigarettes, to exercise regularly, to eat nutritious foods without excessive quantities of fat, salt, sugar, or calories, to deal effectively with stress, and to develop personal support systems

2. Cancer—choosing not to smoke cigarettes, to avoid excessive exposure to the sun's ultraviolet rays, to eat a diet high in fiber, to wear protective clothing in the manufacture of products that are known to be carcinogenic, and to control stress

3. Accidents—choosing to wear a lap belt and shoulder restraint when driving, not to smoke cigarettes in bed, never to drink alcohol and operate a motor vehicle, to control emotions, and to wear safety glasses when operating power tools

It is important to reiterate that primary prevention means not only living a healthy life-style; equally important is the fact that it represents a societal ethic by which pressure is exerted on the individual to work toward such a life-style. For each of the examples just cited, it is more than individual compliance that we are seeking. To be truly effective there need to be social rewards for compliance and social sanctions for noncompliance. The benefits of primary prevention have a "snowballing" effect that transcend the individual to the family, the community, and ultimately the nation.

Secondary prevention consists of those activities that allow for early detection and treatment of a disease. Screening techniques conducted by a health professional among a presumably healthy population often detect the presence of underlying sickness even before clinical symptoms appear, thereby permitting early intervention. Normally, this intervention increases the probability of cure and at a lower financial cost. However, the individual must make the decision to seek further definitive treatment. To illustrate secondary prevention, consider:

1. Cardiovascular diseases—periodic screening for hypertension, atherosclerosis, EKG abnormalities, and cardiac arrhythmias
2. Cancer—periodic breast self-examination, testicular self-examination, Pap smear, oral examination, and continuous monitoring of changes in bodily function
3. Accidents—periodic eye examinations, recertification for driver's license, and checklist for home safety inspection

Secondary prevention is aimed at people who may appear healthy but who, because of age, sex, heredity, or other personal characteristics, might be identified as high-risk candidates for a particular condition. Once the disease is diagnosed, the individual must be encouraged to seek treatment in order to cure or control the illness. As in primary prevention, a community ethic can encourage the individual to continue taking the hypertensive medicine, to stay on the reducing diet, to remain a nonsmoker, or to wear eyeglasses when operating a motor vehicle.

Tertiary prevention refers to the minimization of consequences caused by a disease in order to prevent further complications or reoccurrence. Here, the focus shifts from the individual to the medical care delivery team. Tertiary prevention is also known as rehabilitation. By rebuilding the health of the bodily systems and of the organism itself the medical care delivery team is preventing further harm from the original condition. Obviously, the cost-to-benefit ratio is unsatisfactory, and so is the ethic that permits this kind of procrastination. To illustrate tertiary prevention, consider the following:

1. Cardiovascular diseases—intensive care followed by physical and occupational rehabilitation
2. Cancer—surgery followed by chemotherapy, radiation, and hormone treatments
3. Accidents—intensive care followed by physical therapy

Current Status and Objectives

The surgeon general's 1979 report established five broad goals, each having subgoals to be achieved within the next decade. In the interest of space they are presented here in outline form.

1. A 35% reduction in infant mortality (Fig. 3-1)
   Reducing the number of low birth weight babies
   - Infants below 5.5 pounds are 20 times more likely to die within the first year.
   - Maternal factors such as lack of prenatal care, poor nutrition, smoking, alcohol and drug abuse, and age of the mother are associated with low birth weight.

   Reducing the number of birth defects
   - Birth defects are responsible for about one sixth of all infant deaths.
   - Nearly one third of all hospitalized children are admitted because of genetically determined or influenced disorders.

   Other important problems that need to be considered are injuries at birth, sudden infant death, accidents, inadequate diets, and parental inadequacy.

2. A 20% reduction of deaths of children between the ages of 1 and 14 years (Fig. 3-2)
   Reducing the number of accidental deaths
   - Accidental deaths are responsible for about 45% of childhood deaths.

   Enhancing child growth and development
   - About 100,000 children per year are identified as mentally retarded.
   - Estimates of child abuse range from 200,000 to 4 million cases each year.

   Other important problems that need to be considered are vaccine-preventable diseases and dental illness.

3. A 20% reduction in deaths among adolescents and young adults (Fig. 3-3)
   Reducing fatal motor vehicle accidents
   - More than two thirds of all deaths among people in the 15 to 24-year age group are caused by motor vehicle accidents.

   Reducing alcohol and drug misuse
   - Alcohol and drug abuse are related to increased risk of accidents, suicides, homicides, family disruption, and even unsatisfactory school performance.
   - This age group accounts for 60% of all alcohol-related highway deaths.

   Other important problems that need to be considered are adolescent pregnancy, sexually transmittable diseases, mental illness, suicide, and homicide.

4. A 25% reduction in deaths among adults between the ages of 25 and 64 years (Fig. 3-4)

Reducing the number of heart attacks and strokes

- More than one third of deaths in this age group are a result of cardiovascular diseases.
- Heart disease is the greatest cause of permanent disability claims among workers under the age of 65.

Reducing the number of deaths from cancer

- One in four Americans will develop cancer sometime during their lifetime.

Other important problems that need to be considered are alcohol abuse, mental illness, and periodontal disease.

5. To improve the health and quality of life for older adults by reducing the average annual number of days of restricted activity caused by acute and chronic conditions by 20% (Fig. 3-5)

Increasing the number of older adults who can function independently

- Of American babies born today, three fourths can expect to live to age 65; about half to age 75; and about one fourth to age 85.
- In 1900 only 4% of the population was 65 years of age and older. This has increased to 11% in 1979 and is estimated to be about 17% by the year 2030.
- Currently, the cost of health care for older Americans represents about 30% of the total national health care expenditures.

Reducing premature deaths caused by influenza and pneumonia

- These two diseases are the fourth leading cause of death among the elderly.

Other important problems that need to be considered are costs associated with treatment, relief of pain caused by chronic conditions, institutionalization, and death with dignity.

The broad goals identified by the surgeon general are further delineated in a report entitled *Promoting Health/Preventing Disease—Objectives for the Nation*. It establishes a series of national targets in 15 priority areas. The specific objectives of this report are presented in Appendix A.

The second public health revolution will need to focus on primary and secondary preventive techniques, not only because of the humanistic concern for a healthy person but also because of the economics related to health care. The total cost of health care for 1979 was $212.2 billion. Over the past two decades (1960-1980), health care costs have risen dramatically from 5.3% to 9.0% of the gross national product (GNP). Diseases of the circulatory system cost the nation more than $45 billion; cancer, $19 billion; accidents,

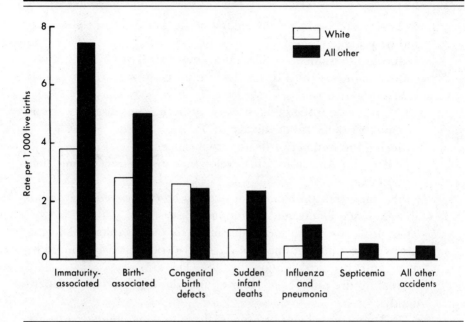

Fig. 3-1. Major causes of infant mortality in United States, 1976. (Data from National Center for Health Statistics, Division of Vital Statistics.)

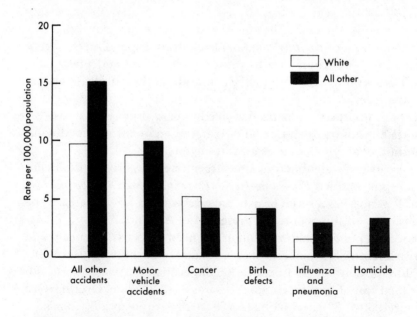

Fig. 3-2. Major causes of death for children age 1 to 14 years in United States, 1976. (Data from National Center for Health Statistics, Division of Vital Statistics.)

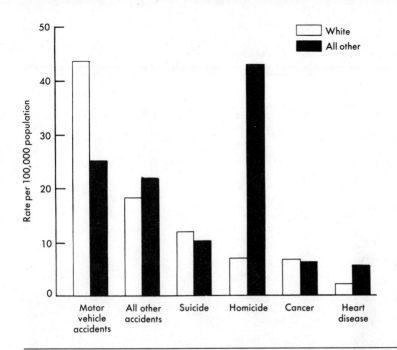

Fig. 3-3. Major causes of death for young adults age 15 to 24 in United States, 1976. (Data from National Center for Health Statistics, Division of Vital Statistics.)

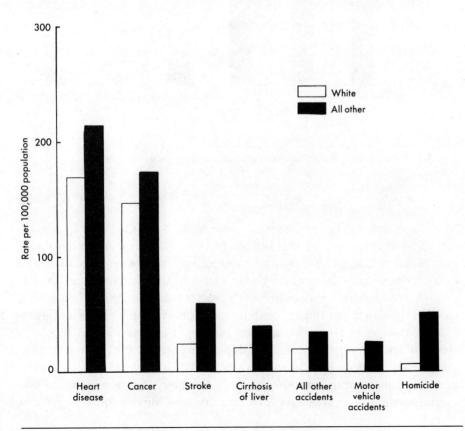

Fig. 3-4. Major causes of death for adults age 25 to 64 in United States, 1976. (Data from National Center for Health Statistics, Division of Vital Statistics.)

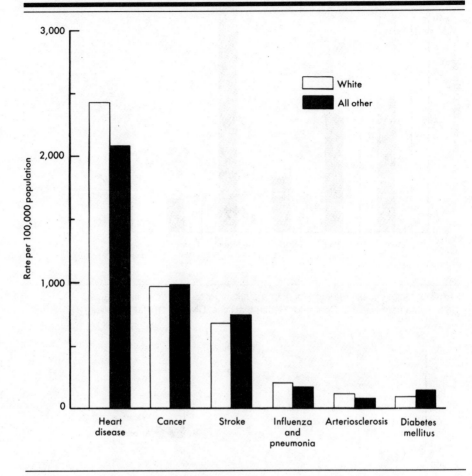

Fig. 3-5. Major causes of death for adults age 65 years and older in United States, 1976. (Data from National Center for Health Statistics, Division of Vital Statistics.)

$27 billion; and diseases of the respiratory system, $18.7 billion.[1] The average cost of a hospital room is roughly $200 per day, with the cost of critical care units approaching five times that amount. Approximately 11 cents out of every federal dollar is spent on health care and the pursuit of health. Obviously, even modest changes in health behavior among 200 million people can have a significant impact on national morbidity and mortality figures and on the expenditures for treating disease. Recognizing that the lion's share of the potential for health is dependent on our way of life, the Department of Health and Human Services (DHHS) has called for an individual and national commitment to health as an alternative to the misery and economic burdens of sickness. As former Secretary Califano concluded, "You, the individual, can do more for your own health and well-being than any doctor, any hospital, any drug, any exotic medical device."[4]

Achieving the Objectives

The rest of this chapter presents a description of how specific segments of society can be involved with health promotion. The subsections include government, communities, schools, employers, voluntary health agencies, and professional associations.

The challenge of health promotion is huge, and meeting it is beyond the capability of any one segment of society. Cooperative efforts, however, can produce a synergistic effect, capable of bringing about drastic changes in the health of a nation. Quality of life is both an ideal and an attainable goal. The essential prerequisite of progress in the quest for a healthy nation is commitment from all segments of society. Our profession can help to raise the level of public consciousness by offering programs that motivate individuals and groups toward healthful behavior.

The Individual. The trend toward healthy life-styles in this country demonstrates the small successes that eventually may pay large dividends in health status. Is it possible that health, like an infectious disease, is communicable? A brief scenario is worth consideration. In your own mind select a person who possesses multiple risk factors associated with his or her life-style. If you could encourage this person to begin with a single change, the benefits might be so rewarding that additional changes might follow. As the balance of that person's life-style shifts from "disease promoting" to "health promoting" a new person may emerge—one who is unwilling to perceive disease as an acceptable state of being. A person who has actually worked at being healthy is not likely to be satisfied with illness at any level.

To continue the scenario, imagine this person has been transformed from someone with a chronic state of low-level health to an effervescent advocate of health. Admittedly, this kind of metamorphosis is rare, but certainly we all know or have heard about people who have been so converted. For the person who feels good, who enjoys life and human relationships, who seems to be effective in adapting to change, the new public image must certainly be attractive. Is it possible that others who witness the zest for life may become at first curious and later personally interested in a healthful life-style? If this is possible, consider the implications. If one person can facilitate behavior change in others by serving as a role model, a whole community of "health seekers" has tremendous potential for encouraging others in the same direction. The practice of overconsumption might be replaced by the practice of moderation. The "hectic roadrunner" syndrome might be replaced by serenity through relaxation. Dependence on others might shift to self-reliance; treatment and rehabilitation might shift to wellness. Accepting responsibility for their own health, individuals might nurture the roots of the second public health revolution.

Government. Responsibility for health lies ultimately with the individual. Nevertheless, much of the emphasis for health promotion has been initiated by agencies of the federal government, notably the U.S. Public Health Service. With each change of administrative leadership in the White House the objectives, priorities, policies, and governmental funding of projects will also change, as witnessed by the change from President Carter to President Reagan and from Secretary Califano to Secretary Schweiker. It remains to be seen how the philosophy of the new head of DHHS, Margaret Heckler, affects funding priorities. A substantial alteration in philosophy creates a ripple effect throughout the entire system. Programs are established, remain in place for a period of time, and then are dropped in favor of more pressing issues. Some examples of governmental programs designed to promote the health of the nation are presented in Appendix B.

DHHS provides a workable structure for national and local efforts by developing key activities grouped into three categories:

1. Measures used by government, industry, and other agencies to protect people from harm
2. Preventive services delivered to individuals
3. Activities that individuals and communities can use to promote healthy life-styles

People normally seek medical treatment for acute conditions or when chronic symptoms become severe enough to warrant a visit to the doctor. Most people see little value in preventive services while they feel well. An important challenge to health promotion is to find ways to change this situation. One successful activity has been to identify the specific risks for a given population and then use screening techniques appropriate for that population and that specific risk. Examples include colorectal examinations, chest x-rays, vision testing, and of course hypertension screening. Appendix C provides additional examples of protection, prevention, and health promotion activities.

Community Involvement. Communities are composed of diverse people who can work together to bring about improvements in health status. Normally, people look to the health care delivery system to solve their health problems. Recently, health care providers have taken an active role in health promotion by helping an already healthy population maintain or improve its health status. Hospitals and health maintenance organizations have begun to establish wellness centers that reach out to the community. They employ

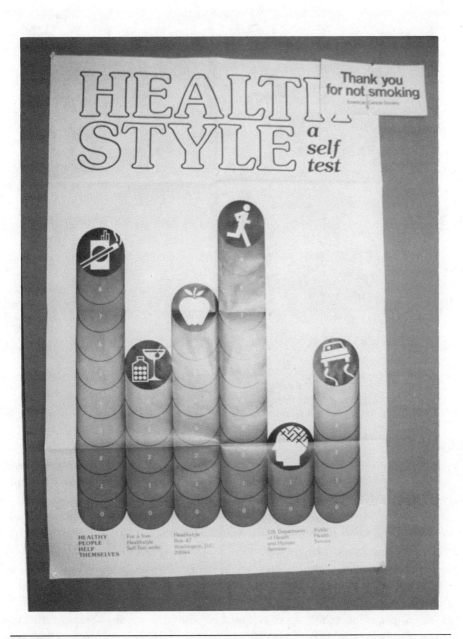

Fig. 3-6. *Healthstyle* is one of many government publications aimed at improving the health of the nation. The easy-to-score pamphlet focuses on individual behaviors that affect health.

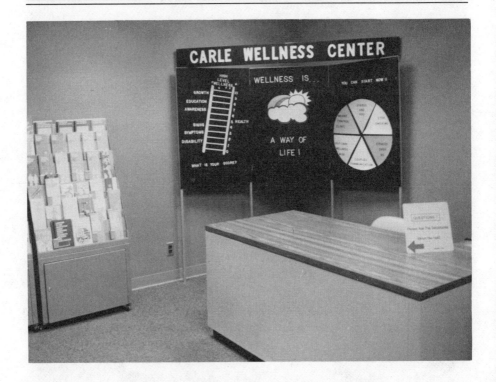

Fig. 3-7. Many hospitals have developed wellness centers to promote the health of the community. Future career opportunities seem to be plentiful for health educators in a hospital-based setting.

health educators to encourage positive health behavior through programs that appeal to the community. Popular programs include stress management, weight control, "quit smoking" clinics, and aerobic exercise.

In most communities, health and social service agencies are plentiful. A few examples will demonstrate that communities can take an active role in promoting health. In Seattle, the American Heart Association sponsored a hypertension program for minority and low-income groups. The program included blood pressure screening, weight loss, exercise, and cooking classes that emphasized ethnic recipes. The Campesino de Salud in Espanola, New Mexico, provides health services and health education that respect the culture, traditions, and language differences of the Chicano population it serves. The Health Education Center of Pittsburgh offers health-promoting activities to an ethnic population in an urban setting, whereas the Rural Environmental Education and Action Project, sponsored by the University of North Carolina, is aimed at health problems of the rural black community.

Similar examples are available at the state level. The Nebraska State Department of Health sponsors the Positive Educational Experiences and Relationships (PEER) program aimed at young people. The New Mexico Health Education Coalition, composed of a broad spectrum of health agencies and health professionals, promotes the health of an extremely enculturated population. The cooperative action of agencies and collective talents can be an effective means of improving the health of the nation.

Schools. Elementary and secondary schools are in a good position to promote healthful life-styles among young people who are in the process of forming opinions, attitudes, and values. School health programs are based on four premises. First, schools have an obligation to help pupils and personnel maintain a high level of health in order to maximize the potential for student achievement. Second, schools can provide learning experiences that encourage young people to appreciate the importance of health in achieving their goals. Third, school health programs provide information with which students can feel confident of their ability to make intelligent decisions regarding personal, family, and community health. Last, by providing a comprehensive health program the school demonstrates in tangible ways its commitment to improving the quality of life for the residents of the community. Collectively, the efforts of the school promote an ethic of responsible decisionmaking and responsible health behavior. A health-conscious child will grow up to become a health-conscious adult.

A comprehensive K-12 curriculum is not the only way to promote health. Another way is through the provision of services that appraise, protect, promote, and occasionally, remedy the health of students. The employment of specialized personnel such as the health educator, school nurse, nutritionist, counselor, athletic trainer, and physical educator demonstrates that schools serve the health needs of students in many ways. A wholesome contact with these people provides the student with perceptions and learning experiences that may last a lifetime. A safe and healthful school environment reinforces the importance of individual well-being. The cafeteria, locker rooms, hallways, home economics suites, playgrounds, and lavatories stimulate impressions that either support or undermine health instruction. The experience of progressing through a health-oriented school system can instill a sense of pride in oneself, one's school, and one's community.*

The school can promote health in many other ways. For instance, the establishment of a school health council may help to bring together members of the community who share common interests. A blood donation day can

---

*A more detailed description of these ideas can be found in Anderson, C.L., and Creswell, W.H.: School health practice, ed. 8, St. Louis, 1984, The C.V. Mosby Co.

stimulate a sense of volunteerism. Health fairs located in a community mall can raise the level of consciousness about issues and problem solving. Career days can encourage young people to consider the allied health professions. Fund-raising activities for charitable organizations can demonstrate the value of people helping people. Evening seminars offered to parents on health-related topics can encourage widespread enthusiasm for the school health program. In many ways the school can promote a healthy way of life for this and future generations.

The Worksite. The worksite appears to be a most appropriate setting in which to conduct health promotion programs. Almost 90 million people come together each day to work in factories, offices, and shops. Workers share specific occupational health risks, their peers provide reinforcement, their jobs play a major role in their lives, and the effects of their work involve home and family.[5] These factors all contribute to making the worksite a logical setting for health promotion.

Several preventive and promotional health programs are currently in existence at the worksite. However, there does not seem to be a particular theme or pattern in corporate decisionmaking that reveals a single motive for initiating a health promotion program. Employer motivation can generally be organized according to four categories:[6]

1. Some programs are offered in the hopes that medical costs for workers and dependents will be lowered because of reduced medical service use.
2. Some employers sense a social responsibility. In this framework, employees are provided with a needed service that previously was not available.
3. Some programs have begun as a result of the personal commitment by a member of senior management, based on individual experience with an illness or the growing recognition that the company can look to health promotion services to reduce employees' health risks.
4. There are also non-health-related factors that further prompt corporate commitment. Some employers assume that offering promotion programs enhances their image. In turn, recruitment is improved. Other employers merely follow the lead of a competitor, and for some, such as insurance companies and hospitals, health promotion programs provide a competitive edge to attract new clients.

Worksite health promotion programs typically consist of screenings for various diseases or risk factors. Health hazard appraisals are often used to identify health behaviors that need to be changed. Based on the results of disease screening and completion of a health hazard appraisal questionnaire, employees can normally select one or more health education programs offered by the company. Establishment of a healthy work environment is also a component of worksite health promotion and serves to reinforce information and healthful behaviors discussed in health education seminars.

The current state of worksite health promotion is hard to describe because programs are new and have yet to establish a single approach that is attractive to many companies. Ideally a program should be comprehensive and include commitment throughout the entire corporate structure. Multiple life-style improvement seminars, peer support groups, improved work environments, employee advisory committees, and a meaningful research design all help to demonstrate corporate commitment to health promotion. Until comprehensive programs have had sufficient operational time and until evaluations are analyzed, it is difficult to determine the full value and cost-to-benefit ratio of worksite health promotion. Logically, it would seem that such programs have tremendous worth, but it is understandably difficult to elicit corporate investment of resources on faith alone. The opportunity for industry to work in cooperation with local voluntary health organizations, public and private health agencies and professionals, and other employers to effect a reversal from a disease care delivery system to a health enhancement delivery system still remains on the horizon. Nevertheless, many employers have begun to move in this direction (see Appendix E). Appendix F provides a list of resources for additional information about worksite health promotion programs.

Voluntary Health Agencies. There are thousands of voluntary health agencies in this country. These nonprofit agencies derive funding from voluntary contributions and depend on volunteers to provide much of the work needed to achieve their stated goals. Usually each agency has a focus that limits its attention to a particular group of diseases. Activities can be grouped into three categories: research, service, and education.

Contributions made at the community level are forwarded to the local chapter, which most often serves a county or group of counties. Some of the money remains with the chapter for the provision of services to those who are afflicted with the disease. Money is also spent to provide both public and professional education. The remainder is sent to national headquarters, which supports large-scale research projects and the development of educational materials that are used by agency personnel and by health educators.

Much of the biomedical research in this country is supported by voluntary health agencies. To illustrate this point, consider that just three voluntary health agencies (the March of Dimes Birth Defects Foundation, the American Heart Association, and the American Cancer Society) spent more than $80 million in a single year on research grants. Collectively, these three agencies have contributed more than $1 billion in research funds. Research money provided by these agencies has led to dozens of important medical breakthroughs.

Films and other visual aids, curriculum packages, pamphlets, and speakers representing a voluntary health agency should be screened before classroom use. Although the information is accurate, the health educator should determine the usefulness of the material in achieving the planned objectives and its appropriateness for the target audience. Some of the materials provided by voluntary health agencies are among the best health education materials available. Nevertheless, they should be considered as supplementing rather than replacing a carefully planned, comprehensive K-12 curriculum. Appendix G provides examples of the many free or inexpensive educational materials available from voluntary health agencies. Health promotion activities carried out by these agencies are presented in the same appendix.

It should be obvious that voluntary agencies have great potential for improving the nation's health. The idea of volunteerism is not unique to America, but implementation of the idea certainly flourishes in our culture. Health educators can serve an important role by volunteering their talents or by choosing employment with such an agency.

Professional Associations and Honor Societies. Professional associations are established to promote the goals of the profession. All associations are political to some extent and lobby for issues they believe are important to the membership. In the case of health education, the professional associations often lobby for issues that affect personal and community health. For the most part, however, professional associations provide a medium through which their memberships can grow and mature. Opportunities are made available to accept the challenge of leadership by serving as officers or committee members or by publishing or presenting papers at conferences sponsored by the associations. Most associations publish journals or newsletters to inform members about important events, current research findings, and successful innovative techniques. The four associations and one national health science honorary most relevant to health education are described below.

American School Health Association (ASHA). In 1927 Dr. William A. Howe and 53 fellow physicians formed the American Association of School Physicians. By 1930 they were publishing the monthly *American Association of School Physicians Bulletin*—324 school physicians received it the first year. In 1936 the association's scope was broadened to include all school health professionals, and the name of the organization was changed to the American School Health Association. The *Bulletin* was changed to the *Journal of School*

Health. Today ASHA has grown to include almost 10,000 members internationally.

ASHA is the only national professional organization whose membership includes all school health professionals—school nurses, physicians, health educators, dentists, and related health service providers concerned with the health of school-aged children. ASHA is a nonprofit educational organization concerned with the development and improvement of school health programs. Since 1927, ASHA has been the only national professional organization concerned solely with the health of the school-aged child. The association promotes comprehensive and constructive school health programs that comprise health services, health education, and a healthful school environment.

ASHA establishes guidelines for standards of excellence and competency for professionals who make up the school health team. It serves as a professional liaison among the disciplines in the field of school health and cooperates with local, state, and national organizations on behalf of all school health personnel. Additionally, ASHA serves as a medium for exchange of information pertinent to child health. Inquiries concerning special problems are referred to members with professional and practical experience for accurate and helpful replies. Its membership develops standards for practice and educational preparation for all school health professionals. Nationally, ASHA represents school health professionals to public and special groups. It cooperates with other national organizations to promote programs that improve the health of children. ASHA publishes the *Journal of School Health* monthly except in June and July. In addition, ASHA offers the following services: a professional referral service, an annual convention, group insurance, teaching and classroom aids and texts, and the opportunity for professional interaction among the various school health professions.

ASHA has been active in supporting programs and regulations concerning aging, the international year of disabled persons, community health education and planning, comprehensive health planning, consumer health education, continuing education, curriculum in health education, dental health education, disease education (communicable and noncommunicable), drug use and abuse, environmental health, family life and sex education, and international health.

Association for the Advancement of Health Education (AAHE). This association, section of the larger American Alliance for Health, Physical Education, Recreation and Dance (AAHPERD), is dedicated to the proposition that health education, as both process and program, seeks the preservation and improvement of health through education. The complexities of living in an age marked by technologic and social change make health education a greater concern in contemporary society than in previous decades. The association's brochure explains that programs of health education involve both individuals and communities at all levels of public enterprise.

> Such activities are envisioned as a vital and permeating force for enhancing the quality of life. An effective, comprehensive program requires the talents and efforts of many individuals and organizations working together in a cooperative manner to achieve common goals. Thus, coordinated effort and group action are imperative to the ultimate success of health education programs. The benefits that accrue from health education can be improved with sound planning and cooperative interaction. This is the premise upon which the Association for the Advancement of Health Education is founded. AAHE publishes six issues of *Health Education* each year. The association lists as its goals the following:
>
> • Provide information, resources, and services regarding health education to professionals and the lay public
> • Promote and interpret research projects relating to school and community health education
> • Promulgate criteria, guidelines, and evaluative procedures for assessing the effectiveness of preservice internship and the continuing education of health education personnel
> • Investigate curriculum needs and develop resources for effective health education at all levels of education
> • Facilitate communication between schools and communities and between professionals and the lay public regarding current health education principles, problems, and practices
> • Provide leadership in health education for the improvement of health through school and community programs
> • Provide leadership in establishing program policies, criteria, and evaluative procedures that will perpetuate effective health education programs
> • Ascertain the relevance of existing legislation and pending lesiglation to AAHE interests and resources
> • Maintain effective liaison with national organizations having allied interests in health education[6a]

American Public Health Association (APHA). The American Public Health Association is a professional society founded in 1872. It represents all disciplines and specialties in public health. APHA is composed of 24 sections concerned with areas such as community health planning, public health education, and school health education and services. The association publishes the *American Journal of Public Health* as well as a monthly newspaper entitled *The Nation's Health.*

In 1982 the APHA leadership was asked to rank the issues or problems of greatest concern to the association. Among the top-ranked issues of interest to health educators were substance abuse among youth, cigarette smoking, automobile accident prevention, community health planning, and promotion of physical fitness.

Society for Public Health Education (SOPHE). The Society for Public Health Education, Inc., is a professional organization whose membership is comprised of persons having specialized preparation and experience in public health education. The Society was formed on October 23, 1949, at the seventy-seventh APHA meeting. Particular concerns were with research in public health education methods and with the development of professional standards. Temporary officers included some familiar names mentioned in Chapter 1: Clair E. Turner and Ruth E. Grout.

Robert D. Patton and others conducted a survey of the 938 SOPHE members in 1978. The entire study is reported in the Spring 1980 edition of *Health Education Quarterly*. A few of the findings are presented in order to help you understand this professional association.

The majority of members were employed in public agencies, followed by private nonprofit and voluntary health agencies. Most members reported that they were college or university faculty members, followed by state, multicounty, county, and city employees. Only six members indicated employment by public schools.

Twenty-five percent of the members had received a baccalaureate degree in education, 20% had earned a degree in natural science, 18% earned a degree in the behavioral sciences, and 8% earned a degree in public health. Approximately half of the membership had earned their first master's degree in public health, while 26% had earned their first graduate degree in education. Nearly one fourth of the members had earned a doctorate: 36% in public health, 31% in education, and 9% in behavioral science.

In response to the question that asked members to identify the primary health education goals that should be accomplished by 1985, nearly one fourth listed the first priority as certification of health educators. Other highranking priorities were funding for state and local health education programs, guidelines for community health promotion and implementation, continuing education, and funding of health education at the federal level.

Eta Sigma Gamma. This professional honor society is dedicated to the elevation of standards, ideals, competence, and ethics of professionally trained men and women in the health science discipline. There are currently 58 active chapters across the United States. *The Eta Sigma Gamman* is published twice yearly. Student manuscripts are of special interest to the journal. Like most professional journals, guidelines for submission of articles are published in each edition. These guidelines detail the submission procedures, including length of manuscript and use of photographs, charts, and illustrations. A meeting of the membership is held each year at the ASHA convention.

Signs of Progress

Clearly, the major threats to health in America are the chronic diseases, conditions that are sometimes easier to prevent than to treat. A recent Harris

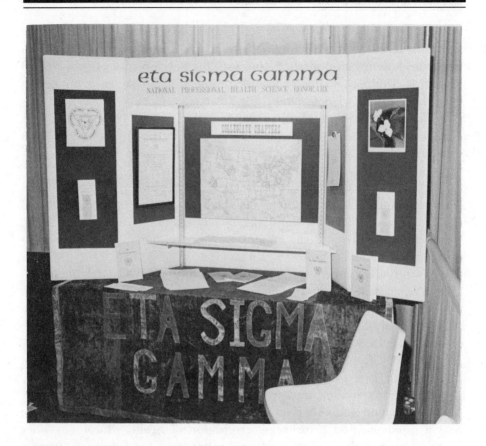

Fig. 3-8. ETA Sigma Gamma booth at a health education conference. (Photo courtesy American School Health Association.)

survey found that half of the U.S. population is much more concerned about preventive health than they had been just a few years before. About three fourths of business executives and union officials indicated they were more concerned with preventive health than they had been 5 years earlier. Within this same group, 80% to 90% stated that the health care delivery system should give more emphasis to preventive medicine and less to curative medicine.[7]

Americans increasingly rate good health as a personal priority. We have begun to change the ethic that sickness is "bad luck," that it is "inevitable," or that "you have to die of something anyway, so why worry about it." The same Harris poll found that 92% of respondents agreed with the statement "If we Americans ate more nutritious food, smoked less, maintained our proper weight, and exercised regularly, it would do more to improve our health than anything doctors and medicine could do for us!" Examples of this changing ethic are numerous. Cigarette smoking is on the decline in every age group, and today there are more than 30 million ex-smokers. (Most recent evidence suggests the rate is also declining among teenage girls.)

Smoking in public places is becoming a socially unacceptable behavior. More people are having their blood pressure checked, are taking their blood pressure medication, and are thereby controlling an important risk factor for heart disease. Many people are joggers. Nutrition and stress control workshops are popular. Many communities have emotional support groups, hotlines, and a network of resources for enhancing the level of health. According to a study conducted by Yankelovich,[8] 46% of American adults reported a recent change in personal and family life-style in the interest of good health. Furthermore, 70% reported that following a good health routine is easy. One in four adults said they were watching their caloric intake more carefully than in 1977, and this same percentage indicated they were eating more nutritious food than they had eaten in 1977.[8] Fig. 3-9 shows some trends in important life-style behaviors.

It appears that the objectives identified by the federal government and the health education priorities identified by the public are quite consistent. The Program and Policies Advisory Committee of the U.S. Centers for Disease Control established the following priorities. Alphabetically, they are alcohol, cardiovascular disease, dental disease, infant mortality, motor vehicle accidents, smoking-related conditions, stress and social disorders, vaccine preventable childhood diseases, and workplace-related diseases.[9] In the same year the American Hospital Association conducted a survey that found the public to be most interested in the following health education programs: stress reduction, home safety, diet, weight control, and consumer health.[10]

To further demonstrate the trend toward a healthy life-style, consider the information gathered from various government documents previously cited.

- Within the past 2 years 59% of the men and 70% of the women have had physical examinations.
- Within the past year 75% of the men and 83% of the women between the ages of 20 and 64 years had their blood pressure checked. Within the past 2 years, 88% of the men and 94% of the women had their blood pressure checked.
- Within the past year 62.5% of the women between the ages of 20 and 64 years had a breast examination performed by a physician. An additional 20% had been examined within the past 2 years. (No mention was given to the percentage of women who practice monthly breast self-examinations—a practice of greater importance than the annual physical examination.)

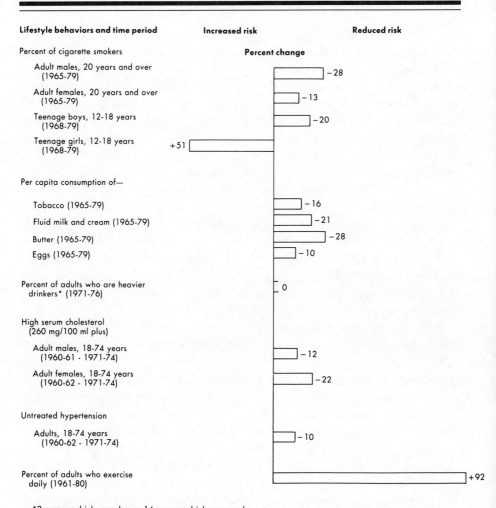

Fig. 3-9. Trends in life-style behavior that affect health.

- Almost 60% of the women had a pap smear within the previous year and 80% had the test performed within the past 2 years.
- Among school children 91% are protected against measles, polio, diphtheria, pertussis, and tetanus; 80% are protected against rubella.
- Between 1968 and 1976 there was a 21% decline in deaths resulting from heart attacks.
- In 1964 more than half of the men in the nation were smokers. by 1975 this figure had dropped to 39%. Overall smoking rates for women have also declined.

- In 1972 only half of the people with high blood pressure knew they had it, whereas in 1979 in some communities the percentage had risen to 70%.
- In 1972 only 16% of people with hypertension had their disease under control. By 1979 the figure had doubled. Patient visits for high blood pressure have increased by 50%.
- Since 1970 there have been only 76 cases of polio reported in the United States. Smallpox has been eradicated worldwide.
- Accidental poisoning deaths among children under 5 years of age have decreased substantially since the 1970 federal legislation that required poison prevention packaging.
- Since enactment of the national 55 m.p.h. speed limit, highway fatalities have dropped 20% which translates into 10,000 fewer deaths per year.

On January 13, 1983, President Reagan nominated Margaret Heckler to replace Richard Schweiker as Secretary of Health and Human Services. It will be interesting to see the direction and priorities of the largest cabinet department. It is hoped that the progress that has been observed in the nation's health during the past decade will continue to receive encouragement from an agency that spent $275 billion in 1982.

Editors' Remarks

Health promotion consists of all of those planned activities that have a positive influence on the health of individuals, communities, and the nation. Some of these cannot be conducted by the individual; therefore governments or institutions such as schools, hospitals, and industry must take an active role in the protection of health. Schools establish policies that are directed toward health and safety issues. Examples include restricting students who are suffering from communicable diseases in order to prevent the further spread of infection. Fire drills, clean shower rooms and lavatories, sanitary cooking facilities, and rules regarding student conduct are only a few of the many ways that schools protect the health and safety of the school community.

Hospitals provide protection to patients and visitors by establishing regulations that affect hospital security, maintenance and storage of medical equipment, radiation, medical records, laboratories, and operating rooms. Industry protects its workers by requiring the use of safety equipment, providing preservice training of employees for the safe operation of machinery, color-coding of dangerous areas, and monitoring dust, particulate matter, or radiation. Similarly, all levels of government establish rules, standards, policies, guidelines, directives, and regulations that are intended to protect the health of its citizens.

There is not much opportunity for health educators in these protection activities. In schools, decisions are made by the administrative staff, although health educators may be asked to provide input. In the hospital such decisions are made by the hospital administrator, the medical director, or the department heads of radiology, medical records, laboratories, and nursing. In industry, decisions are made at the corporate level and implementation is carried out by specialists in occupational health. In the government, bureaus are established to enforce the existing legislation. Other than making people aware of the need for protection, health educators are rarely involved in this type of activity unless they have additional training at the graduate level.

Prevention of disease overlaps somewhat with protection because any efforts aimed at protection will also help to prevent illness or trauma. Whereas protection usually involves procedures or standards, prevention activities are more behaviorally oriented. Obviously, there is a niche for health education in this area. Using a few of the examples just given, school health educators can help students and faculty see the logic behind protective measures and encourage compliance that is motivated by a concern for their well-being. Fire drills, clean lavatories, and control of communicable diseases have direct implications on health; however, the school community must perceive and appreciate these benefits.

In the hospital setting, education might take the form of inservice programs to keep the staff apprised of important changes in health care. Another type of education consists of educational programs for patients and their families. A physician may prescribe an educational package specific to the nature of the illness, the treatment method, the restrictions after the patient leaves the hospital, or the psychosocial concerns likely to be encountered.

Industry used to be concerned exclusively with safety issues. Safety specialists were employed to provide in-service education, to monitor and investigate accidents, and to recommend changes that would prevent accidents. Today, industry is employing health educators because of the many ways that illness negatively affects productivity. For instance, health educators may be in charge of an "employees assistance" program that attempts to help employees with alcohol-related problems. Also, health educators are employed to develop and implement educational programs that inform workers of the health-related aspects of their job. For example the availability of respiratory equipment is of no value unless the employee wears it to prevent exposure. Wearing such equipment is facilitated when the worker perceives the seriousness of the disease, recognizes his or her susceptibility, and appreciates the benefits of its use.

Community health education has traditionally focused on prevention. The primary responsibility of the health educator employed by governmental or private agencies was to develop educational materials and programs to inform citizens about steps they could take to reduce the risk of illness. Historically these programs were directed at communicable diseases such as tuberculosis, sexually transmitted diseases, influenza, and the infectious childhood diseases. More recently program interest has shifted toward chronic diseases, with content related to health risks from pollution, carcinogens, toxic waste, and radiation.

In the same way that protection overlaps with prevention, so too, prevention overlaps with promotion. Prevention seeks avoidance of disease. Health promotion activities are intended to encourage healthful decisions that improve an individual's or a community's level of health. It is not the activities as much as the focus of the message that makes the difference between prevention and promotion. School health educators deal with self-esteem, interpersonal relationships, decision making, values clarification, and appreciation for the zest of living. Hospital-based health educators encourage participation among the community on topics of public interest that enhance the quality of life. Coping skills, effective parenting, low-cost menu planning, aerobic exercise, and effective use of the medical care system are popular offerings. Industry accepts the "quality of life" premise in recognition that a healthy, happy employee will be more productive. Communities recognize that quality of life issues have an important bearing on the provision of other governmental services. Presumably, a healthy and happy citizenry will reduce the level of mental illness, suicide, homicide, divorce, and institutionalization in its many forms.

This is not to suggest that health promotion can secure all of these benefits merely through health education. Rather, the sum of collective activities is necessary to make a significant contribution to health. The establishment of policies that protect and programs that prevent, and the work of people who can facilitate an appreciation of health (physical, mental, social, and spiritual), can make a beneficial difference. In fact, the final section of Chapter 3 demonstrates that these activities have already made a substantial difference in the health of the nation.

Career Opportunities for Health Educators

As will be indicated in Chapter 4, the anticipated responsibilities of an entry-level health educator are quite similar, regardless of occupational setting or job title. The following analysis describes the nature of employment in a variety of settings for individuals who have earned at

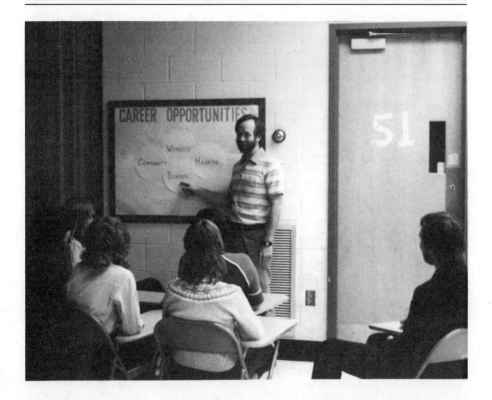

Fig. 3-10. There are many career opportunities in health education. The future looks bright as work settings continue to expand.

least a baccalaureate degree in health education. Presented below are the major areas of responsibility identified by the Role Delineation Project as being common to the profession. These responsibilities can be applied to each of the employment settings described in this section.

1. Communicating health and health education needs, concerns, and resources
2. Determining the appropriate focus for health education
3. Planning health education programs in response to identified needs
4. Implementing planned health education programs
5. Evaluating health education
6. Coordinating selected health education activities
7. Acting as a resource for health and health education

School Health

The school health setting may be the one most often associated with the profession. Traditionally after graduation, health educators were certified by the state to provide instruction in the public schools. In the past, certification was formally attached to physical education. More recently, however, in response to changing needs of school curricula, recognition of the complexity of health behavior, and changes in state laws that recognize, encourage, or require separate certification, colleges and universities have been preparing students with a major in health education. Many individuals are choosing to specialize in school health education and seek employment as full-time school health specialists. These people also may coordinate school health programs that consist of instruction, maintenance of a healthful school environment, and provision of school health services.

During the past decade the public schools have experienced a decline in student enrollment. The practice of "furloughing" teachers is common. But simultaneously, there has been an ever-increasing demand for curricular time and resources allocated to health education. Because certification normally limits teaching to a given area of curricular responsibility, the furloughed teachers cannot teach health education unless their certification permits them to do so. This means that although teaching jobs are hard to find, there still may be opportunities for certified health educators. And although the number of openings may be limited, so too is the availability of people who are certified and able to compete for the openings.

Individuals who are certified as school health educators can definitely search for careers outside of the public schools. Although their preparation will not be as comprehensive as a person who specialized in community health education, it is often better than the background of people who currently are employed as "community health educators." In order to expand their job potential beyond the school setting, students should select courses in community organization, public health, sociology, epidemiology, and behavioral psychology.

Hospital-based Health Education

It was not too long ago that people perceived the hospital as a place to die. More recently it has been perceived as a place for medical treatment and rehabilitation, with patient education considered to be an important part of the total treatment. Within the past 5 years, hospitals have begun to offer health education in what have become known as "wellness centers." In these centers, hospitals offer educational programs to an essentially healthy population of employees and to members of the community. In order to meet the particular needs of the community the offerings are diverse. Although some of the programs are contracted with local providers, such as the American Cancer Society, American Red Cross, or March of Dimes Birth Defects Foundation, many are conducted by the hospital staff. This includes the wellness center staff and other hospital employees such as nutritionists, physicians, nurses, and allied health personnel.

Obviously, this type of effort requires someone to administer the program. Because there are no programs of professional preparation that lead to certification as a "wellness coordinator," individuals from a variety of professional backgrounds are hired to perform this role. Health educators would seem especially well suited for such a job because they are familiar with needs and interests studies, health content, program planning, classroom teaching strategies, and evaluation. Additional coursework that would make health educators even more attractive candidates include marketing, hospital or business administration, public relations, communications, and management.

Hospitals are especially sensitive to their public image. In fact, wellness centers are often established to create a marketing edge with competing facilities. By demonstrating its concern for personal and community health the hospital hopes to attract public support for all of its services. The administrator of the wellness center needs to be constantly aware of the fact that programs offered through the center are a primary source of exposure for the institution. The overall quality of wellness center programs can dramatically affect the community's perception of the institution itself. For some people the only visible activities of the hospital are the outreach efforts conducted by the wellness center.

Worksite Health Education

Employers pay most of the health insurance premiums in this country as a fringe benefit to the employee. When an employee becomes ill the employer loses even further because of "sick days" with pay, on-the-job recuperation time, and lowered productivity from the employee. Many business, commercial, and industrial firms have become interested in employee health promotion programs as ways of reducing disease care costs and increasing corporate profit.

There are a number of special concerns that must be acknowledged by a worksite health educator. First, it may be difficult to motivate employees to attend health-related programs, especially on their own time. If the program is administered "in house" through the medical or personnel office, the issue of confidentiality is always present. Who will have access to information obtained through these programs? If labor unions are involved, the establishment of a health program can easily become a collective bargaining issue. That is, who is entitled to take part in the programs and who is required to take part in the programs? Who will pay for the programs? If it is the employer, would employees benefit more from increased insurance coverage or higher wages to pay for medical services?

As in the hospital setting, the health educator in the worksite needs to be aware of the surrounding political issues and the implications of offering health-related programs. The most obvious example is a program for employees who are addicted to alcohol. Effective programs serve the best interests of both employer and employee. Good health, positive morale, and increased productivity can result from worksite health promotion programs. But if these programs are to succeed they will need to demonstrate their worth. Continuous measurement of the cost-to-benefit ratio is especially important in this setting because business is conditioned to analyze the "bottom-line" budget figure. However well-intentioned an employer may be, if the cost exceeds the benefits, the program is in jeopardy.

Additional coursework that may prove helpful to worksite health educators includes marketing, business administration, research and evaluation, computer science, labor relations, and small group facilitation.

Voluntary Health Agencies

Voluntary health agencies typically have three major areas of concern: financial support of research, provision of services, and education. Usually the paid staff are few in number compared to the volunteers who serve the organization. For this reason the job descriptions and the day-to-day activities of the staff member may not coincide. People who work for voluntary health agencies may spend part of their time performing their specific roles and part of their time helping others perform their roles. The health educator, most often referred to as a programming specialist, probably will be involved in most of the ongoing activities of the agency regardless of job title.

The voluntary health agency has a variety of target audiences. First, there is a need to provide in-service education to the volunteers so that they are competent in the delivery of educational programs. This increases their level of satisfaction and keeps them active as volunteers. Second, the general public is concerned about the goals and activities of the organization. Civic and community groups often request educational programs. Effective programs can actually recruit new volunteers, enhance fund raising, and stimulate advocacy for the organization within the community. The third area of educational programming is professional education. Although the health educator may not actually conduct the program, he or she probably will be responsible for organizing it.

This job setting, more than the others, requires a willingness to accept unusual working hours. Programs are normally held when it is convenient for the participants. Often, this means evenings or weekends. Offsetting this concern, however, is the benefit of autonomy. Assuming that programs are well run, the health educator is rarely restricted in carrying out his or her responsibilities.

Most agencies employ an executive director of a local chapter, unit, or affiliate. Once again, there is no academic program of study that prepares a person to assume this role. Health educators are certainly competitive by virtue of their undergraduate training. Additional coursework that might prove helpful includes personnel management, accounting, fund raising, community development, and marketing.

Government

Most health educators probably think of county health departments when considering government employment. Certainly there are opportunities for health education specialists, particularly in the more populated urban and suburban areas. But remember that many federal and state-funded programs specifically call for the education of clients. A good example is the WIC program that requires nutrition education as part of the services offered to qualifying women, infants, and children. Tax-supported family planning clinics are another example. Clients need to be informed about their options and should be instructed in the proper use of contraceptive devices. Small group facilitation and counseling skills are especially important to health educators who work for government-funded projects.

As with the voluntary agencies, government programs have a diversity of employment opportunities. This is especially true of middle management and administrative positions. Obviously, health educators cannot expect to start out at this level of employment, but they can use previous professional experience over time to qualify for administrative positions within a health-related agency. An individual with a health education background and management experience would seem to be highly competitive. If the person also has done coursework in health administration, budget planning, and public health, his or her employment prospects would be greatly improved.

In conclusion, it should be apparent that having an undergraduate degree in health education enables you to pursue a variety of careers in both the public and private sector. The academic preparation permits entry-level employment. By making the most of your professional experiences and by carefully selecting in-service or graduate coursework to meet the need for advanced skills, it is possible to fill roles that never would have been anticipated as an undergraduate student. Many administrative jobs go to individuals who are less qualified than others but who nevertheless apply for those positions. Health educators need to expand their thinking about career opportunities. The seven responsibilities identified by the Role Delineation Project describe many jobs that are both professionally and financially rewarding. A health educator who can fulfill these seven responsibilities will always have abundant career options.

Summary

This chapter describes the major risk factors for disease in each of the five age groups. The federal government has identified long-range goals for improving the health of Americans across the life span. Analysis of these goals demonstrates that their attainment will depend on effective health education. Health promotion is a larger concept, consisting of a variety of activities, but all efforts at health promotion require health education. This is true because health promotion seeks to enhance the quality of life by enabling people to make healthful choices in their daily living. Healthful choices depend on accurate information and appropriate attitudes. Health educators will play a prominent part in the achievement of governmental goals.

A number of preventive services are being delivered to individuals, such as family planning, immunizations, and high blood pressure control. Measures to protect people from harm, such as toxic agent control, occupational safety, and water fluoridation, are also currently being provided. These prevention and protection services all require the skills of a health educator to facilitate the acceptance of these services. There is already mounting evidence that health promotion can be effective. In areas such as cigarette smoking, alcohol and drug abuse, nutrition, fitness, and stress control the short-term evidence is positive. For instance, fewer people currently smoke cigarettes, and more people exercise regularly and incorporate stress management techniques into their life-styles. It will take time, but if current trends continue we will see a decline in diseases such as lung cancer, heart disease, and stomach ulcers. When that happens the current health promotion efforts will be seen as cost-effective and the outcome will justify the notion that "an ounce of prevention is worth a pound of cure."

Questions for Review

1. How would you respond to the claim that health educators are "warriors against pleasure"?
2. How has the changing nature of disease in this country affected school and community health education?
3. Other than routine responsibilities, what activities can school health educators and community health educators organize in order to promote the health of others?
4. In what ways do health educators use the behavioral sciences in their work?
5. What evidence is available to suggest that the medical model is neither the most effective nor the most cost-efficient route to good health?
6. What are some examples of primary, secondary, and tertiary prevention activities in the areas of communicable diseases, drug abuse, family living, birth defects, accidents, cancer, and cardiorespiratory diseases?
7. How would you describe the current social ethic for each of the health concerns just listed?
8. What are the major obstacles that stand in the way of the five broad goals established by the surgeon general?
9. In certain health-related areas the issue is raised about how far the government should be allowed to interfere with individual rights. How would you address this issue with regard to the health problems mentioned in question 6?
10. What health promotion activities have been conducted in your hometown? Who sponsored them? Were they successful?
11. Consider the following questions about worksite health promotion: Who should pay for the services? Should time off be given so employees can attend? Should the company offer incentives for attendance? What issues could be raised in a management/union work place? Will worksite health educators need special skills not needed by the school or community health educator?
12. What evidence can you cite that demonstrates the worth of health promotion activities?
13. What do you consider to be the advantages and disadvantages of working as a health educator in each of the settings discussed in Chapter 3?
14. In what ways can health educators in each of the settings work together to link professional expertise in order to enhance community health?

References

1. U.S. Department of Health and Human Services: Health: United States, 1980, U.S. Public Health Service, Office of Health Research Statistics, and Technology, DHHS Pub. No. 81-1232, Washington, D.C., 1980, U.S. Government Printing Office.
2. Scheffler, R.M.: The economic evidence on prevention. In U.S. Public Health Service: Healthy people: background papers, Pub. No. 79-55071A, Washington, D.C., 1979, U.S. Government Printing Offce.
3. Califano, J.A., Jr.: A message to participants, In U.S. Public Health Service: Promoting health: issues and strategies, Pub. No. 0-301-263, Washington, D.C., 1979, U.S. Government Printing Office.
4. Califano, J.A., Jr.: Healthy people, the surgeon general's report on health promotion and disease prevention, U.S. Public Health Service, DHHS Pub. No. 79-55074, Washington, D.C., 1979, U.S. Government Printing.
5. U.S. Department of Health, Education and Welfare, Public Health Service, Regional Forums on Community Health Promotion: Promoting health: issues and strategies, Washington, D.C., 1979, U.S. Government Printing Office.
6. Washington Business Group on Health: Health promotion in the community: a guide to working with employees, Washington, D.C., 1980.
7. Harris, Lewis and Associates, Inc.: Health maintenance, Newport Beach, Cal., 1978, Pacific Mutual Life Insurance Co. (As cited in Health: United States, 1980.)
8. Yankelovich, Skelly, and White, The General Mills American family report, 1978-79, family health in an era of stress, Minneapolis, 1979, General Mills, Inc. (As cited in Health: United States, 1980.)
9. U.S. Department of Health, Education and Welfare, Centers for Disease Control, Programs and Policies Advisory Committee (ad hoc): Recommendations for a national strategy for disease prevention: report to the director, Atlanta, Ga., 1978, Centers for Disease Control. As reported by Gloria Ruby in Background papers for the surgeon general's report.
10. American Hospital Association: Health: what they know, what they do, what they want— a national survey of consumers and businesses, Chicago, 1978, The Association. (As cited in Healthy people: Background papers.)

Additional Readings

Averson, D.C., guest editor: Promoting health through the schools, Health Education Quarterly 8(1):5-117, 1981 (entire issue).

Balog, J.E.: The concepts of health and disease, Health Values: Achieving High Level Wellness 6(5):7-13, 1982.

Baranowski, T.: Toward the definition of concepts of health and disease, wellness and illness, Health Values: Achieving High Level Wellness 5(6):246-256, 1981.

Becker, M.H., guest editor: The health belief model and personal health behavior, Health Education Monographs 2(4):324-473, 1974 (entire issue).

Brennan, A.J., guest editor: Worksite health promotion, Health Ed. Q. 9(3):5-91, 1982 (entire issue).

Crosby, R.: Psychosomatic wellness, The Eta Sigma Gamman 13(1):17-20, 1981.

Deeds, S.G., and Mullen, P.A., guest editors: Managing health education in H.M.O.'s, Health Education Quarterly 8(4):279-372, 1982 (entire issue).

Deeds, S.G., and Mullen, P.A., guest editors: Managing health education in H.M.O.'s, Health Education Quarterly 9(1):3-95, 1982 (entire issue).

Dunn, H.L.: What high level wellness means, Health Values: Achieving High Level Wellness 1(1):9-16, 1977. (Reprinted from Canadian Journal of Public Health 50:447-457, 1959).

Faden, R.R., and Faden, A.I., guest editors: Ethical issues in public health policy: health education and lifestyle interventions, Health Education Monographs 6(2):177-257, 1978 (entire issue).

Green, L.W., Wilson, R.W., and Bauer, K.G.: Data requirements to measure progress on the objectives for the nation in health promotion and disease prevention, American Journal of Public Health 73(1):18-24, 1983.

Hatch, J.W., Renfrow, W.C., and Snider, G.: Progressive health education through community organization: a case study, Health Education Monographs, 6(4):359-371, 1978.

Kreuter, M.W., Parsons, M.J., and McMurry, M.P.: Moral sensitivity in health promotion, Health Education 13(6):11-13, 1982.

Laughlin, J.A.: A wellness approach to health in the workplace, Health Values: Achieving High Level Wellness 6(2):5-9, 1982.

McClure, D.L.: Wellness, a holistic concept, Health Values: Achieving High Level Wellness 6(5):23-27, 1982.

Ross, C.R.: Factors influencing successful preventive health education, Health Education Quarterly 8(3):187-208, 1981.

Rustia, J.: Rustia school health promotion model, Journal of School Health 52(2):108-114, 1982.

Simonds, S.K., guest editor: Health manpower, Health Education Monographs 4(3):204-284, 1976 (entire issue).

Wallace, B.C.: Organizing the community for health education and health promotion, The Eta Sigma Gamman 13(2):18-20, 1981.

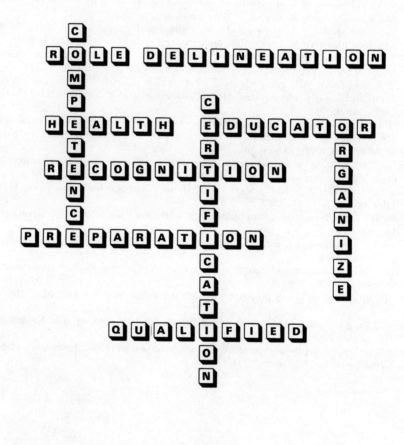

4 Professional Competencies of the Health Educator

Introduction

This chapter is divided into three major sections. The first section describes the characteristics of a profession, and uses these characteristics to evaluate the position of health education. The second section offers an overview of the roles, functions, and responsibilities of health educators. The third section deals with competency-based education as it relates to the preparation of health educators.

In the opening section of the chapter Professor Neutens presents the steps that ordinarily occur as a field of specialization seeks professional status. Against this backdrop, he provides a brief chronology of health education's movement toward this goal. It appears that our current status is that of an aspiring profession. Although we have made definite progress, considerable effort lies ahead. Professor Neutens is optimistic that we are moving in the right direction and that we have within our midst the talent necessary to achieve public recognition and professional status.

The keystone of all professions is the quality of the membership who represent it. The public is often confused or misinformed about what health education is and what roles are performed by health educators. Consequently, many important job opportunities have been filled with people who possess no professional identity as health educators and who have limited abilities to perform the tasks required by their employer. This places the burden of the development of health educators squarely on the shoulders of the more than 250 academic programs of professional preparation. If health education is going to fulfill its potential it must do so with people who are capable. But that has been the question from the beginning: Capable of what?

Briefly stated, competency is the possession of an acceptable level of skill or proficiency required to carry out an activity. Theoretically, it is a simple matter to develop and test individual competency. This chapter reveals, however, that competency-based education is a complex issue. The identification of skills determined to be essential, and the use of a test situation to evaluate an individual's status with respect to these skills, pose significant challenges. For instance, there are decisions about (1) what skills to require, (2) the minimal level of acceptable performance, (3) whether minimal cmopetence is really what you want, and (4) establishment of criteria that are able to locate a person on the pass or fail side of a continuum.

Although there are problems associated with competency-based education, there are also advantages. Recognizing that the process is imperfect, that competency requirements may vary from institution to institution, and that flaws exist in evaluating performance, competency-based education does at least force the creation of some standards. If nothing else, competency-based education requires a look ahead to determine what skills are needed by the entry-level health educator. It happens all too often in professional preparation programs that individuals are trained without regard to the actual skills that are necessary to do the job. Competency-based education is not an end in itself. Rather, it can serve as a means for standardizing professional preparation for health educators assuming entry-level positions.

The final section of the chapter examines what the entry-level health educator should be able to do. This helps the prospective employer know what to look for in selecting the best candidate from among the applicants for the job. It also ensures a pool of applicants who can meet the expectations of the employer. The Role Delineation Project is seeking to identify the threads of unity that will eventually become the fabric of the profession. This project has provided seven broad areas of responsibility common to all health educators, regardless of whether they are working in a school, a hospital, or a community-based agency.

It should be pointed out that the Role Delineation Project is also discussed in other chapters of this text. We believe the project is of monumental importance to health education's quest to gain public recognition and ultimately to achieve professional status. In the chapters that discuss the Role Delineation Project the material is relevant to the chapter itself. The information presented in this chapter is not duplicated elsewhere in the text.

A Sense of Professional Growth

Since its inception, health education has been described as being at a crossroads. The underlying problem seems to have been caused by a persistent lack of identity for the profession. More than a decade ago this concern was prominent in the literature.[1,2] In his discussion of *What's in a Name?* Governali[3] reflects on this dilemma, as does Hurster,[4] both labeling it as the first and foremost problem confronting health education. The passage of time has done little to improve the situation. Until the profession develops a recognized set of competency requirements, standardized entry routes that it controls, and a formalized code of ethics, health education will remain at the crossroads and will be continuously subjected to the pressures of outside forces.

As more and more employment positions begin to open for health educators, a greater number of applicants are invidiuals with wide and diverse backgrounds.[5] Many of these jobs are being filled by outsiders because employers are uncertain about the profession and its constituents. Further, there is little doubt that attempts to attract funding for training programs have suffered because of this lack of understanding about the professional competency of those who have the title "health educator."[6] At the Conference of the Preparation and Practice of Community, Patient, and School Health Educators, Cleary[7] demonstrated that perhaps this ignorance was rampant within the profession as well as extraneous to it. In attempting to establish the parameters of the profession, she recognized three possible classifications for health educators. These classifications were discussed in Chapter 2. Please refer to p. 43 for review.

It is possible that these classifications of professional identity can be subdivided even further. For instance, those who see themselves as "teachers" may identify with community health education or school health education. Their own sense of identification may be as a sex educator, death educator, or alcohol educator rather than as comprehensive health educator. Similarly, they may see themselves as a biology teacher, a home economics teacher, or a physical education teacher rather than health educator. Those individuals who identify with the role of school health education planner may call themselves "curriculum specialists." The curriculum specialist may have been trained as a health educator or as a science teacher. Community-based health education planners may call themselves "community specialists," or "adult education specialists." The community specialist may have been trained as an educator, a nurse, a psychologist, or a social worker. Those people having a professional identity outside of health education will undoubtedly view the role of health education differently from those who are trained as health educators. It is a concept that has entirely different meanings to those who perform one or more functions of a health educator. The question that remains is What is a health educator? Ware[8] and Hochbaum[9] believe that external forces are bringing about a renewed interest in health education because of the potential of health education to affect current social issues. Some of these issues are consumer rights and responsibilities, the rising cost of medical care, the proliferation of the allied health professions and employment of paraprofessionals and nonprofessionals in health care, problems in adherence to medical regimens, informed consent, the increase in medical malpractice suits, and the recognition that an individual's level of health is largely dependent on his or her own life-style.

The role of health education is becoming more and more important in American society. Employment opportunities are becoming more and more diverse, as evidenced by the number of health educators who currently work in hospitals, health maintenance organizations, industry, and governmental agencies. This diversity of role and function necessitates the establishment of common philosophic, ethical, and preparatory foundations for health education.[10,11] Now, more than ever before, it is important for health education to develop a unifying philosophy and a set of competencies that characterize all health educators regardless of their job setting. The past has witnessed intraprofessional competition among associations for members, money, and recognition.[12] Recently an attempt to bring health education professionals together by means of a state organization failed to materialize because the potential members were involved with other competing associations.[13]

According to 25 national leaders representing universities, government and private agencies, and professional societies, between the years of 1985 and 1995 there will be one monolithic society of health educators that will reflect unity, common philosophy, and common knowledge.[14] Taub[15] found that although members of the New York Federation of Professional Health Educators placed health education at a midpoint between a profession and a nonprofession, they would support activities leading to further professionalism.

Leaders from several health organizations are currently working toward this end through the efforts of the Role Delineation Project. This is a project of the National Center for Health Education through a contract with the Bureau of Health Manpower. The intent of the Role Delineation Project is to define and verify the role of the health educator and to develop a curricular guide for academic programs preparing health educators, as well as self-assessment tools and continuing education materials for practitioners.

What is a Profession?

There still exists the pervasive question of what constitutes a profession. Moore[16] describes the professional as having

1. A full-time occupation
2. A commitment to a calling (treatment of the occupation and all of its requirements as an enduring set of normative and behavioral expectations)
3. Membership in an organization for all
4. A specialized training or education
5. A service orientation
6. Autonomy restrained by responsibility

Upton[16a] states that each profession seems to

1. Provide a unique and essential social service
2. Require of its members an extensive period of preparation
3. Have underlying its practice a theoretical base
4. Have a system of internal controls that tend to regulate the behavior of its members
5. Have a culture peculiar to the profession
6. Be sanctioned by the community
7. Have an occupational association that is representative of and can speak on behalf of all members of the occupation.

Employing these criteria in the Taub study,[15] the New York Federation of Professional Health Educators categorized health education as a semiprofession or an aspiring profession. This poses an interesting question: If health educators view their status as a semiprofession, how should they expect others outside the field to view their status?

According to Elliott[17] and Wilensky,[18] professionalization takes place in recognizable stages:
1. Functional specialization
2. Formation of professional association
3. Public recognition
4. Standardized entry routes
5. Formalized code of ethics

Following the natural history of professionalization, it is possible to tract the progression of health education. At the outset a service orientation is most likely to be found among members of an organization, but as the group emerges, full-time workers focus on a particular set of problems. The basis for this group concern is usually a result of functional specialization. Historical foundations of health education demonstrate that our roots are similar to the beginnings of other professions. We evolved from educators who saw the need for specialization as a result of the tremendous amount of information related to health.

The next stage is the formation of a professional association to assist in the continuing process of revising qualifications, defining occupational functions, establishing internalized standards and norms, and managing relationships with competing groups. As time goes by and the process of professionalization continues, standardized qualifications for entry and formalized entry routes for employment become established. Needless to say, an occupation with professional intentions cannot afford to become a refuge for the unqualified. Over the past several years health educators, through associations such as SOPHE, ASHA, APHA, AAHPER, and the Role Delineation Project, have been generating preparation lists for institutions to consider. The National Center for Health Education, by means of the Role Delineation Project (1980), views credentialing as a process of demonstrating evidence of qualification. The three avenues available are accreditation, licensure, and certification. Although professionalization of this type is now occurring in health education, common standards for professional preparation have yet to be adopted by all preparatory facilities.

The presence of myriad health associations representing three seemingly disparate branches of health education makes this stage look distant. However, Sliepcevich[19] noted at the Conference on Preparation and Practice of Community, Patient, and School Health Educators that there are indeed many commonalities among these occupational settings.

Further growth occurs when a professional association strives for public recognition and legal support to control program entry and entry into the profession. In regard to the schools, education is in the domain of the states, many of which have passed legislation supporting the teaching of health and the separate certification of health educators. Although most efforts have been piecemeal in approach, such as requiring specific curricula on venereal disease or drug abuse, some legislatures have recognized the advantages of having a comprehensive health education program. In addition to stipulating topical areas, a few states have designated the establishment of training centers for teachers as well as minimal requirements for teachers.

In community education, three major legislative packages (PL 93-641,

PL 93-222, and PL 94-317) are serving to advance the growth of health education. The National Health Planning and Resources Development Act of 1974 (PL 93-641), through Title XV, directs the development of "effective methods of educating the general public concerning proper personal health care and effective use of available health services." Title XIII of the Public Health Services Act, (PL 93-222) also indicates the need for health education and specifies the importance of patient education. Title XVII of the Public Health Services Act, (PL 94-317) is a three-part package entitled the National Consumer Health Information and Health Promotion Act of 1976. This act has helped to demonstrate the potential for health education in the public sector.

The culminating stage suggested by Elliott and Wilensky[18] is the elaboration of a formal code of ethics. In 1978 the Association for the Advancement of Health Education (AAHE) sponsored a conference devoted to the philosophy of health education, and in March 1979 AAHE held a Conference on Ethical Issues in Health Education. The ethical issues raised by participants were categorized into philosophy of ethics, professional preparation, methodology, role modeling, content selection, research, accountability, and political activities. There is little doubt that health education has much distance to travel in its efforts to fully reach the status of profession, although progress has been evident. Functional specialization, the formation of associations, and (to an extent) public recognition have been achieved. Standardized entry routes and a formalized code of ethics are on the horizon.

Elliott[17] has diagrammed the essential features of professionalism along a series of continua (see box). In the right-hand column, Elliott attempted to show how these features link to form a self-supporting whole. In examination of this diagram consider for yourself whether health education should be granted professional status.

Employing this schematic, the field of health education does appear to be moving in the direction of full professional status. It possesses broad, theoretical knowledge, frequently tying together pieces from related disciplines. As new settings emerge and themes of wellness and holism replace disease orientation, this knowledge will be applied more and more to non-routine situations. This will require innumerable decisions, particularly in behavior modification, if the populace is to shift to health-inducing activities. Authority is increasing as accountability and evaluation expand. Identity is being established through a concerted effort as a greater number of health educators make a career out of their position and others retrain to meet entry requirements. Health education is becoming an activity wherein both related fields and the public are beginning to recognize and accept the potential of the profession.

Although the natural history previously outlined is clearly not the only possibility for professional evolution, it is interesting to note that health education may be following a path analogous to already established professional occupations. The comparison reflects both direction and progress. Although overnight success is not to be expected, the near future holds many answers to health education questions—if they are allowed to come forth. The challenge is large, but the abilities of individuals within the profession and the strength of our professional associations appears to be equal to the challenge. Some traditions may have to be surrendered as new ways are forged, but as pointed out by Hochbaum,[9] "When one generation feels proud and superior because of what is has accomplished since the previous generation had done its work, it should remember that it can look down on its forefathers only because it stands on their shoulders."

Continua in the Professional Ideal Type*

Nonprofessional		**Professional**
Technical, craft skill	Knowledge	Broad, theoretical knowledge use in ↓
Routine	Tasks	Nonroutine situations to reach ↓
Programmed	Decision making	Unprogrammed decisions according to ↓
Ends decided by society (or other institution)	Authority	Ends (derived from knowledge) decided for society (or institution within it) and supported by ↓
Other or nonwork	Identity	Occupational group because work and occupation are ↓
Means to nonwork ends	Work	Central life interest and are also the basis for ↓
Occupational/class advancement	Career	Individual achievement, which involves meeting initial entry qualifications through ↓
Limited	Education	Extensive education, showing skill, and meeting other latent status requirements involved in the ↓
Specific	Role	Total role (that is, expectations extend beyond expertise and work situation)

*From Elliott, P.: The sociology of the professions, New York, 1972, Herder & Herder.

Identification of Competencies
Steps in Deriving Competencies

If professional preparation in health education is thought of as an instructional system designed to achieve common purposes, it is necessary to determine what those purposes should be. In system terminology, what is the expected output of the program? In most instances, the principal intention is to produce health educators who possess certain knowledge, appropriate attitudes, performance skills, and the ability to put these together to bring about desirable learning, attitudes, and behavior among the target population. Nevertheless, a number of questions must still be asked, such as: Exactly what knowledge, attitudes, and skills should the prospective health educator possess? What changes should they be able to bring about in the various target populations?

The answers to these questions largely establish the direction for professional preparation programs. In other words, to determine the output of the system, that is, the types of health educators the program wishes to produce, a set of assumptions must be developed from which goals can be generated. From these goals more specific objectives can be derived that define the competencies a health educator will need in order to achieve the goals of the program.

Today there are over 250 programs on college campuses with health education majors or specialities[20] and there is little doubt that most have failed to develop sets of assumptions or goals about either health educators or the requirements of preparation programs. Further, programs that operate from a variety of basic assumptions and goals will certainly function in different ways, thereby producing health educators who operate in different ways. For too long, graduates in health education have been the product of individual program interests rather than the product of a unified set of experiences common to everyone who has the title of health educator.

The need is clear. Professional preparation programs in health education must develop a common set of assumptions and goals based on a clear definition of the roles of the health educator. Only then can specific objectives and competencies be developed.

Roles, Functions, and Goals

Bowman[10] has reviewed the literature in an attempt to observe the role of community health educators over time. His examination revealed that health educators are moving away from functions concerned with dissemination of information and toward functions of community organization, program planning, evaluation, and personal forms of communication, (such

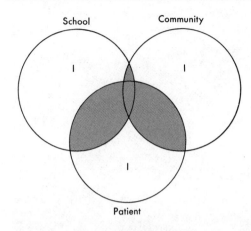

Fig. 4-1. Role commonalities and differences. Shaded area identifies overlapping functions among health educators. *I.* Represents potential interaction through creation of communication channels and through resource sharing and mass media use. (From The proceedings of the Workshop on Commonalities and Differences: preparation and practice of community, patient, and school health educators, U.S. DHEW [HRA] Pub. No. 78-71, Washington, D.C., 1978, U.S. Government Printing Office.)

as roles of facilitator, resource person, coordinator), with special emphasis on the behavioral approach in order to effect changes in health behavior as they concern individuals, groups, or organizations. These latter functions have also become the concern of school and patient health educators.[4,11,21,22] This shift of functions or roles common to all three branches of health education was acknowledged at the 1978 workshop on Commonalities and Differences. Fig. 4-1 illustrates the relationship among health educators in school, community, and patient settings. The shaded area identifies the overlapping functions among health educators and the "I" represents potential interaction through the creation of communication channels and through resource sharing and media use.

After reviewing these commonalities the workshop participants described three functions that are instrumental to health educators in all settings of the profession. The first function is "to assess health and educational needs and interests of the target population."[19] This fundamental function is germane to the development of an educational strategy because the health educator must determine not only the health needs of the individual or group in question but also the educational needs.

According to the Workshop on Commonalities and Differences, the second function common to all health educators is to "design, implement,

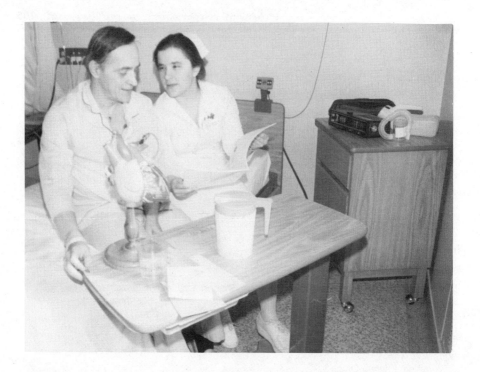

Fig. 4-2. Patient education in a health care facility, Urbana, Illinois. (Photograph by Lyn Lawrance.)

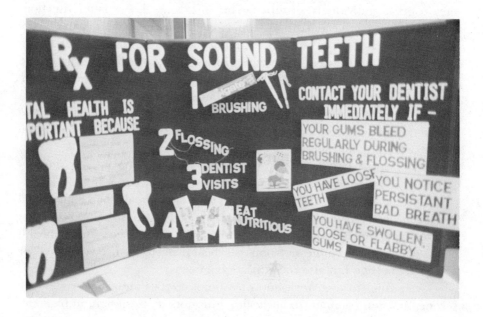

Fig. 4-3. Classroom bulletin board during National Dental Health Week. (Photograph by Lyn Lawrance.)

coordinate and evaluate health education activities to meet the goals of health education."[19] This function involves the development of an all-encompassing educational strategy. Further, it outlines the various tasks demanded by such a strategy, indicating the areas in which a health educator may participate. The point at which the health educator becomes involved will vary according to the educator's background and preparation.

The third common function is to "coordinate multidisciplinary resources to enable an educational planning implementation process to exist."[19] Those in attendance concurred that a health educator frequently functions as a central agent, bringing together a wide variety of resources to attain a goal. These resources may include personnel, materials, or facilities. It is interesting to note the consistency between the functions developed at the workshop and those observed by Bowman[10] and others.

The tasks or functions specific to community, school, or patient health educators were found to vary according to the setting, target population, and motivation of the groups or individuals to whom the health education was directed. Table 4-1 elaborates on the factors distinguishing the functions.

Table 4-1
Factors differentiating the functions throughout community, school, and patient health education

	Community	**School**	**Patient**
Target Population	At risk population as defined by particular health concern	Young school-age population (5-18 years, generally healthy)	Direct: medical care professionals within health care facility—medical content oriented
	Problem solving–oriented, generally noncaptive audience	Health promotion and disease prevention–oriented, captive audience	Indirect: patients or families of patients
Setting	Community in general	Classroom/school system	Health care facility
Motivation	Community health–related problems	School attendance required by law	Direct: health care professionals need for educational process assistance when instructing patients on health maintenance and disease management
	General health promotion interests of community members	Health and disease knowledge and health values	Indirect: presence of disease presence of illness

From The Proceedings of the Workshop of Commonalities and Differences: Preparation and Practice of Community, Patient, and School Health Educators. (U.S DHEW (HRA) Pub. No. 78-71), Washington, D.C., 1978, U.S. Government Printing Office.

From the discussion of the commonalities and differences, a clearer idea of the roles of the health educator emerged. This allowed the workshop participants to develop several assumptions about the professional preparation of health educators. That in turn resulted in three preparatory statements:

Preparation Statement I

A common core curriculum for all health educators needs to be established, followed by specialized curricula at the advanced levels for the various areas of health education.

Preparation Statement II

At the entry level of preparation, a common core of skills and knowledge should be established and adopted that contain, at a minimum: behavioral and social sciences, biological sciences, educational theory, and an effective field experience, all of which integrate health education concepts.

Preparation Statement III

Specialized preparation should be established, primarily at the advanced levels, for specific health education settings and functions.[20]

It was assumed that a common core program would enable the entry-level health educator to function effectively in a variety of settings. From the roles and functions observed, the framework for that core was suggested in the second preparatory statement. The last statement reflects the assumption that at advanced levels of preparation the commonalities appear less frequently.

The participants at the Workshop on Commonalities and Differences made great strides toward the clarification and unification of roles of health educators. Fortunately, their efforts were not forgotten. One of the recommendations made was that the planning committee for the workshop "be charged with responsibility for developing a plan of action leading to a credentialing program within a specific time frame for the total field of health education."[23] In September 1978 a contract between the Center for Health Education and the Bureau of Health Professions Division of Associated Health Professions, DHHS, was signed to

initially specify the responsibilities, functions, skills, and knowledge of entry-level health educators; to define entry-level into health education; and to identify levels of supervision required for entry-level personnel.[24]

All of this came to be known as the Role Delineation Project.

To provide direction, and to build on the accomplishments of the previous workshop participants, the working committee and project staff of the Role Delineation Project agreed to operate on the assumption that common functions or roles exist among health educators, regardless of whether the setting is the community, medical facility, or school. The strategy therefore was to delineate the role of the generic entry-level health educator, beginning with the general areas of responsibilities that would lead to the specification of functions, skills, and knowledge required to meet those responsibilities. This is akin to the development of goals, subgoals, and objectives that define the competencies a health educator will need to achieve the goals.

The three functions outlined at the Workshop on Commonalities and Differences were adopted by the Role Delineation Project members to serve as starting points. From these functions broad areas of responsibility were developed, each within inherent functions. Together these areas of responsibility make up the role of an entry-level health educator. Resources for this part of the project included (1) expertise from members of the Role Delineation team, (2) literature about professional preparation and publications of professional standards by various organizations, and (3) approximately 600 job descriptions from 300 individuals who had been identified as contacts in the field of health education. The perceptions of practicing health educators were not a part of the initial process but are to be included during refining and verification activities.[24]

The broad areas of responsibility, which may be perceived as goals, and the functions or subgoals they encompass are presented below.

Area of Responsibility I

The entry-level health educator, working with individuals, groups, and organizations, is responsible for communicating health and health education needs, concerns, and resources.
Functions:
Providing information about health
Interpreting health information
Facilitating communication
Disseminating information about health education programs
Advocating health education in policy formulation

Area of Responsibility II

The entry-level health educator, working with individuals, groups, and organizations, is responsible for determining the appropriate focus for health education.
Functions:
Collecting information about populations of interest
Analyzing information to determine areas of need

Area of Responsibility III

The entry-level health educator, working with individuals, groups, and organizations, is responsible for planning health education programs in response to identified needs.
Functions:
Participating in the educational planning process
Participating in developing program objectives based on information acquired as part of the planning process
Designing educational programs consistent with specified educational objectives

Area of Responsibility IV

The entry-level health educator, working with individuals, groups, and organizations, is responsible for implementing planned health education programs.
Functions:

Assisting in mobilizing personnel needed to carry out the plan
Securing operational resources necessary to carry out the plan
Carrying out the educational program for sharing information, influencing behavior, and resolving problems

Area of Responsibility V

The entry-level health educator, working with individuals, groups, and organizations, is responsible for evaluating health education.
Functions:

Participating in developing an evaluation design
Assembling resources required to carry out evaluation
Helping to implement the evaluation design
Communicating results of evaluation

Area of Responsibility VI

The entry-level health educator, working with individuals, groups, and organizations, is responsible for coordinating selected health education activities.
Functions:

Assisting personnel to carry out health education activities
Promoting awareness of health education's contributions to achieving goals
Carrying out designated administrative activities

Area of Responsibility VII

The entry-level health educator, working with individuals, groups, and organizations, is responsible for acting as a resource for health and health education.
Functions:

Gathering information from various sources regarding needs, concerns, and interests
Responding to requests for information
Initiating opportunities for consultation
Seeking consultation from others
Providing consultation to others
Preparing others to perform health education–related skills
Providing educational resource materials[28]

Although not everyone may concur with these efforts, it must be realized that the assumptions, goals (areas of responsibility), and subgoals (functions) were obtained by a group of people representing the profession. This in and of itself has helped to alleviate the fragmentation that has plagued health educators for years. On the other hand, although they provide direction for professional preparation programs, in no way should it be construed that the assumptions and goals should forever remain fixed, with no possibility of change, extension, or even replacement.

The parameters have now been set, based on a definition of the roles of the health educator. The next step is to identify competencies and objectives consistent with the roles.

Professional Preparation and Competencies

Over the years, all the professional societies have prepared statements on the professional preparation of health educators. The School Health Division Task Force of AAHPER published a document in 1974 for baccalaureate preparation. According to this document, the prospective health educator must show competency in the following major areas:

1. Health content
2. Allied health fields
3. Professional education
   Curriculum
   Methodology and materials
   Evaluation and measurement
   Organization and administration
   Public relations
4. Personal qualifications
5. Practicum[25]

This document was written to show both objectives and competencies to be employed in a competency-based program.

In 1976 ASHA published a report by the ASHA Committee on Professional Preparation.[30] The report, unlike the AAHPER document, was not competency oriented because the participants felt that "because of the current difficulty agreeing on a definition of competencies it was decided to speak about 'skills and knowledge' rather than competencies."[26] The key areas involved were:

1. Content areas in health education
   Direct health content
   Related health content
2. Educational skills
   Learning theory applied to health behavior
   Verbal and nonverbal communication
   Curriculum planning and implementation
   Methodology applied to direct and related health content
   Resources applied to direct and related health content
   Evaluation techniques
3. Orientation to the profession
   Philosophy
   Organization/administration
   School health program
   Community health program
   Process skills
4. Demonstration of skills and knowledge
   Student teaching
   Community health practicum[26]

In the same year, SOPHE published *Guidelines for the Preparation and Practice of Professional Health Educators*.[27] Although written somewhat differently than the AAHPER document, it is competency oriented and identifies six major areas to be achieved by both the baccalaureate and master's candidate.

1. Foundations of health education
2. Administration of health education
3. Program development and management
   Planning for change: planning process for health education
   Health education methods
      Training theory and skills
      Group dynamics theory and skills
      Community organization
      Information and media
4. Research and evaluation
5. Professional ethics
6. Special applications

Analysis of the statements from the three associations reveals that the underlying assumptions for which the listed competencies and objectives were originally intended are quite different. The AAHPER and ASHA documents emphasize preparation of the school health educator, while the SOPHE document leans in the direction of health educators in community settings.

As would be expected, the skill and knolwedge objectives developed by members of the Role Delineation Project[28] attempt to avoid this separation of school and community health education through the assumption of a generic role. As noted previously, each broad area of responsibility contains a list of functions that must be performed to fulfill those responsibilities. In sequence, each function encompasses a skill (an ability to do or to apply something) and several knowledge objectives. An example is given below.

Area of responsibility I: Communicating health and health education needs, concerns, and resources
Function B: Interpreting health information
Skill 3: The health educator must be able to explain the purposes and resources of the organization employing the health educator.
Knowledge: The health educator must be able to:
1. Identify the purposes, objectives, and resources of his or her employer (such as statements of goals, legal status, statements of position on issues, history of the organization, features of its activities)
2. Describe methods and materials used to inform selected audiences (such as professional meetings, pamphlets, films, annual reports, civic club meetings)[28]

A brief discussion of some of the issues pertaining to professional preparation can be found in the Editor's Remarks at the end of this chapter.

Competency-based Education: a Debatable Vehicle to Professionalism

Although the belief is stronger than ever that health education must be professionalized, a definite approach has yet to be established. The competency-based method is seen by some observers as the most promising vehicle for achieving such a status.[29] This is especially true for arriving at entry-level qualifications. On the other hand, Glass[30] observed that "a common expression of wishful thinking is to base a grand scheme on a fundamental, unsolved problem." A review of the literature brings a deluge of reports, speeches, conferences, research, and position papers that can build a case either for or against competency-based education. The underlying theme in the mass of paper that has been produced is the recurrent question Just what is competency-based education?

The Meaning of Competency-based Education

The obvious temptation now is to present a neatly packaged definition of competency-based education. After all, is it not merely professional preparation based on competencies? Perhaps, but the inherent difficulty is arriving at a definition for *competence*. According to Pollock[31] the word *competence* is akin to *motherhood* and *patriotism;* the words are so familiar and so well accepted that definitions seem unnecessary. This is also true for the word *health*. Meanings appear to be self-evident. A close review of any of these words reveals that they are abstractions—ideas—and as such they defy succinct definition. For example, if the health educator in question is competent, does it mean that he or she is *adequate, able, effectual, capable, qualified* or all of these? Each of these terms conjures a kaleidescope of images that can only be sorted by specifying the knowledge or task in which one is to be competent.

A competency-based educational program must specify the competencies to be demonstrated by the learner as well as the criteria to be employed for evaluation. The competencies and subsequent criteria should involve (1) knowledge to assess cognitive components, (2) performance to assess the acquisition of skills, and (3) product (that is, target population) to assess effectiveness and accountability. The latter competencies and criteria are a necessity for evaluating field work, whether it be in the classroom or in the community.

Competency-based education is not, however, an end in itself. Rather it is a process that can move preparation from an ambiguous state to a clearly articulated program of professional education.[23] Further, whether it is viewed as a nuisance or a desirable addition to education, it is a growing part of the current educational scene, a part that contains many challenges for the health educator.

Challenge of Competency-based Education

To assess the existence of competency-based health education programs in 1976, Pigg[33] surveyed 178 institutions from the National Directory of College and University School and Public Health Educators developed by Eta Sigma Gamma. Of the 157 responses he found that 29% of the programs had some type of competency-based program while another 25% were planning to move in this direction. Of the 76 institutions responding to another question, 47% indicated that they had established a list of health-related competencies and 53% replied negatively. It appears that health education preparatory institutions are to some extent already involved in some type of competency-based education. However, not unexpectedly there appeared to be a lack of consensus among the health educators as to what actually constitutes competency-based education. This finding underscores one of the major challenges confronting health educators: the need to establish a common direction.

Yet even if this direction is agreed on, the discipline must search for the ever-elusive health education competencies they wish their graduates to possess before entry into the professional field. Whether they are written as competencies or as behavioral objectives, it will be a time-consuming and demanding task. To be effective they must be functional. Assuming this challenge is met, the setting of standards for minimal competence holds the dual problem of method and meaning. That is, what is going to be the minimal degree of competence required, and how will the cut-off point be determined?

Finally, the profession must consider how all of this will be enforced. The usual choices are accreditation, in which an agency or organization evaluates and approves the institution and its program of study; licensure, in which a government agency grants permission to individuals to engage in health education once they have obtained minimal competence; and certification, in which a nongovernmental agency or association grants recognition to an individual who has met the predetermined qualifications specified by the agency or association.

Conclusion

Once again, the field of health education is at a crossroad. Unlike the past, however, action must be taken with deliberate speed if we are to progress as a profession, and to prevent the usurping of positions, grant money, and public recognition. Although numerous events are pushing health education to center stage in the health care system, it is our responsibility to prove that we belong there. To accomplish this task health educators must unify and present an image that is both unique and accountable.

Although this is a demanding task, especially because our roles are changing as new settings emerge, the attributes and abilities within the field are present to fulfill the mission. One possible vehicle is a competency-based professional preparation program in which both new and traditional assumptions and goals may be blended to guide us as a monolithic group. The criticisms and challenges of this approach are many but alternatives are few. Recent efforts by educators representing all facets of health education give evidence that commonalities are considerable enough that professional preparation programs can be based on a definition of the roles of health educators. Once this definition is established we are only a short way from identifying the competencies needed by the profession.

The myriad techniques available to derive competencies are waiting to be employed. Although mistakes will be made and wrong avenues will be taken from time to time, it is a great feeling to know that our future is in capable hands—our own.

Editors' Remarks

In Dr. Neuten's discussion of competencies and professional preparation he mentions that the AAHPER and ASHA documents deal with preparing the school health educator, while SOPHE's document deals with preparing community health educators. The Role Delineation Project attempts to avoid this separation and proposes that *health education* and *health educator* become generic terms. Although that is one of the major issues confronting the preparation of health educators, there are additional ones:

1. Certification of individuals not prepared in health education
2. Screening of prospective health education majors
3. Content in the professional program
4. Separation of health education from physical education
5. Dual preparation of school and community health educators
6. Increase in the number of professional preparation programs

This list is certainly not complete but it does provide a general sense of a few of the issues and problems facing health education professional programs.

Certification of Individuals Not Prepared in Health Education

Mandated health education requirements can be met in a number of ways that do not necessarily lead to becoming a qualified health educator. This is especially true concerning school health educators who are certified to teach by gaining credit through in-service courses, correspondence courses, and proficiency examinations. The usual circumstance is one in which a health educator is needed in a public school, and the physical educator is chosen by the principal to teach the required health education course.

This type of situation may lead to dissatisfaction among teachers who now must be retrained, the possibility of inadequate health education teaching, and a resentment toward health education by students, teachers, and administrators.

Screening of Prospective Health Education Majors

In the late 1970s, programs for professional preparation in both school health education and community health education, realized increases in enrollments. At the present time the number of students entering school health education programs has declined, probably as a result of the limited number of teaching positions that become available. However, community health education programs have grown and will continue to do so, especially if options in health administration, health promotion, patient education, and worksite education continue to proliferate. Screening of potential students may become commonplace in the very near future so that quality can be maintained in all professional preparation programs.

Other popular fields, such as finance, computer technology, and engineering have had to use screening programs or have had to limit the number of students by imposing unusually high admission standards. These are some alternatives that some professional preparation programs have begun to adopt (at Towson State University, The Ohio State University, and the University of Illinois) and other programs might have to consider.

Content in the Professional Program

Most programs that prepare undergraduates have a core of courses, and these allow a certain degree of latitude in course selection for the student. Students usually choose content area courses and may, at some institutions, specialize in an option area as noted above. The questions concerning course content revolve around the amount of choice a student encounters. Are students mature, self-directed, and far-sighted enough to choose those courses most commensurate with their skills and interest areas? Furthermore, programs might want to appear flexible and adaptable to attract students in light of the predicted declining enrollments.

In any case, this issue may be resolved if the Role Delineation Project is completed and is able to disseminate its resultant documents.

Separating Health Education from Physical Education

Although the struggle has been for the two professions to separate themselves, these areas of study, as perceived by outsiders, tend to be synonymous. As health educators for many years, we on several occasions have had to be explicit (to those outside the traditional health, physical education, recreation complex) as to where health education is located. Consider a typical conversation with an associate dean of engineering:

> Dean: "Health education? Oh, is that part of physical education? Ball games, right?"

> Author: "No, not part of physical education, but akin to it. No, we do not teach ball games."

And the conversation continues.

Separation of the fields has at times caused its own problems, such as the double major and the major/minor issues. Can a student be prepared to teach two subjects equally well after 4 years of undergraduate education? Will the student with a minor in physical education really be able to teach a full load of physical education classes, or even want to?

The disadvantages that have arisen from separating the disciplines are not insurmountable and appear to be outweighed by the advantages both professions have enjoyed since the separation. However, please keep in mind that there are many states that do not have a separate certification requirement for health educators.

Dual Preparation of School and Community Health Educators

The process of dual preparation probably came about as a result of a decline in the number of students in the school health education option, which could cause programs to be terminated. Furthermore, school health education preceded the option of community health education and had a more stable record. Dual preparation offers many advantages: enabling both types of health educators to better understand the functions of each domain, allowing the educator a wider choice of employment opportunities, and enabling the options to be housed within the same administrative structure.

However, the idea of dual preparation has caused some problems in recent years. The market for school health educators is limited, few student teaching and prestudent teaching positions are available, and other options have come into existence, such as worksite health care administration and environmental and safety education.

Increase in the Number of Professional Preparation Programs

There appears to be an excess of professional preparation programs. At last count (1983), the AAHE's directory indicated approximately 260 undergraduate programs within the United States. Although many of these programs have long histories, several were initiated during the 1970s. Are these programs viable? Are they producing too many health educators?

The preceding discussion attempted to review some of the basic issues concerning professional preparation of health educators. You are presently in a program, or have graduated from one, that has probably wrestled with these problems and issues. Students, professors, and administrators within a program must constantly evaluate and examine their goals, objectives, and methods so that the field of health education will continue to grow and expand in ways beneficial to society.

Summary

Professor Neutens correctly observes that health education lacks identity. This problem appears to have been a result of the emergence of health education from several disciplines, such as education, nursing, medicine, and the behavioral sciences. Although external forces have created a strong public interest in health education, this interest must be viewed as a mixed blessing. On the positive side it represents job opportunities, research funding, and the potential for recognition. On the negative side, because health education lacks professional status, the roles, functions, and responsibilities of people employed as health educators often fall outside of the academic preparation and work experience of the individual.

Health education has struggled with this identity crisis for decades. Journal articles, textbooks, conferences, and professional associations have addressed the issue, thereby serving as catalysts for self-examination. But in order for health education to achieve full professional status it will need to establish unity within the field. Until we can agree on what health education is, how we prepare individuals to become health educators, and how we evaluate their performance in that role, our progress will be stymied.

The self-identified health educator often has professional training in another field and professional commitment to that field. The Role Delineation Project has the potential to provide us, and others, with an understanding of the skills, knowledge, and responsibilities that individuals must have in order to perform the role of a health educator and that can be found only among those individuals who are trained as health educators. Ultimately this will engender a sense of cohesion and unification of purpose that can lead to the expression of a common philosophy.

The Role Delineation Project has encouraged voluntary credentialing. Credentialing is a mechanism by which the profession determines its own standards, prepares individuals to meet those standards, evaluates performance against established standards, and recommends individuals to employers as being competent. Accreditation sanctions those programs that adequately prepare individuals to meet a preestablished set of skills. This serves as an internal approval of the program and, by extension, of the person seeking licensure. Licensure or registration ensures that only people who are qualified (graduates of accredited programs) can be employed as health educators. Credentialing would appear to be the most appropriate route in establishing a professional niche for health education. If only licensed or registered people receive employment as health educators, the level of employer satisfaction should increase, and with it the public acceptance of health education as a true profession.

Questions for Review

1. This chapter indicates that health education is striving toward full professional status. What activities need to be completed in order for this status to be achieved?
2. Reconsider the important historical events presented in Chapter 1. To what end have they helped health education in its quest for professional recognition?
3. What obligations do individual members have with regard to the enhancement of the profession?
4. Most programs of professional preparation are fairly standard in their methods and curriculum. Are there creative techniques that could be used to prepare health educators? Can we borrow some techniques from other professions and use them in training health educators?
5. What can be done about the many people who have no formal training but nevertheless have the title of health educator?
6. Are there generic competencies of health educators that are required in all job settings? How would you evaluate yourself using the seven areas of responsibility identified in the chapter?
7. What problems are associated with implementing the procedures of accreditation, licensure, and certification?
8. In what ways should health educators be held accountable for their activities? What about students in programs of professional preparation?
9. What are the similarities and differences found in competencies identified by AAHPERD, ASHA, and SOPHE?

References

1. Burt, J.: Health Science in the professional preparation of health educators, School Health Review 2(4):22, 1971.
2. Slocum, H.M.: Teacher preparation in health education, School Health Review 2(1):8-10, 1971.
3. Governali, J., and Sechrist, W.: What's in a name? Health Education 9(9):31, 1978.
4. Hurster, M.: Critical issues in health education, Journal of School Health 47(1):42, 1977.
5. Grosshans, O.R.: Traditional outlooks for a new century, Health Education 11(2):18-19, 1980.
6. Green, L.W.: Impressions of an overviewer, Proceedings of The Workshop on Commonalities and Differences, Preparation and Practice of Community, Patient, and School Health Educators U.S. DHEW (HRA) Pub. No. 78-71, Washington, D.C., 1978, U.S. Government Printing Office.
7. Cleary, H.P.: Health education, the state-of-the-art, parameters of the profession, Proceedings of The Workshop on Commonalities and Differences, Preparation and Practice of Community, Patient and School Health Educators U.S. DHEW (HRA) Pub. No. 78-71, 1978.
8. Ware, B.G.: Directions for health education: new spokes in the wheel . . . or a new wheel, Health Education Monographs 4(3):247-253, 1976.
9. Hochbaum, G.M.: At the threshold of a new era, Health Education 7(4):2-4, 1976.
10. Bowman, R.A.: Changes in the activities, functions, and roles of public health educators, Health Education Monographs 4(3):226-246, 1976.
11. Simonds, S.K.: Health education today, issues and challenges, Journal of School Health 47(10):584-593, 1977.
12. Grosshans, O.R.: Traditional outlooks for a new century, Health Education 11(2):18-19, 1980.
13. Olsen, L.K.: Problems faced in developing a state constituent organization, J. School Health 51(3):168-170, 1981.
14. Toohey, J.V., and Shirreffs, J.H.: Future trends in health education, Health Education 11(2):15-18, 1980.

15. Taub, A.: Health education: a profession? Health Education **11**(2):26-27.
16. Moore, W.E.: The professions: roles and rules, New York, 1970, Russell Sage Foundation.
16a. Upton, L.A.: A study of secondary school counselor's perceptions of school counseling as a profession and their desires for the professionalization of school counseling, doctoral dissertation, Buffalo, 1970, State University of New York at Buffalo.
17. Elliot, P.: The sociology of the professions, New York, 1972, Herder & Herder.
18. Wilensky, H.L.: The professionalization of everyone, American Journal of Sociology **70**:371-80, 1964.
19. Sliepcevich, E.M.: Impressions of an overviewer, Proceedings of the Workshop on Commonalities and Differences, Preparation and Practice of Community, Patient, and School Health Educators, U.S. DHEW (HRA) Pub. No. 78-71, Washington, D.C., 1978, U.S. Government Printing Office.
20. Deeds, S.G.: SOPHE at the crossroads, SOPHE presidential address, Presented at the Twenty-ninth Annual Meeting of the Society of Public Health Educators, Los Angeles, November 3, 1979.
21. Howell, K.A.: Visions on the future of health education, Health Education **11**(2):24-25, 1980.
22. Zimmering, S., and McTernan, E.: The role of the clinical health educator, Health Education Monographs **4**(3):266-275, 1976.
23. U.S. Department of Health and Human Services, Public Health Service: Health education and credentialing: the role delineation project, Focal Points, Atlanta, July 1980.
24. Henderson, A.C., McIntosh, D.V., and Schaller, W.E.: Progress report of the role delineation project, J. School Health **51**:373-376, 1981.
25. AAHPER, School Health Division Task Force: Professional preparation in safety education and school health education, Washington, D.C., 1974, American Alliance for Health, Physical Education and Recreation.
26. American School Health Association Committee on Professional Preparation and College Health Education: Professional preparation of the health educator, Journal of School Health **46**:418-421, 1976.
27. Society of Public Health Educators Task Force on Professional Preparation and Practice of Health Education: Guidelines for the preparation and practice professional health educators, San Francisco, 1976, The Society.
28. Henderson, A.C., Project Director: Initial role delineation for health education: final report, U.S. DHHS (HRA) Pub. No. 232-78-0154, Washington, D.C., 1980, U.S. Government Printing Office.
29. Houston, R.W., and Howsam, R.B.: CBTE: the ayes of Texas, Phi Delta Kappan **55**(5):229-300, 1974.
30. Glass, G.V.: Standards and criteria, J. Educational Measurement **15**(4):237-261, 1978.
31. Pollock, M.B.: Speaking of competencies, Health Education **12**(1):9-13, 1981.
32. Rosner, B., and Kay, P.: Will the promise of C/PBTE be fulfilled? Phi Delta Kappan **55**(5):290-295, 1974.
33. Pigg, M.: National study of competency based health education programs, Health Education **7**(4):15-16, 1976.

Additional Readings

Andrew, B.J., and Hecht, J.T.: A preliminary investigation of two procedures for setting examination standard, Educational and Psychological Measurement **36**:45-50, 1976.

Bradley, C.E.: Health education: a planning resource for Wisconsin schools, Madison, 1977, Wisconsin State Department of Public Instruction.

Burns, R.W.: Behavioral objectives for competency based education. In BUrns, R.W., and Klingstedt, J.L.: Competency based education, Englewood Cliffs, N.J., 1973, Educational Technology Publications.

Crase, D.: Needed: comprehensive profiles of school health educators, J. School Health **51**(6):391-393, 1981.

Ebel, R.L.: Essentials of educational measurement, Englewood Cliffs, N.J., 1972, Prentice-Hall, Inc.

Fodor, J., and Dalis, G.: Health education: theory and practice, Philadelphia, 1983, Lea & Febiger.

Gonder, P.: The competency challenge: what schools are doing, Arlington, Va., 1978, National School Public Relations Association.

Hall, G.E., and Jones, H.L.: Competency-based education: a process for the improvement of education, Englewood Cliffs, N.J., 1976, Prentice-Hall, Inc.

Hamburg, M.: Credentialing: implications for school health education. In National Conference for Institutions Preparing Health Educators, DHHS Pub. No. 81-50171, Washington, D.C., 1981, U.S. Government Printing Office.

Henderson, A., Wolle, J., Cortese, P., and McIntosh, D.: The future of the health education profession: implications for preparation and practice, Public Health Reports **96**(6):555-559, 1981.

Henderson, A.C.: Development of the essential competencies of school and college health educators, Unpublished doctoral dissertation, Los Angeles, 1976, University of California at Los Angeles.

Johnson, C.E., and Shearron, G.F.: Specifying assumptions, goals, and objectives. In Andersen, D.W., Cooper, J.M., DeVault, M.V., and others, editors: Competency based teacher education, Berkeley, 1973, McCutchan Publishing Corp.

Linn, R.L.: Demands, cautions, and suggestions for setting standards, J. Educational Measurement **15**(4):301-308, 1978.

Maxwell, D.W.: PBTE: a case of the emperor's new clothes, Phi Delta Kappan, **55**(5):306-311, 1974.

Meskauskas, J.A., and Webster, G.W.: The American board of internal medicine recertification examination process and results, Ann. of Intern. Med. **82**:577-581, 1975.

Nedelsky, L.: Absolute grading standards for objective tests, Educational Psychological Measurement **14**:3-19, 1954.

Popham, W.J.: As always, provocative, J. Educational Measurement **15**(4):297-300, 1978.

Trivett, D.A.: Competency programs in higher education, ERIC/Higher Education Research Report No. 7, Washington, D.C., 1975, ERIC.

Watche, G.A.: Educational accountability: the issue of competency based education, Madison, Wisc., 1977, Wisconsin State Legislative Reference Bulletin.

Weller, R.B.: Identification and evaluation of knowledge competencies in health education, Unpublished doctoral dissertation, Urbana, 1977, University of Illinois at Urbana-Champaign.

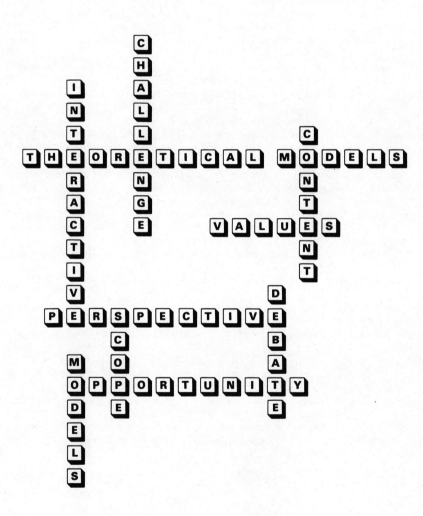

5 Health Education Issues

Introduction

Issues represent differences of opinion of near equal merit; therefore satisfactory justification may be provided for a variety of positions on a particular issue. In discussing five major issues and several subissues, Dr. Creswell provides information without leading the reader to adopt one position or another. Instead, the relative merits of each issue are presented for consideration. Quotations from professional journals and reports of commissions, committees, task forces, and agencies support the legitimacy of the opposing sides.

The major challenges the profession must address are the following:
1. The need to specify the goals and purposes of health education
2. The need to establish theories and guiding principles
3. The need to clarify content and methodology
4. The need to articulate professional preparation with the realities of the work place
5. The need to assess the status of health education

Dr. Creswell covers the issues in chronologic order. These issues however, are interrelated; decisions that affect any one of them will therefore affect the remaining four. As a practical matter each issue must be resolved before health education can make significant strides toward unification and full professional status. The issues are the very heart of what we are and where we are going as professionals. You are encouraged to consider the definition of health education; to judge whether health education is more beneficial when presented as a categoric area of interest or as a comprehensive field of study; to decide whether health education is a process that disseminates information or whether interactive models of instruction should be endorsed as a way of facilitating healthful behavior; and to determine whether professional preparation should produce specialists or generalists.

The central issue that seems to be present throughout the chapter is the need to establish a professional identity, an issue also discussed in Chapter 4. Throughout the history of our country health education has been endorsed by educational leaders and by governmental bodies. A review of these endorsements would lead one to believe that health instruction is firmly entrenched in the school curriculum. Unfortunately, health education suffers as a low-priority area of instruction; it receives inadequate funding and is often taught by teachers who are not fully prepared as health educators. In order for this situation to change the general public will need to better understand our profession and certainly will need to have more realistic expectations of what we can and cannot accomplish. Therefore we shall need to specify the goals and purposes of health education, to establish theories and guiding principles, to clarify content and methodology, and to articulate professional preparation with the realities of the work place.

According to the dictionary, an *issue* is a matter or question, such as a political question, that is disputed by contending parties. Characteristically an issue is of considerable importance either to the general public, as in the case of political issues, or to a specific group, as in matters of professional issues. The controversy over an issue, and the implications arising from the decision reached can have a profound effect on the individuals involved.

Any growing and dynamic profession committed to public service is bound to be confronted with issues of critical importance. Questions over public service policy, the goals of research, or the standards for professional training are likely to stir much discussion and debate.

The individual professional member should feel both an obligation and an opportunity to share in the deliberations and in the decision making—a prescription for continued growth of both the individual and the profession. The health and vitality of any profession are dependent on this participation. For health education, or any other field, the results of this process ultimately determine the nature and scope of programs, the type of services to be rendered, the requisite skills and technical knowledge that will be important to the practitioner, and the code of ethics that will govern the actions of the membership. Ultimately, the decisions that prevail may well determine whether the profession achieves a place in the mainstream of society or moves in a direction of isolation and eventual extinction.

Health education is a relatively new and emerging field. The outline of its form and character are still not clear. Is it a profession per se or is it, as a national task force (1976) has stated, not a single discipline but rather a field of interest that draws on the knowledge of biomedical, biostatistical, and behavioral sciences as well as various administrative, planning, and research skills?

Surely no one can deny the fact that there is much vitality and activity reflected in the number and variety of health education programs now being offered. These include programs for hospitals, clinics, schools, industries, voluntary and commercial agencies, and the mass communication media. The health education issues are further complicated by the problem of identifying those individuals responsible for the programs. The categories of those actively working to achieve health education goals continue to grow with the growing interest in disease prevention and health promotion. Included at this time are nurses, dentists, anthropologists, educators, economists, psychologists, sociologists, social workers, and political scientists, to say nothing of practitioners in the newer areas of specialization such as health psychology, behavioral health, and behavioral medicine.

Examining the Issues

It is important to recognize at the outset that an issue represents a difference of opinion or disagreement supported by arguments of equal or near equal merit. Persons of reputation and recognized authority may be aligned on either side of the question. Therefore it is important to proceed on the assumption that strong justification may exist for adopting any of the positions being represented in the argument or controversy. Moreover, mature and intelligent handling of a controversial issue requires that the nature or type of problem must first be carefully defined. For example, is the question a philosophic, political, or scientific one? Is it an issue containing strong moral overtones? In most instances, benefit may be gained from rigorous debate and objective discussion, but it must be recognized that debating questions that in some way relate to religious dogma may simply complicate matters and serve no useful purpose. The long-standing controversy over abortion is a case in point.

Several areas have been identified for issue analysis and discussion, based on the experience of professional practice and the information obtained from the literature of health education. Some of these issues have already been the subject of much debate and discussion, while others have yet to satisfy the criteria of a genuine issue and remain on the periphery of professional interest. However, the topics presented here are considered to be of increasing importance to the field; actions growing out of these deliberations will have a major impact on the future of health education. What are some of the dilemmas facing health education?

Selected for further analysis and discussion are questions or issues relating to (1) the goals or purposes of health education, (2) the theories or guiding principles for health education, (3) the content and method of health education, (4) the nature of professional preparation or training needed by the health educator, and finally (5) an assessment of the status of health education.

Goals or Purposes

One of the problems affecting the health education field is the apparent disagreement on the purposes of health education. The Task Force Report on Consumer Health Education[1] raised a number of questions and issues about the goals and the objectives of health education as well as the role it is to play. The following statements offer varying definitions of health education:

1. A learning experience for the purpose of developing the individual's health knowledge, attitudes, and practices
2. A means of guiding individuals and groups toward healthful behavior
3. The bridge between health knowledge and health practice

4. An integral part of health care, including the improvement of health care and the use of health services

In addition to these differing definitions, a number of questions have been raised about the function and purpose of health education, such as the following:

1. Is health education a part of health care or is it a separate activity?
2. Is health education the same as health promotion? If not, what is the distinction?
3. How should health education be conducted? Is it primarily a series of structured learning experiences or is it any activity or experience that guides individuals or groups toward more healthful actions?
4. What does health education include? Are knowledge, attitudes, and practice the essential bases or are information and policies also included?

These questions develop from the general confusion or lack of agreement over what the goals or purposes of health education should be. This difference of opinion is illustrated by the report of the President's Committee on Health Education.[2] The committee conducted a series of public hearings throughout the nation for the purpose of clarifying the role of health education. It became apparent that two approaches were being advocated by those offering testimony before the committee. One group thought that the goal of health education was to achieve the optimum level of health—a concept of health similar to that embraced by the World Health Organization. The other group favored a problem- or disease-oriented approach aimed at preventing diseases or managing specific conditions. Recent legislation that created the U.S. Office of Disease Prevention and Health Promotion, and recent publications of the U.S. Public Health Service (PHS) issued under a similar title, indicates that the federal government is attempting to circumvent this controversy by including both concepts, positive health and disease prevention, in its concept of the goal of health education.

The fact that health education had its origins in two fields, health and education, may explain this difference in orientation or philosophy. The field of health education has long been dominated by the influence of medicine, with its focus on the treatment and control of disease. The other major influence on the field is education, focusing on the nurturing of the individual's growth and development, or health promotion.

Objectives: School Perspective

How are the goals of health education selected or defined? School programs, responsible for many different curricula and program specialties, maintain an on-going process of selecting or defining goals. In order to be assured that a particular school program's goals are consistent with those of the larger mission or purpose of the educational enterprise, a careful survey of the educational literature pertaining to the fundamental purpose of schooling is first conducted. Sources that may be consulted when writing or selecting program goals include the following:

1. State and federal legislation (especially that which is mandatory)
2. Literature pertaining to local and national concerns
3. Goals of other programs, especially those considered to be exemplary
4. Parental concerns, requests, and special study reports on program needs

In general terms, the purposes or goals of education focus on the development of cognitive abilities and positive habits of the individual. In American society, schools play a major role in helping to establish an ideal democratic society in which respect, justice, and fair play provide firsthand experiences with ethical values. As a result, a general goal of education is the opportunity to learn the responsibilities of adulthood and citizenship.[3] Although these general goals of education may not be specifically identified as health goals, health education is nevertheless an essential component of the achievement of such aims.

Other goals of education stress personal, intellectual, creative, social, moral, emotional, and physical development. Here the relationship to health education is more obvious. Such general concepts as personal development, including a social consciousness, convey clear implications for health education.[4]

Undoubtedly one of the most important and influential statements affecting the development of health education in American schools was the 1918 statement issued by the NEA Commission on the Reorganization of Secondary Education, *The Cardinal Principles of Education*. These principles were intended to serve as the general goals of all secondary schools and are frequently cited in the health education literature. The following areas are included:

1. Health
2. Command of fundamental processes
3. Worthy home membership
4. Vocation
5. Citizenship
6. Worthy use of leisure
7. Ethical character

This statement has been of singular importance because of its influence on and widespread recognition by educational leaders. Because of its historical significance, the NEA appointed a special commission to reexamine and restate the seven cardinal principles. The results were issued as a part of the nation's bicentennial celebration in 1976. Members of the commission were among the nation's most prominent leaders, representing such fields as business, industry, and labor, as well as the professional and scientific fields. The commission reaffirmed the validity of the cardinal principles and their value as goals for all secondary schools. However, in their review of the original statements, the commission restated and reinterpreted each of the goals in order to make them more relevant to the needs of today's society. For example, the commission's interpretation of the goal of health was as follows: "The scope and importance of health as an educational objective has become even more important than it was in 1918."[5] Accordingly, the commission called for greater emphasis to be placed on "the need for healthy interpersonal and intellectual attitudes." The commission encouraged open discussion of unhealthy life-styles and of environmental conditions in the

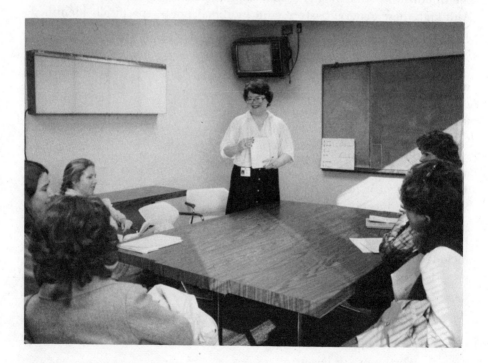

Fig. 5-1. Adult education workshop. (Photograph by Lyn Lawrance.)

United States. The commission also called attention to the importance of a world view of health and the worldwide challenge such a view entails. They supported a broad concept of health, including total mental, physical, and emotional health, for each individual. The commission called for support of the efforts to improve drug education and encouraged frank discussions of family living. This aspect of education, the commission argued, is necessary if youth of today are to be guided toward acceptance of responsible citizenship in their role as tomorrow's leaders.

Although it is evident that the goals of education have included health and health education as an important purpose of the schools, the vagueness or generality of the goals make them difficult to achieve. As Ralph Tyler pointed out during the progressive education movement of the 1930s, the goals of education were so vague that something had to be done in order to clarify the school's role. Tyler ushered in what has since been popularized by Robert Mager as the behavioral objective movement.

Others hold that health education has remained too theoretical and perhaps too impractical. For example, Green[6] contends that the practice of health education has remained ideologic, with many practitioners holding beliefs about the correct way to practice health education that are based more on the philosophy and ideology of the institution in which they work or were trained than on a careful assessment of educational needs.

A review of statements drawn from several school health education developments illustrates the range of these goals. The proposed rules and regulations of the Health Education Act of 1978 (PL 96-541) state that a comprehensive school health education program should provide learning experiences based on the best available scientific information to promote the understanding, attitudes, behavioral skills, and practices that prepare and motivate elementary and secondary students to (1) prevent illness, disease, and injury and (2) enhance the physical and mental health of themselves, their families, and their communities.

The major goal of this school health education legislation is the use of learning experiences based on scientifically valid information to achieve student health education outcomes.

Examination of the School Health Curriculum Project,[7] one of the most widely adopted programs in the United States, reveals the emphasis that is given to cognitive or knowledge objectives, although the major goal statement is couched in attitudinal and behavioral terms:

> . . . to help the child realize that the body is each person's greatest natural resource in life, that is is exquisitely beautiful and complex in its structure and functions, that it is influenced by one's own choices made throughout life.[7]

Moreover, it is the project developer's point of view that

> by knowing about oneself, the individual is therefore much more likely to care about his/her self; and that this attitude of caring for oneself will continue throughout life. And finally, that the individual comes to believe that actions to preserve one's personal health are worth doing.[7]

Another example is the nationwide School Health Education Study[8] developed during the 1960s and 1970s. This program advocated a conceptual approach to curriculum design and was one of the most comprehensive and detailed representations of the school health education curriculum ever developed. Although the long-range goals of this program recognized the three major domains of knowledge, attitude, and actions or behavior, the curriculum is organized around a conceptual structure that reflects the cognitive or knowledge basis.

Objectives selected from the area of food and nutrition illustrate the importance of the cognitive area and also show how attitudinal and behavioral objectives are integrated into this curriculum. Two objectives from the senior high school level illustrate these points:

1. The student analyzes various influences that affect one's diet.
2. The student *applies* criteria for selecting foods and planning meals that provide for a balanced diet.[8]

In the first statement the behavior of analysis, a cognitive skill, leads the student into an awareness of his or her own emotions and feelings about foods as well as an appreciation for the role of cultural values in dietary choices—the affective or attitudinal influence. In the second statement the verb *applies* calls for sophisticated student understanding and knowledge skills of evaluation that lead the student into behavior such as selecting and purchasing of foods to be included in the diet.

Objectives: Community Health and Health Care Perspective

Traditionally, health education has been characterized by its threefold objectives of health: knowledge, attitudes, and behavior. However, the degree to which these objectives are emphasized is to a large extent determined by the particular point of view held regarding the purpose of health education and the theory of learning and behavior change.

Two recent publications, the surgeon general's report entitled *Healthy People*[9] and its companion publication entitled *Disease Prevention and Health Promotion: Objectives for the Nation,* have both placed great emphasis on the role of education in developing health-promoting and disease-preventing behavior. It is apparent that health education is expected to play a key role in helping the nation to achieve its health goals. Perhaps this is best illustrated by the following statement from *Healthy People*[9]:

> Personal habits play critical roles in the development of many serious diseases and in injuries from violence and automobile accidents.
> Many of today's most pressing health problems are related to excesses—of smoking, drinking, faulty nutrition, over-use of medications, fast driving and the relentless pressure to achieve.
> In fact, of the ten leading causes of death in the United States, at least seven could be substantially reduced if persons at risk improved just five habits; diet, smoking, lack of exercise, alcohol abuse and use of antihypertensive medication.

Moreover, analysis of the various health problems posing serious threats to the different age groups in American society, infants, children, adolescents, and adults, unmistakably calls for changes in behavior or life-style. It is clear that health education programs committed to reducing many of these problems are attracting widespread support. The childhood accident problem is a case in point. With some 10,000 children below the age of 14 years killed annually, the need for remediation of this problem can hardly be questioned. The accident problem, it is argued, is in large part a result of environmental and social factors. As such it is not amenable to medical care or to methods of medical intervention.

This same point of view is expressed in the late Governor Nelson E. Rockefeller's (New (York) report on social problems and health and hospital services and costs: "Prevention and sound maintenance are as much an individual responsibility as they are a medical responsibility."[10]

Is health education a part of health care? At least a partial answer to this question is provided in the *Discursive Dictionary of Health Care*,[11] which was prepared for the use of the Subcommittee on Health and Environment of the United States Congress. The following statement has been excerpted from this report's definition of preventive medicine:

> It is now operatively assumed that most if not all problems are preventable at some stage of their development. Preventive medicine is also concerned with general preventive measures aimed at improving the healthfulness of our environment and our relations with it through such things as avoidance of hazardous substances, modified diet and family planning. In particular, the promotion of health through altering behavior, especially by health education, is gaining prominence as a component of preventive care.

Returning to the question of What should be the objectives of health education? the importance of disease prevention and the role of education in this regard has attracted increasing support. As Ogden[12] has observed:

> The sudden emergency of health education as a high priority item is based more on a dissatisfaction with the high costs of therapeutic medicine and the attractiveness of the idea of prevention than it is on any solid evidence that health education can produce results.

Nevertheless, there has been an unmistakable trend toward greater public awareness and interest in health-promoting activities. This interest is reflected in a variety of ways that range from individual activities such as jogging and recreational pursuits to organized group efforts to promote health through wellness centers and holistic health care programs.

During the 1970s increased interest in health education was evidenced within government at the national level through legislation, organizational development, and public policy statements. An amendment to the Public Health Service Act, Title XVII, created a new mechanism within government, the Office of Health Information and Health Promotion, which was devoted specifically to these activities. These developments are also reflected in the 1981 change in the title of the U.S. Bureau of Health Education to that of the U.S. Center for Health Promotion and Education. Additionally, two reports, the surgeon general's *A Forward Plan for Health,* and the National Academy of Sciences statement, *Perspective on Health Promotion and Disease Prevention in the United States,* are examples of this interest in disease prevention and health promotion. Whether this is a genuine change in public attitude and public policy in the United States is unclear at this time.

In analyzing the role of school health education, many medical and public health leaders recognize that certain circumstances and constraints placed on the school limit what can be accomplished and restrict the extent of the schools' contribution to the achievement of the nation's health goals. At the same time, however, society's expectations of the schools' role are very high indeed, as expressed in the APHA policy statement on school health:

> The school, as a social structure, provides an educational setting in which the total health of the child during the impressionable years is of priority concern. No other community setting even approximates the magnitude of the grades K-12 school educational enterprise and the millions of children enrolled.[13]

Guiding Theories

Perhaps part of the difficulty in determining goals for health education stems from the differences that exist in the philosophy of the foundational disciplines of health and education and the way in which these two fields have become manifest in professional practice. The field of health education may be suffering from a kind of philosophic schizophrenia that precludes the acceptance of the theoretical framework that is necessary for the development of a clear delineation of purpose and goals.

Such a difference seems to have been recognized by the delegates at

the Role Delineation Conference, held for the purpose of developing strategies for promoting health for school-aged children and youth. They expressed the following concern:

> The difference in opinions between health and education professionals should be ac-
> knowledged. While the mission of the education professions is to help prepare children
> and youth for life decisions through education, the mission of the health profession is
> preventing illness and disability through environmental and life-style modification and in
> the early identification, referral and effective follow-up care for disease. The disagreements
> over program priorities caused by these different missions must be recognized and com-
> promises worked out.[14]

Still others have observed that health education, unlike most fields, has
been and remains very much practice oriented, focusing on problems and
applications without having a well-developed theory. Moreover, the lack of
theory has led to still more problems, including the failure to follow sound
scientific procedures. This condition, together with the inherent difficulty
of measuring long-term outcomes in health education, has seriously under-
mined the credibility of the field in the eyes of the biomedical and behavioral
sciences communities.[15]

Theory of Learning and Behavior Change Process

Although there may be no formal commitment to a particular theory,
characteristic practices of the profession seem to point to certain unstated
assumptions about the theory of learning and the behavior change process.
Rabinowitz[16] points out that health education programs have for years been
dominated by what he calls a pedagogic model that has strongly stereotyped
a teacher-pupil relationship that is conceived as a unilateral flow of information in which the teacher is the dispenser and the child is the recipient.
Instead, he would argue, a true teaching-learning situation is one in which
there is a reciprocal effect or influence exchange taking place between the
teacher and the student.

Examination of health programs reveals that the knowledge-attitude-
behavior consistency model is widely used in the field. Undoubtedly, the
early work of Hochbaum, Rosenstock, and others in developing the health
belief model, which draws heavily on communication theory, as well as the
research of Katz and Lazarsfeld[16] in diffusion theory, have had a major
influence on the field. As Wallack[17] has observed, common sense tells us that
if we want a change in behavior, a model that focuses on increasing knowledge or changing attitudes reflects a real world relationship—namely, a
change of attitude will ultimately lead to a change in behavior. Hence, an
assumption that is widely used by program developers conducting health
education through the mass communication media tholds that "an increase

in knowledge will lead to a change in attitude and will result in a change in behavior."[17]

If such an assumption is widely held by communication specialists, is it not also a viable theory for the practicing health educator? Although lacking in the technical skills and the usual resources available in the field of mass communication, the health educator does have other advantages, such as additional opportunities and time to clarify and to reinforce the health message through close personal contact with the student or target audience. In fact, experience as well as research has often demonstrated the superiority of the person-to-person communication over that of impersonal mass media methods.

Despite the widespread acceptance of the attitude-behavior consistency model, there is also a general awareness of the fact that people who apparently know frequently fail to act in accordance with their knowledge. In fact, among the examples most often cited are health professionals whose actions belie their teachings, such as the overweight nutritionist, the physician who smokes, or the nonexercising health educator. This lack of consistency between knowledge, attitude, and behavior has been the subject of much research.

Many educators believe that interest and attitudes are a natural outgrowth of increasing information. If this is the case, then it would seem that major emphasis should be placed on developing information and knowledge; the attitude development will then take care of itself. However, other educators[18] have argued that it is the particular learning experience that determines the relationship between knowledge and attitude. Thus one set of learning experiences may produce a high level of knowledge achievement and at the same time cause a disinterest in or a distaste for the subject. In another situation both high-level knowledge and interest development may occur simultaneously. Finally, the experience may result in little knowledge gain but stimulate an interest in or liking for the subject.

McGuire[19] suggested that in addition to the

commonsense view of attitude change leading to behavior change, at least three other relationships exist: attitude change following behavior change, attitude change and behavior change exhibiting a lack of relationship, and attitude and action changes as alternative responses.

Two examples show how the results from research appear to offer support for different aspects of this issue. First, a study conducted by LaPiere[20] was designed to test the relationship between what people say and what they actually do. In this study the requests for hotel accommodations by a Chinese couple traveling in the United States were compared to the responses given by the same proprietors in a follow-up survey 6 months later. In actuality the Chinese couple were refused accommodations only once. However, in responding to the survey question "Would you provide hotel accommodations for a Chinese couple?" over 90% of the proprietors said no. In this instance there was a clear lack of consistency between what people said and what they did.

On the other hand, Festinger's[21] theory of cognitive dissonance offers support for a consistent relationship between the individual's cognition (knowing) and behavior (doing). This relationship was investigated in a number of studies involving persons who believed that sodium fluoride in drinking water would produce toxic effects if ingested. When persons holding such beliefs were confronted with having to drink water from fluoridated water supplies, they were faced with a cognitive dissonance or a conflict between what they believed and how they behaved. In order to resolve the dissonance or conflict the subjects tended either to change their beliefs about the toxic effects or to refuse to drink the water, in either case demonstrating the influence of knowledge on behavior and the importance of restoring a consistent relationship between the two.

Nevertheless, health education is currently under fire because of what critics believe to be too heavy an emphasis on information. They argue that much of what is called health education is nothing more than information dissemination. According to these critics, this approach is based on an overly simplistic view of the health behavior change process. Other critics state that these health messages have seldom been pretested to determine their relevance for the intended audience, hence the message may be too technical to be understood by the recipient. These critics state that even when the health communication was received and apparently understood, the complexity of the resulting behavior suggests that cognitive changes may have little or no effect on the individual's health attitudes and behavior.

Effect of Communication

Despite the criticisms, other authorities in the field contend that effective communication can stimulate new thoughts and feelings that in turn create the conditions that bring about the desired behavior. Hochbaum[22] and Rosenstock,[23] in expanding on the earlier concepts of communication theory, have stressed that motivation is the key to the application of health information. In this regard they have identified three factors in order to explain health behavior:

1. A readiness to act that is determined by the individual's perceived susceptibility to and the perceived severity of a given condition,
2. The individual's perception of the benefits to be gained in comparison to the perceived barriers to the health behavior

3. A cue mechanism, which is needed to bring about the behavior change

The success of the Stanford Heart Disease Prevention Program research[24] in achieving effective health results through the use of mass communication media has stimulated a renewed interest in communication theory among health education professionals. In a three-community study, two experimental methods were tested: (1) mass communication media alone and (2) mass communication media plus intensive instruction for individuals with a high risk of cardiovascular disease. The third community served as a control. Those persons who received both mass communication media and intensive individual instruction showed the greatest change, with a 30% reduction in their risk of cardiovascular disease. Those individuals who received only the mass communication media instruction showed reduced risks ranging from 8% to 10% to more than 20%.

However, as Bauer[25] has pointed out, the approaches used in this study were quite different from those of the usual public information campaigns. The media materials used in the Stanford program were designed to teach behavior skills as well as to present informational and motivational messages. In fact, Maccoby and Farquhar[26] have stated that although they were interested in informing and motivating people to do something about their cardiovascular risk factors, in the case of smoking, most persons with whom they were working were already informed of the dangers to their health. In fact the smokers by and large wanted to stop. What they needed was not an exhortation to quit but rather to "learn the skill of not smoking."

Cohen and Cohen[27] have argued that the significant changes achieved in the Stanford Heart Disease Prevention Program are in part a function of the large numbers. They also assert that the reduction in cigarette smoking was so small that it is not likely to have any meaningful effect on the morbidity or mortality caused by smoking. Leventhal[28] has also criticized the Stanford study on the basis of research design and statistical analysis rather than the theoretical formulations on which this study was based. One contention is that the special biomedical measures employed, rather than the educational interventions, may have influenced the changes. Perhaps these effects, rather than the educational intervention, caused the difference between the experimental and control groups. Also, because the intensive-instruction groups were given information about their personal risk factors, this knowledge may have contributed to their greater risk reduction scores and higher knowledge scores.

Leventhal[28] and others also cited weaknesses in the Stanford study's design, which failed to provide the control necessary to evaluate the effects of the intensive instruction only, without the added effect of mass communication media. Because the mass media–only group showed a change in knowledge with no apparent effect on smoking behavior, interpretation of study results, according to these reviewers, has been seriously weakened.

Nevertheless, results of the Stanford study have created a new public awareness as well as widespread interest in health education. Moreover, this

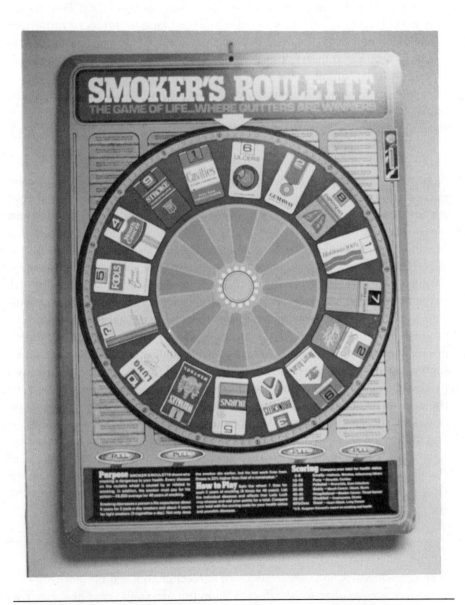

Fig. 5-2. Educational workshop to stop smoking. (Photograph by Lyn Lawrance.)

project has helped to focus attention on a number of issues that are of importance to the future of health education. For example, information gained from this study points to a more significant role for mass communication media in educating the public about health. The long-running controversy over the relationship between knowledge, attitudes, and health behavior has been further enhanced by the results of this study. Despite the general failure of mass communication media alone to influence important behavior change, the Stanford researchers remain strongly committed to the proposition that mass communication media, when "appropriately used, can successfully influence behavior."[29]

Moreover, analysis of the educational intervention employed in the Stanford study highlights the issue of learning theory. For example, the strategies employed in the various methods demonstrate an important blending and unique application of the principal learning theories characteristic of the associational or behavioral and cognitive traditions. The interpretation of learning, as revealed in Bandura's social learning theory,[30] goes beyond the narrowly defined associations between stimulus and response and stresses the importance of the social environment. For example, through the social environment a vicarious reinforcement is provided, such as observing a role model in order to learn self-control or techniques of self-management.

Health educators as a group have tended to reject behavior modification methods on the grounds that its failure to recognize the subjective nature of the individual is a serious weakness. Such elements as feelings, aspirations, values, and attitudes are important determinants of health behavior. The most serious objection to behavior modification centers on its seemingly insensitive and mechanistic methods of controlling human behavior by manipulating the environment in order to reward and reinforce the desired behavior. This controlling or manipulating of human behavior has placed the behaviorist in an undesirable and unethical position. However, the demonstrated success of behaviorists in reducing risks and undesirable behaviors and in developing behaviors essential to healthier life-styles has caused many health educators to reassess this position. In particular, the work of Bandura[30] and the social learning theory seem much more attractive to health educators than when presented earlier. This is discussed in more detail in the Editorial remarks at the end of this chapter.

Content and Method

The probelms arising from selection of subject matter and methodology are of course not peculiar to health education but affect all areas of the curriculum. However, health education, a comparatively new field, does suffer from some special problems. The study and practice of medicine has a long history and tradition, but this is not the case with the study of health. It is not as well defined as medicine and other traditional fields such as mathematics, history, or the physical sciences. There is a wide difference of opinion concerning the content of the health education curriculum. In addition, there is the more fundamental controversy over whether health education should even be included in the school program. Today's curriculum developed from the experience and research of the past. It is interesting, as well as instructive, to review nineteenth-century education and examine what the leaders of that time said about the purposes of schooling in America. According to Kliebard,[31] at the turn of the century four different interest groups exercised a major influence on the school curriculum. First were the humanists, who thought that curricula should be constructed around the finest resources of western culture. This group saw their task as a reinterpretation of western culture and preservation of those traditions and values. One of the leaders of this group, William T. Harris, contended that this cultural heritage could best be preserved by studying those courses that he called the "windows of the soul": art, mathematics, geography, and history. Education scholars thought that Harris was influenced by the earlier ideas of Johann F. Herbart, a German philosopher and psychologist, who contended that the major purpose of education was the development of social and moral character. According to Herbart, this could best be done through the study of history and literature.[32]

Other groups having a major effect on the curriculum included the social efficiency reformers, the child study movement, and the social meliorists. The emphasis of the social efficiency group was on the development of a smoothly running society, which according to their views could be achieved by eliminating waste and by applying the techniques of business and industry to education.

The influence of the child study and social meliorist groups helped to bring health education into the schools. In fact, the child study group helped to establish many of the early child health programs in America. The work of this group led to the creation of the American Child Health Association, which played an important role in establishing the field of health education.

The influence of these groups on the school became evident in the early 1900s. These leaders believed that schools should play an important role in promoting the health and well-being of individuals and communities. The child study group contended that the most appropriate curriculum should be determined by a scientific study of the various growth and developmental stages of childhood and adolescence. The social meliorists viewed education as the remedy for social and political evils. According to their view, a new generation of children should be educated and equipped to handle or solve such social problems.

Problems of Interpretation

As previously stated, statements of definition have contributed to variations in perception and to disagreement over the nature of health education programs. For example, in the early development of health instruction (or what was then called hygiene instruction) great emphasis was placed on memorizing and reciting the anatomic names of body parts. Students were expected to know the names and number of bones and muscles in the body. This emphasis changed when educators and the public realized that knowledge of anatomy was not necessarily equated with the achievement of good health.

The program then broadened to include, in addition to anatomy (structure), the study of function (anatomy and physiology). In addition to learning all the anatomic terms, students were expected to know the physiologic processes. Hygiene courses placed heavy emphasis on technical and factual material but fell into disrepute because of the emphasis on the memorization of technical and factual material that seemed to have little relevance to the needs and interests of students. As a reaction to this overemphasis on facts, the pendulum of hygiene instruction swung back to a more functional approach: the rules of health. These rules of health behavior were developed for all aspects of life, including a prescribed set of practices for grooming, bathing, and diet, and rules for rest, sleep, exercise, and elimination. In order to attain good health, the student was required to learn the rules for living instead of memorizing facts about the body.

Comprehensive versus Categoric Approach

During the period of the curriculum reform movement in the 1960s, leaders in health education sought to develop a comprehensive approach to the teaching of health education. The guiding theory behind this method held that the study of health could be organized into a conceptual structure, that in turn could be presented as a curriculum plan to be taught in an articulated sequence of learning experiences, beginning in the elementary school and continuing through high school. The goal of this approach was the development of a health-educated citizenry.

As expressed in PL 95-561, the Health Education Act of 1978, the comprehensive school health program provides learning experiences based on the best available scientific information in an effort to promote the understanding, attitudes, behavioral skills, and practices of students with respect to their health. The principal long-range goals of the program are to prepare and to motivate elementary and secondary school students to (1) prevent illness, disease, and injury and (2) enhance the physical and mental health of individuals, their families, and their communities.

The act identifies some 21 different health topics that are to be organized into a progressive sequence of activities taught through the elementary and secondary school years. A number of states, including California, Florida, Illinois, Michigan, and New York, have adopted the comprehensive health education program approach.

Proponents of the comprehensive approach contend that health-promoting principles and theories of disease causation can be generalized and that such principles may be transferred and applied by the learner to all conditions and circumstances of health and disease. According to this view, health is a quality of life involving a dynamic interaction and interdependence among the different aspects of health. These include the physical, mental-emotional, social, and spiritual dimensions of health. Thus it is argued that if the individual is to be truly healthy, health must be understood in its totality.[8]

This theory holds that approaching health education from a categoric disease perspective is both limiting and artificial. Teaching about health by focusing on health problems is a negative orientation that falls far short of the goal of health education. Moreover, taking a disease or health problem approach is inefficient because the emphasis is placed on the disease manifestation rather than on the more positive and productive approaches of disease prevention and health promotion. Further, it is argued that there is not enough time in the curriculum for health education if every health problem must be covered. Instruction can be generalized from these experiences. This approach tends to focus on correcting the cause of the problem rather than the effect and is analogous to someone trying to get rid of water on the floor by mopping instead of turning off the faucet. Finally, a categoric disease approach is poor pedagogy. Teaching about specific diseases, apart from the general study of health and disease, is like teaching the concepts of multiplication apart from the context of mathematics.

Perhaps Green's[6] analysis, *The Cycle of Poverty*, helps to explain, at least in part, why the comprehensive program has not been successful. According to this analysis, the cycle begins with (1) inadequate support and is further complicated by (2) objectives that are diffuse, which in turn lead to (3) programs, methods, and procedures that are also diffuse and lacking focus. As a consequence, the program produces (4) little or no positive effects. This chain of events completes the cycle, resulting in a kind of self-fulfilling prophecy that began with a lack of commitment and ended with a verification of the program's ineffectiveness, which justifies the lack of support in the first place.

There are many critics of the categoric approach; according to them it is health education by crisis. Such programs are usually launched with little planning and often without adequate resources or support. Typically, the program wafts back and forth between each new development or issue, vacillating from one crisis to the next, with health education being forced to draw its support from whatever problem has temporarily captured the public's interest. For example, in the 1960s the smoking problem was a primary concern of the public, followed by the drug abuse crisis of the 1970s, the problem of teenage pregnancy, the venereal disease problem, and the immunization problem. This means a constant shifting of priorities as well as program activity. Programs therefore lack the stability essential to long-range planning and the systematic progress necessary for achieving long-term goals.

However, with respect to the comprehensive program, critics argue that it is too general and too vague to be meaningful or to communicate effectively. Instead, they argue for a specific problem approach because it does communicate to people and it takes advantage of their natural interest and motivation to solve problems. In support of this approach they point to the many voluntary and governmental organizations that deal successfully with categoric problems. Further, it is argued that organizing health education around a problem approach need not fall into the trap of overemphasis on the disease entity to the exclusion of the health concerns. Instead, this approach can also develop the students' understanding of general principles of disease prevention and health promotion that are applicable to all aspects of life. Also, directing the health education effort to the most important health problems for a particular age group offers the advantage of concentrating limited resources where the need is greatest and where the greatest benefits may be achieved.

Finally, they argue that the failure of states to implement effective comprehensive school health education programs, even when such programs have carried the force of mandatory legislation, indicates the weaknesses and impracticality of this approach. Comprehensive programs represent a major undertaking and commitment on the part of the school. In an era of limited budgets, state and local school systems lack the resources to implement a program of such magnitude.

On the other hand, several voluntary, commercial, and governmental agencies have developed a number of excellent curriculum modules around

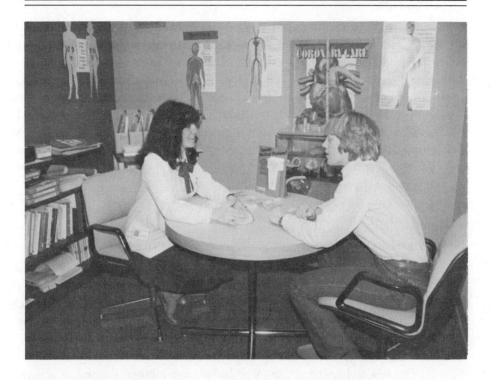

Fig. 5-3. Adult counseling sessions for breast self-examination. Carle Wellness Center, Urbana, Illinois. (Photograph by Lyn Lawrance.)

specific or categoric problems. Because there are high-quality materials already available, the school can implement specific health topic programs at relatively low cost. The fact that such programs are targeted for a specific problem often means that they are more likely to be undertaken by a school. Visibility of a categoric problem approach also may attract support from a community agency whose goals are closely related to those of the school. Instead of languishing on the shelf of the curriculum writer, these categoric programs have shown steady and consistent growth. In particular, those health education curricula relating to cardiovascular disease, cancer, and personal risk behaviors such as smoking, diet, and alcohol use are being implemented in a growing number of schools.

Teaching Methods

The emphasis on information dissemination is evident from past public health education and school health instruction efforts. This approach is based on the assumed validity of the traditional communication knowledge, attitude, and behavior model and holds that the public (or students) should be informed about the importance of the desired health behavior or the health hazards that are to be avoided. Although the particular method of the presentation or communication may not be stressed, it is assumed that, whatever the message, it must be clearly and effectively communicated. The challenge to the health educator is to make effective use of educational methods. Being able to communicate effectively may be more complex than is generally understood or appreciated. At the minimum, persuasive communication requires (1) a creditable source, (2) a message that is capable of arousing emotion, and (3) a message that is appropriately directed to the needs and interests of the target audience.

Information Dissemination—Didactic Methods

Green[33] has observed that virtually every experimental study has confirmed the efficacy of the lecture method in conveying factual information. Also in this regard, McGuire,[19] an authority on communication research, points out that professionals often assume that the public or target audience lacks motivation to change behavior when in fact a lack of information is more often the problem.

The health hazard appraisal technique is a method that is based on the assumption that if the correct information is communicated to the indivdiual about his or her health status, together with information about habits that create a health risk, the individual will make the appropriate decisions and changes in health behavior. The critical questions for health education are Does the evidence support the hypothesis? Are people changing their behavior in order to reduce their risks?

An analysis of the public's health habits with respect to exercise, diet, and smoking habits seems to indicate that people are adopting healthier lifestyles. Moreover, the recent decline in deaths caused by heart and blood vessel disease strongly suggests that public health education campaigns are effective. The evidence shows that more people are making an effort to control their weight through diet and exercise, and an increasing number of adults are making an effort to stop smoking. It is also evident that more people are aware of the danger of high blood pressure and are making efforts to control their blood pressure.

Perchacek[34] credits the antismoking campaigns with causing the significant reduction of adult smokers that has occurred since the first surgeon general's report on *Smoking and Health,*[35] in 1964. This reduction in smoking is also believed to be a factor in the reduced rate of death from cardiovascular disease. Given these facts, a number of leaders have urged that health education in schools concentrate more on teaching students about the hazards of smoking and the importance of proper diet, regular exercise, and the dangers of drug abuse in order to prevent the onset of major chronic diseases, such as cancer and cardiovascular diseases, in later life.

Despite the apparent success of mass communication media and public information campaigns, community educators have long recognized the limitations of didactic methods and simple information-giving approaches. Specifically, the lecture may not be effective because the individual or group to whom the information is being directed does not require the learner to become actively involved. Because of this lack of involvement, the students or target audience frequently make little or no effort to receive the message. In fact, there is a general criticism that the lecture method is overused, especially in schools.

Although health educators agree that it is important to stress prevention of major health problems such as heart disease and cancer, they strongly disagree with the methods of educating the public (students or the community) that are often proposed. Perry[36] and colleagues have stated that it is not surprising that school curricula that focus on the health hazards of smoking have not been effective. Although the approach of making people more aware of the hazards of smoking seems to be effective with adults, this technique has often not been successful for adolescents. Instead of declining, the rate of adolescent smoking has remained unchanged; in the case of teenage girls, smoking has increased to an all-time high. These investigators contend that teaching about long-term health hazards is not effective because it fails to consider the social factors shaping the adolescent's behavior.

Recent experiences with the issue of teenage smoking, drug abuse, and sex behavior have raised a number of questions about those teaching methods that have emphasized the formal scientific and factual approach. In discussing the successes that have been achieved in reducing youth smoking by the use of the peer leader to create a positive nonsmoking teenage role model, Fisher[37] has raised a troublesome question: "To what extent is it necessary to teach any factual information?"

Program planners should also be aware of communications research that points out that the knowledgeable health professional is not necessarily the best person to communicate the health message. Studies have shown that uninformed lay persons, including adolescents, tend to be more persuaded by the experience of people similar to themselves than they are by the knowledge of experts.[19] In addition, Halpin and Whiddon[38] in a study of high school drug education programs, also challenge the validity of programs that are confined to information giving methods. The results of their investigation showed that those students who had the most knowledge about drugs were also the students who tended to misuse drugs, including beverage alcohol. These findings, they concluded, call for a reappraisal of drug education programs.

Socratic Methods of Interactive Models

What must be kept in mind is the age-old axiom of education: the objective is one thing, but achieving the objective in its most complete sense is quite another. Nearly four decades ago Kurt Lewin[39] conducted what has since been recognized as a classic study in the social and behavioral sciences. In this research, conducted for the National Research Council during World War II, Lewin studied methods of changing the food habits of women. His objective was to get them to use certain foods such as organ meats, which are a rich source of nutrients. However, these were foods that the women were not accustomed to using. Lewin found that the use of the lecture method, explaining the merits of these rarely used foods, produced little or no change in the actual food habits of the women. However, after he conducted group discussions about the foods, including problems of food preparation, and received verbal commitments from the women about using the new foods, a significant number of the women changed their food habits.

Krathwohl,[18] in analyzing this research and other studies with consistent results, explained that for any major reorganization of an actual practice or behavior to take place the educational method employed must allow the individual to do several things. The student or the learner must be able to examine his or her own feelings and attitudes on the particular subject, must bring these feelings and attitudes out in the open, and must compare them with the feelings and attitudes of others. According to Krathwohl, it is this process or method that enables the individual to move from a point of intellectual awareness to one of behavior change or practice and ultimately to actual commitment to the new behavior.

This position holds that if specific changes are to take place in the learner there must be a two-way experience such as is provided in the Socratic method of education. Krathwohl describes this as an interactive relationship between teacher and student, as opposed to the didactic model in which the teacher presents something to be learned by the student.

Further support for this method of education may be drawn from Wagner's[40] review of the sex education literature, which implies that the more formal teaching methods, such as lectures on factual and technical material, seem to have little effect on an adolescent's heterosexual development. What appears to be more effective in leading adolescents to accepting responsible sexual behavior is communication with significant others.

A review of the literature on teaching and curricula reveals that no single method or approach is effective for health educators in all cases. McGuire[19] has observed that "what is involved in effective communication" is an extremely complex question; so also is the determination of elements in the complex teaching-learning process. Moreover, it is no doubt the very nature or complexity of this issue that explains in part the inconsistencies and the new questions that are raised by the following conclusions that may be drawn from the literature on teaching and learning:

1. Achievement of complex learning objectives requires not only a powerful environmental influence but also the coordinated efforts of the entire faculty and curriculum.
2. A single hour of classroom activity involving a peak experience may bring about major knowledge and attitudinal changes in the student.
3. Despite the many studies that have investigated the effects of teaching methods, no one single method has been found to be consistently superior to another.
4. Although the teacher and the curriculum constitute a major influence on the child's learning, relatively speaking this influence may be much less than that of the home and the community.

Professional Preparation

The nature of the professional training or preparation of the health educator is determined to a large degree by such factors as the philosophy, program goals, and particular theory of health behavior change held by those who plan and administer the program. For example, if the curriculum developers see the role of the health educator as primarily that of a disseminator of heath information, it is logical that their program would place emphasis on training in mass media communication techniques. On the other hand, if the curriculum developer's perception of the health educator's role emphasizes individual instruction, then the importance of developing skills in counseling techniques and the ability to write self-instruction materials become most important.

From the standpoint of professional preparation, the critical question is Are the differences in the role of the health educator of such a magnitude as to require special attention in order to prepare the specialist to the requisite level of competence and effectiveness? Of equal importance is the question Are there commonalities or areas of similarity that can serve as the common core of preparation for all health educators, regardless of their particular function or work setting?

Since the mid-1960s, health education professionals have recognized the need to evaluate the role and functions of practitioners. Because of the growing interest in health promotion and disease prevention, many have argued that there is an urgent need to accept a common basis for professional practice and a more systematic approach to the preparation of the health educator. Reaching agreements about role and function is essential to establishing qualitative standards for health education practice. Further, it is argued that this will ultimately be in the public's best interest by assuring quality service, which in turn serves to justify the field of health education in American society.

A group of professionals representing all aspects of health education met at the Workshop on Commonalities and Differences in 1978 to develop a set of recommendations for future action in achieving quality assurance for health education practice. This group's analysis of professional preparation programs indicated that there is no guarantee that any two programs offering a major in school or community health education will have the same or even similar curriculums in health education.[41] Although diversity in academic training has often been valued in American higher education, the advancement of professional discipline or practice rests on the recognition and acceptance of a common core of knowledge and skill defined by the profession at large.

However, recognizing that there is a need to standardize preparation and practice in order to establish quality control is one thing; it may be quite another to reach agreement on what that preparation should be. Again, the perception of what the health educator's role is to be determines the nature of the training. Examination of professional preparation programs for the school health education specialist indicates clearly that emphasis thus far has been placed on the professional as a communicator of health information. As an example, the goal of teaching people how to improve their diets would require preparation of the health educator in the area of nutrition. Also, emphasis on methods of communication in a one-to-one, small group, or large group lecture-discussion format would be required. Knowing the what and how of communication is central to training, according to this perspective.

At the other end of the spectrum of professional preparation is the community health educator. Here the specialist is seen as one who works behind the scenes, planning, organizing, and arranging an environment that will facilitate health behavior change. For example, it is often pointed out that some adults may already have factual knowledge or content information about a certain health problem. Yet because of certain factors in their physical or social environment, they are unable to apply their knowledge. Enabling an adult to achieve success in a weight control program may require the creation of a supportive environment in the home or a re-shaping of the individual's work schedule in order to control calorie intake.

In considering the training of the health education specialist, there is the question of apportionment of time to be spent developing the process skills and time to be spent learning about the health content areas. This is-sue of balance between content and process was discussed at a national conference (1981) on professional preparation. However, the issue was not resolved but its importance was underscored (see Chapter 4).

There are differences in emphasis between the so-called traditional health education approach and the recommendations coming from the Role Delineation Project. An AAHPER report calls for devoting approximately 30% of preparation effort of the health educator to the development of competencies in the health content areas. In contrast, the new Role Delin-eation Report[14] recommendation calls for about 8% of the training effort to be devoted to what is described as "providing" and "interpreting" health information or health content.

Although it is generally recognized that the health educator will need skill and understanding in both process and content, the issues of how much emphasis should be given to the professional preparation and the degree of skill the professional health educator should have in each of these areas remain unresolved.

Assessment

Health education is like motherhood and love of country—everyone seems to be in favor of it. However, the failure of achieve an effective level of implementation suggests that there is a lack of commitment or perhaps a lack of agreement on what is to be done. There is little doubt that health education, as an idea, has long been accepted. Efforts aimed at preventing disease and promoting health have been recognized as making good sense for reasons of good health and sound economic policy. Health education has generally enjoyed at least tacit support from the public at large. State-ments recognizing the importance of what may be considered health edu-cation as it is recognized today can be found throughout recorded history.

Support of the Idea

For example, proponents of health education in the schools have often cited statements of the famous philosopher John Locke concerning health and hygiene that were included in his classic publication *Some Thoughts About Education*[42]: "A sound mind in a sound body is a short but full description of a happy state in this world. He that has these two has little more to wish for."

The emphasis on health education as an important part of both public health and public education was expressed by early leaders. Shattuck wrote in his now famous *Report of the Sanitary Commission of Massachusetts,*[43] issued in 1850, that "every child should be taught, early in life, that to preserve one's own life and his own health and the health of others, is one of his most important and abiding duties." Shattuck also called on the schools to adopt procedures that would encourage both teachers and pupils to make personal applications of the laws of health and life.

Horace Mann, as first secretary of the Massachusetts Board of Education, frequently emphasized the importance of hygiene and physical training in his annual reports to the board.

From the mid-nineteenth century to the present, recurring statements of support for the concept of health education can be found. During the 1950s the Commission on Building America's Health[44] issued its report to President Harry S Truman, calling for major changes in the country's health care system. In setting forth its recommendation, the importance of health education was stressed. The commission pointed out that "the individual effort of an informed person will do more for his health and that of his family than all the things which can be done for them."

The decade of the 1970s was ushered in by two related and important health education developments: (1) the report (1971) of a steering committee commissioned by then New York Governor Nelson Rockefeller on Social Problems and Health and Hospital Costs, and (2) the report of the President's Committee on Health Education (1973). Rockefeller's committee consisted of a blue-ribbon panel of leaders representing business, education, management, and labor. Because some of the same persons served on both the Rockefeller committee and the President's committee, the contents of these reports reflected both a consistency and continuity in the planning and recommendations presented.

The combined impact of the two reports triggered a series of developments that resulted in a decade of unparalleled activity in health education. A quotation from each report may serve to capture something of their essence and illustrate the importance these committees attached to health education. The Committee on Social Problems and Health and Hospital Costs stated

> The responsibility of the individual for his own health and well-being is a vital factor in any rational approach to health. The fact is, the nation does not have the resources, no matter how great a portion of the GNP is allocated for health to provide sufficient services after the patient becomes ill.[10]

However, it was a statement in The President's Committee report that helped to create widespread interest in health education.

Of the more than 75 billion dollars being spent annually for medical, hospital and health care, about 92 to 93 percent is spent for treatment after illness occurs. Of the remainder 4 to 5 percent is spent for biomedical research, 2-2½ percent for preventive health measures and ½ percent for health education.[2]

This interest is reflected in the growth of health education, especially within the federal government, in which two major offices have been created: (1) the Office of Health Information and Health Promotion (OHP) and (2) the Center for Education and Health Promotion.

Perhaps of greater significance is the increased emphasis and recognition that have been given to disease prevention and health education in the form of officially published statements, as represented in a series of reports, *A Forward Plan for Health, FY* 77-81, FY 78-82, and FY 79-83*.[45] Also, Congress has rewritten the missions of two institutes, the National Heart, Lung and Blood Institute (NHLBI) and the National Cancer Institute (NCI), in order that research on disease prevention and health education might be encouraged and supported in addition to traditional support of biomedical research.

This increased emphasis on health education was also apparent in the form of several major legislative developments occurring in the 1970s. Examples include the Occupational Health and Safety Act, the Health Planning and Resources Development Act, the Health Maintenance Organization legislation, the creation of the OHP, and finally the Health Education Act of 1978, which is an amendment to the Elementary and Secondary Education Act.

Current Status

All of this might lead to the conclusion that the status of health education is very strong. But is this in fact the case? Ironically, it was statements issued by the Rockefeller and the President's committees that helped to dramatize the gap between the theory and the practice of health education. The increase in public awareness of the lack of support and resources devoted to prevention and health education served to arouse the public's interest. In fact, this heightened interest on the part of the public and the health care industry is in part creating another issue for the field of health education: the problem of unrealistic expectations for health education.

What is the reality of health education today? Has this rebirth of public interest and increased attention been translated into significant progress

*Fiscal year.

toward achieving the goals of health education? What is the status of health education? Is there a basis for optimism about its future? What assessments are being offered as to the state of the art for health education? Because it is generally acknowledged that the 1973 report of the President's Committee on Health Education was a landmark event, awakening new interest in the field and providing much of the impetus behind contemporary developments in the field, what were the conclusions drawn by the committee from its year-long study of health education?

Although public demand for improved health status and health care services has been increasing, the field of education has been neglected and largely unevaluated. At the time of the President's committee report there was no agency inside or outside of government responsible for establishing or assisting with the setting of goals or the maintaining of performance criteria. In addition, the report states

> It is a frustrating paradox, given their relative effectiveness in effecting change, that while health information has grown year by year in volume and in excellence, health education has developed much more slowly.[2]

The committee was even more specific in its criticism of the status of school health education. The quality—even the existence—of health education in the classroom varied greatly throughout the country. And at the time of the committee's report, the situation was described as one of antiquated laws, indifferent parents, unaggressive school boards, teachers poorly prepared to teach the subject, lack of leadership from government or the public, lack of funds, lack of research, and lack of evaluation. All of these factors have seriously handicapped the ability of health educators to provide an effective, comprehensive program of health education for the nation's children. The committee offers little in the way of evidence of recent progress in school health education. In fact, the opposite seems to have been the case.

> Our findings are that school health education in most primary and secondary schools is not provided at all, or it loses its proper emphasis because of the way it is tacked onto another subject such as physical education or biology, assigned to teachers whose interest and qualifications are elsewhere.[2]

According to the committee, evidence shows that much of the health education offered in schools is not effective. The committee pointed to such specific problem areas as nutrition, where studies reveal that teenagers, especially girls, often damage their own health and deprive themselves of vitality because of poor eating habits. Young people who once urged their parents not to smoke have become cigarette smokers as teenagers. The high and rising incidence of venereal disease and the spread of drug abuse among teenagers are two of the most urgent reasons for assigning a special priority to health education among school children.

The Task Force report on Health Promotion and Consumer Health Education apparently concurred in this assessment of school health education.

School health education programs are faced with three major constraints: a) a tradition of low visibility and low priority; b) a narrow definition of the appropriate content and jurisdiction for health efforts; and c) a shortage of adequately trained health educators.[1]

Gap Between Theory and Practice

Again, however, it is the gap between the present status of health education and what is seen as the potential of schools for preventing illness and injury and for promoting the health and well-being of children and youth that has led to the impatience and disenchantment on the part of public health and medical leaders with the school health education effort. These same leaders contend that there is nothing wrong with the goals nor with the philosophy of school health education. Rather, they argue, the problem lies at the program action level, with the failure on the part of school officials to adopt sound procedures and to provide the resources to implement programs that are known to be effective. Instead, school health education has been allowed to languish in a fantasy land, remaining out of touch with real problems and issues.

Silver,[46] a nationally known authority in child health, states that school health services are hedged with so many restrictions that the prerogatives of the home, the school, and private medicine are all given priority over those of the child's health needs. Teacher, supervisors, and school administrators tend to take the position that a consideration of the child's health needs is an intrusion on more important teaching duties. Silver contends the "new morbidity" problems of smoking, drugs, alcohol and other substance abuse, venereal disease among the young, and teenage pregnancies are areas requiring official school action. These problems cannot be solved or even addressed without a joint effort of the schools, the parents, and the health authorities. All these conditions have a direct effect on education. Even though they may accept the more conservative position that the school's primary role is to develop student learning in the area of the cognitive or knowledge domain, public health and medical officials contend that there is still a serious health problem. Schools have largely defaulted on their responsibility for providing the public with the basic health knowledge that is essential to responsible citizenship and to conduct public health and medical care in a modern society.

In support of their argument, the medical and public health leaders point out that despite the fact that schools have been required by law for over a half century to teach the harmful effects of tobacco, and despite the fact that great effort and public health funding have been directed to help schools strengthen their antismoking education programs since the surgeon general's report on *Smoking and Health* in 1964, recent national polls (1980) show that 31% of smokers in the United States are unaware that smoking increases the risk of cancer. Some 27% to 38% of the smokers surveyed stated that they were unaware that smoking causes lung cancer. Even more startling is the fact that 13% to 17% of these individuals did not know that smoking was hazardous in any way.

The late John H. Knowles,[47] former president of the Rockefeller Foundation, has argued that the behavior of Americans might be changed if there were adequate programs in primary and secondary schools and colleges. But, as he observed, they simply do not exist.

> School health programs are abysmal at best. With respect to the teaching of health knowledge, there is a lack of careful evaluation—there are no examinations to determine if anything's been learned.

Is it possible that these evaluations of school health education are in error or unfair? Are these school programs as bad as they appear to be? Several of these evaluations have been offered by groups outside of the schools. Could it be that a part of the problem is a lack of understanding or perhaps a fundamental difference of opinion over the purposes of schooling? Are these evaluations confirmed by leaders from within the educational family?

A recent task force report to the Education Commission of the States,[48] although not as negative as some, does call attention to several major problems affecting school health education program development and implementation. They are:

1. The school health education curriculum is often assigned a low priority because of a lack of understanding of the program's content, scope, and methods.
2. Because of this lack of understanding, a lack of confidence in health education results and inadequate resources are allocated for the program.
3. People hold unrealistic expectations for health education. This results in part from a failure to understand the complexity of health behavior.
4. Many teachers have been assigned health teaching responsibilities without adequate preparation.
5. Health education programs suffer from an inadequate level of resources for designing, implementing, and improving programs.

The Health Educator's Side of the Argument

A number of writers appear to be in substantial agreement with at least two of the problems cited by the Education Commission of the States: (1) the lack of understanding of health education, which also contributes to the second problem, that of (2) unrealistic expectations that people hold for health education, as well as their failure to appreciate the complexity of the behavior change task.

As Kreuter and Green[49] have stated, unless steps are taken to clarify the functions of the school health education program, there is the likelihood that programs will be judged on outcome criteria that are both inappropriate and unrealistic. Further, they have warned that it is naïve to expect health education to produce health behavior changes that will result in significant improvements in health. Instead, they argue that school health education can make its most important contribution in the development of specific knowledge and skill.

Bartlett[50] and Immarino and others[51] after extensive reviews of the research literature on school health education, have reached conclusions similar to those reported earlier by Krueter and Green.[49] They conclude that there is little evidence to show that school health education programs are likely to achieve significant improvement in health behavior. However, even among those leaders who argue for a more realistic and perhaps conservative role for the school, there are also those who have urged the schools to accept a more aggressive stance in preventing disease and in promoting the public's health.

This raises the question By what criterion should school health education be held accountable for its expenditure of schools' limited resources and time in the curriculum for health education? Although recognizing the difficulty of changing health behavior, Green and others[52] argue that settling for an improvement in student knowledge alone is not a satisfactory answer to the question.

If school systems are held responsible for preparing children to achieve specific levels of performance by age and grade level, what are the health education responsibilities? This task, according to Green, is to help children acquire the health knowledge and skills necessary to maintain their health and to cope with the potential threats to health at each age and developmental level. Accordingly, the criteria of success for school succeed in helping children acquire these fundamental health knowledge and health maintenance skills.

Hochbaum[53] has challenged the most fundamental core concept—behavior change as the goal of health education. To be more exact, he is challenging the premise that health behavior change is the central goal of health education. Instead, Hochbaum argues that health educators must be more precise about what can be accomplished. The more appropriate mission is to promote health-supportive behaviors and to fortify the already existing health-supportive behaviors in order to prevent them from deteriorating into health-threatening behavior. The health behavior change goal not only fails to recognize the complexity of this task but also overlooks the need to help people (at all age levels) to resist the internal and external influences that cause people to adopt behavior detrimental to their health.

Still another concern raised by Hochbaum is the ethical question of advocating health behavior changes that often turn out to be ineffective or even detrimental to one's health. This smacks of a kind of professional arrogance that not only claims superior knowledge of what is good for everyone but also tends to mold the behavior of others in one's own image.

Whether or not an individual ultimately adopts a given health practice or behavior depends on innumerable factors, some of which are outside the control of the educator; still others are outside the control of the individual.

Evaluative Studies. Although a number of medical and public health leaders have expressed dissatisfaction with the level of success, or rather with what they perceive to be a lack of success in changing health behavior, there are a number of successes to consider.

Several evaluative studies of well-developed programs have shown that school health education programs have been successful in increasing knowledge, somewhat successful in improving attitudes, and occasionally successful in facilitating life-style changes.[50-52] Podell[54] conducted an experiment in which a high school biology course served as the educational intervention. He was able to demonstrate an improvement in the students' knowledge and also to show a more positive attitude toward eating foods low in cholesterol. An analysis of school-based heart health education programs conducted by Immarino and others[51] revealed similar results; an increase in student knowledge and more positive attitudes toward health.

In one of the most comprehensive reviews undertaken, Green and others[52] critically analyzed the results from 24 different evaluative studies that had been conducted to test the effectiveness of the School Health Education Curriculum Project. As a consequence of this review, the following conclusions were offered:

1. Each of the three major grade level units that characterize this project, the respiratory, circulatory, and nervous systems (grades 5, 6, and 7), is effective in increasing student knowledge.
2. Each of these units is also effective in increasing positive health-related attitudes among students exposed to this curriculum.[52]

This chapter attempted an examination of some of the major issues facing health education. Examples including the school, community, clinical, and worksite settings were used where appropriate. These issues are challenges for all members of the profession and especially for those newest colleagues, you, the students. With foresight and diligence it is very probable that these challenges will be successfully met.

Editors' Remarks

As noted earlier, other disciplines interact with health education. One of these is psychology, and the following provides an example of that interaction.

Recently, social learning theory has become an important facet of health education programs, which will be illustrated within these comments. As Dr. Creswell so aptly pointed out, Bandura (the father of social learning theory as we know it today) stresses the importance of the learner's environment as well as intrinsic motivation.

Social Learning Theory—A Brief Explanation

Bandura's social learning theory can best be described as a process of reciprocal determinism. Behavioral, environmental, and cognitive (personal) factors interact to determine an individual's behavior. The theory involves three important aspects: vicarious learning, use of cognitive symbols, and principles of self-management.

Vicarious learning involves imitation of behavior and modeling. An example of this type of learning is language development in children. Symbols are used to foresee the effects of our actions, enabling us to change our behavior if necessary. Symbols allow us to react in different or new ways and to plan and create. Most importantly, symbols guide our future behavior. The third component of this theory, self-management principles, enables us to exercise some control over our own behavior. This is accomplished by (1) the arrangement of environmental inducements, (2) the generation of cognitive supports, and (3) the production of consequences pursuant to our actions.

Application in Health Education

Although the social learning theory may seem complex, it has been easily used in health education programs. When the theory has been incorporated into research programs, usually only one of the three components seems to have been adopted by the health educators. The following are a few examples of how this theory has been incorporated into health education in an attempt to explain and predict behavior.

Aspects of Bandura's social learning theory were used in a major study conducted by Evans and others at the University of Houston in its social psychology doctoral program. The study was designed primarily to prevent youngsters from smoking cigarettes. Junior high school students were trained to cope with immediate social pressures and other social influences to smoke.

The program specifically involved psychologic inoculation against peer pressure, in which the student is taught how to deal with the pressures to smoke in the form of posters. In addition, the students viewed a videotape concerning the immediate effects of smoking on their health and appearance. The researcher's interventions used the vicarious process of observation of the film and symbolic interaction through communication for inoculation against peer pressure.

A well-known community health program involving alcoholic treatment is Alcoholics Anonymous (AA). The basic principles used by AA are self-control and the setting of goals. Their slogan "one day at a time" indicates their use of Bandura's self-regulatory principles. Bandura has proposed that self-control principally operates through two sources of motivation: proximal goal setting and the representation of future consequences in thought. The first principle operates through goal setting and self-evaluation of one's performance. This is the principle used by AA and its success has been well documented.

Several popular diets and diet centers have appeared in recent years, some of which use a self-management or regulatory approach. One program has their clients meet with a trained health educator or counselor. A complete history of eating habits, responses, stimuli, and patterns is taken by the counselor. The client and the counselor then set about the task of working out a plan (self-management program) whereby the client regains control of her or his eating habits. The program is aimed at having the client achieve success early in the program by meeting short, well-defined goals. This type of program has been attempted at worksite settings whereby the employer contracts with the diet center to meet with those employees in need of such a program.

As you can imagine, there are numerous ways that social learning theory has and will be used. Programs at all levels and in many settings can be based on the principles set forth by Bandura.

Summary

Dr. Creswell began this chapter by recognizing that the vitality of a profession is dependent on the willingness of its members to meet the challenges brought about by an ever-changing world. All professions are confronted with a continuous barrage of new issues that need resolution. Health education suffers from a unique problem for two reasons: (1) it is still an emerging profession and (2) it was given birth by the established fields of education and health care. This means that the issues of current interest are also the foundations on which a profession is built.

The issues described in this chapter appear to be natural outgrowths of the historical, philosophic, and competency-related concerns discussed in earlier chapters. Initiatives directed toward resolving these issues can be viewed by the health educator as a responsibility for action and an opportunity for satisfaction. Although it is never directly stated, Dr. Creswell certainly implies that health education will accept the challenge and, having done so, will come away from the struggle as a more unified profession.

Questions for Review

1. What do the professors in your department consider to be the goals and purposes of health education?
2. Dr. Creswell has written a chapter about what he considers to be some of the central issues facing health education. From your reading of the first four chapters can you add other issues that need to be resolved?
3. Do you think the profession is moving toward a resolution of these issues? Explain.
4. To what extent do the *Seven Cardinal Principles of Education* (developed to guide secondary education) define the responsibilities of community and worksite health education?
5. To what extent were the *Seven Cardinal Principles* evident in your school health education experience?
6. Why is it difficult for health education to provide "solid evidence" of positive results?
7. How would you respond to someone who said that "much of what is called health education is nothing more than information dissemination"?
8. What are the relative merits of using the "expert" to communicate health information as opposed to a member of the target audience who serves as a peer educator?
9. The chapter uses many quotes from individuals, committees, commissions, and professional associations. What three quotes do you consider to be the most important to the profession?

References

1. Preventive medicine, U.S.A., health promotion and consumer health education: a task force report. Sponsored by the John E. Fogarty International Center for Advanced Study in the Health Sciences, National Institutes of Health and The American College of Preventive Medicine, New York, 1976, Prodist.
2. The report of the President's Committee on Health Education, New York, 1973, Xerox Corp.
3. Tyler, R.N.: Reconstructing the total educational environment. In Hass, G., editor: Curriculum planning: a new approach, Boston, 1977, Allyn & Bacon, Inc.
4. Saylor, G.J.: Humanistic education: the minimum essentials. In Hass, G., editor: Curriculum planning: a new approach, Boston, 1977, Allyn & Bacon, Inc.
5. The seven cardinal principles revisited, Today's Education **65**(3):67-72, 1976.
6. Green, L.W.: Evaluation and measurement: some dilemmas for health education, American Journal of Public Health, **67**(2):155-161, 1977.
7. U.S. Department of Health, Education, and Welfare: The school health curriculum project, HEW Pub. No. (CDC) 78-8359, Washington, D.C., 1977.
8. Health education: a conceptual approach to curriculum design, Washington, D.C., 1967, School Health Education Study, Inc., St. Paul, Minn., 1968, (Published by 3M Education Press.)
9. Healthy people: the surgeon general's report on health promotion and disease prevention, U.S. Department of Health, Education, and Welfare, DHEW (PHS) Pub. No. 79-5507, Washington, D.C., 1979, U.S. Government Printing Office.
10. Governor's Steering Committee on Social Problems: Report from the governor's steering committee on social problems on health and hospital services and costs, New York, 1971, State of New York.
11. A discursive dictionary of health care, Prepared by staff of the House Subcommittee on Health and the Environment of the Committee on Interstate and Foreign Commerce, U.S. House of Representatives, Washington, D.C., 1976, U.S. Government Printing Office.
12. Ogden, H.G.: Recent developments in health education policy, Health Education Monographs Supplement **6**(suppl. 1):67-73, 1978.
13. American Public Health Association: Education for health in the school community setting, Position paper of the School Health section of the APHA, New Orleans, October 23, 1974.
14. U.S. Department of Health, Education and Welfare Focal Points, Health Education and Credentialing: The Role Delineation Project. PHS-ODC Bureau of Health Education. Atlanta, Ga., July 1980.
15. Dwore, R.B., and Matarazzo, J.: The behavioral sciences and health education, disciplines with a compatible interest? Health Education **12**(3):4-7, 1981.
16. Katz, E., and Lazarsfeld, P.F.: Personal influence: the part played by people in the flow of mass communications, Glencoe, Ill., 1955, The Free Press.
17. Wallack, L.M.: Assessing effects of mass media campaigns: an alternative perspective, Alcohol Health and Research World **4**:18-34, 1980.
18. Krathwohl, D.R., Bloom, B.S., and Masia, B.B.: Taxonomy of educational objectives, the classification of educational goals, handbook II: affective domain, New York, 1956, David McKay Co.
19. McGuire, W.J.: Behavioral medicine, public health and communication theories, Health Education **12**(3):8-13, 1981.
20. La Piere, R.T.: Attitudes versus actions, Social Forces **13**:230-237, 1934.
21. Festinger, L.: A theory of cognitive dissonance, Stanford, Cal., 1962, Stanford University Press.
22. Hochbaum, G.M.: What communication can and cannot achieve. Communication and behavior change: factors of active participation of the population for attainment of better health, Proceedings of the Seventh International Conference on Health and Health Education, Buenos Aires, 1969, International Journal of Health Education **12**(3):142, 1969.

23. Rosenstock, I.M.: The health belief model and preventive health behavior, Health Education Monographs **2:**354-386, 1974.
24. McAlister, A., Perry, C., Killen, J., and others: Pilot study of smoking, alcohol and drug abuse prevention, American Journal of Public Health **70**(7):719-721, 1980.
25. Bauer, K.G.: Improving the chances for health: lifestyle change and health evaluation, San Francisco, 1980, The National Center for Health Education.
26. Maccoby, N., and Farquhar, J.W.: Communication for health: unselling heart disease. In Health promotion and consumer health education, Preventive Medicine, U.S.A., New York, 1976, Podist.
27. Cohen, C.I., and Cohen, E.J.: Health education: panacea, pernicious or pointless? The New England Journal of Medicine **299**(13):718-720, 1978.
28. Leventhal, H., Safer, M., Cleary, P., and Gutman, M.: Cardiovascular risk modification by community-based programs for life-style change: comments on the Stanford study, Journal of Consulting and Clinical Psychology **48**(2):150-158, 1980.
29. Meyer, A.J., Nash, J.D., McAlister, A.L., and others: Skills training in a cardiovascular health education campaign, Journal of Consulting and Clinical Psychology, **48**(2):129-142, 1980.
30. Bandura, A.: Social learning theory, Englewood Cliffs, N.J., 1977, Prentice-Hall, Inc.
31. Kleibard, H.: Education at the turn of the century: a crucible for curriculum change, Educational Researcher **11**(1):16-23, 1982.
32. Butts, R.F.: A cultural history of education: reassessing our educational tradition, New York, 1947, McGraw-Hill, Inc.
33. Green, L.W., Heit, P., Iverson, D.C., and others: The school health curriculum project: its theory, practice and measurement experience, Health Education Quarterly **7**(1):4-34, 1980.
34. Pechacek, T.F.: Modification of smoking behavior, In Smoking and health, a report of the surgeon general, DHEW Pub. No. (PHS) 79-5066, Washington, D.C., 1979, U.S Government Printing Office.
35. Smoking and health, a report of the surgeon general, U.S. Department of Health, Education and Welfare, Public Health Service, Office of the Assistant Secretary for Health, Office on Smoking and Health, Washington, D.C., 1979 U.S. Government Printing Office.
36. Perry, C., Killen, J., Slinkard, L.A., and McAlister, A.L.: Peer teaching and smoking prevention among junior high students, Adolescence **15**(38):227-281, 1980.
37. Fisher, E.B., Jr.: Progress in reducing adolescent smoking, American Journal of Public Health July 1980, Vol, 70, No. 7 ISSN: 0090-0036.
38. Halpin, G., and Whidden, T.: Drug education: solution or problem? Psychological Reports, Vol. **40:**372-374, 1977.
39. Lewin, K.: Group discussion and social change. In Newcomb, T.M., and Hartly, E.L., editors: Readings in social psychology, New York, 1947, Holt.
40. Wagner, C.A.: Sexuality of American adolescents, Adolescence **15**(59):62-66, 1980.
41. Cleary, H.: Preparation and practice of community, patient, and school health educators, Proceedings of the Workshop on Commonalities and Differences, February, 1978, Washington, D.C., 1978, U.S. Department of Health, Education and Welfare.
42. Locke, J.: Some thoughts concerning education, London, 1705, A. & F. Churchill.
43. Shattuck, L.: Report of the Sanitary Commission of Massachusetts, (fasc. ed.) Boston, 1850, Dutton & Wentworth.
44. Building America's health: president's commission on the health needs of the nation. Vol. I. Findings and recommendations, Raleigh, N.C., 1953, Health Publishing Institute, Inc.
45. Forward plan for health, FY 1977-81, U.S. Department of Health, Education, and Welfare, Washington, D.C., 1975, U.S. Government Printing Office.
46. Silver, G.: Redefining school health services: comprehensive child health care as the framework, Journal of School Health, **51**(3):157-162, 1981.
47. Knowles, J.H., editor: Doing better and feeling worse, New York, 1977, W.W. Norton & Co.

48. Recommendations for school health education: a handbook for state policy makers, Education Commission of the States, Report No. 130, Boulder, Colo., March, 1981.
49. Kreuter, M.W., and Green, L.K.: Evaluation of School Health Education: identifying purpose, keeping perspective, J. School Health **48:**228-235, 1978.
50. Bartlett, E.E.: The contribution of school health education to community health promotion: what can we reasonably expect? American Journal of Public Health **7**(12):1384-1391, 1981.
51. Immarino, N.K., Weinberg, A.D., and Holcomb, J.D.: The state of school heart health education: a review of the literature, Health Education Quarterly **7**(4):298-320, 1980.
52. Green, L.W., Kreuter, M.W., Deeds, S.G., and Partridge, K.B.: Health education planning, a diagnostic approach, Palo Alta, Cal., 1980, Mayfield Publishing Co.
53. Hochbaum, G.M.: Behavior change as the goal of human education, The Eta Sigma Gamman **13**(2):3-6, 1981.
54. Podell, R.N., Keller, H.K., Mulvihill, M.N., and others: Evaluation of the effectiveness of a high school course in cardiovascular nutrition, American Journal of Public Health **68**(6):573-576, 1978.

Additional Readings

Bandura, A.: Social learning theory, Englewood Cliffs, N.J., 1977, Prentice-Hall, Inc.
Bandura, A., and Simon, K.M.: The role of proximal intentions in self-regulation of refracting behavior, Cognitive Therapy and Research, **1:**177-193, 1977.
Evans, R.I.: Smoking in children: developing a social psychological strategy of deterrence, Journal of Preventive Medicine **5**(1):122-127, 1976.
Evans, R.I.: Training social psychologists in behavioral medicine research. In Eiser, J., editor: Social psychology and behavioral medicine, New York, 1982, John Wiley & Sons, Inc.
Hall, C., and Lindzey, G.: Theories of personality, New York, 1978, John Wiley & Sons, Inc.

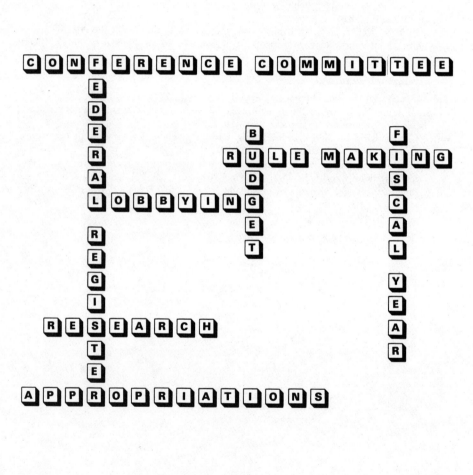

6 Understanding and Influencing the Legislative, Appropriations, and Regulatory Processes

Introduction

In this chapter Dr. Iverson presents a concise description of the legislative, appropriations, and regulatory processes, with parallel descriptions of how to become an advocate for health education. The focus of this chapter is on the activities of the federal government. Procedures at the state, county, and municipal levels vary so widely that a discussion of processes at these levels would be useless. You are urged to make inquiries into legislation and appropriations at the state level. The best source of information is your local representative to the state legislature. This individual can keep you apprised of bills that affect health and education.

Advocacy can begin even before a bill is introduced by making congressional members aware of issues that affect the nation's health. As a bill makes its way through the Senate and the House of Representatives there are opportunities for input from individuals and from professional associations at each step of the process. There are six committees in the House of Representatives that most frequently deal with legislation of interest to health educators: agriculture; appropriations; education and labor; ways and means; aging; and narcotics abuse and control. In the Senate there are four committees of interest: agriculture, nutrition and forestry; appropriations; labor; and human resources and aging.

The appropriations process provides funding for federal programs. The process begins between 18 and 24 months before passage of an appropriations bill. During this period of time about 12 months of discussions have occurred within the executive branch between the various departments and the Office of Management and Budget (OMB). Then, 8 months before the beginning of the new fiscal year, the proposed budget is delivered to Congress. Extensive hearings are conducted by Congress and the public has an opportunity for input. The House and Senate issue their reports around the middle of May. A conference committee composed of members of both houses resolves the differences that exist within the two reports. House and Senate approval normally take place between June and September 30 before the fiscal year, which begins on October 1.

The regulatory process is the implementation of legislation. This activity occurs almost exclusively within the domain of the executive branch of government. Although Congress can veto proposed regulations, it rarely does so. The department in question prepares a written plan that describes how the legislation is to be implemented. The public is informed of the proposed regulations through the *Federal Register* and ordinarily 60 days are allowed for public comment.

The final section of the chapter describes how to get information from the federal government (see also Appendix D). A brief description of the Public Health Service is offered along with the names of the units that make up this service. Descriptions are also provided for 11 other agencies of interest to health educators.

The federal government is directly and indirectly involved in numerous disease prevention and health promotion activities (see also Chapter 3 and

Appendix A). The individual and collective impact of these activities is such that federal disease prevention and health promotion policy is often altered. In addition, the legislative and appropriations processes in Congress affect the scope of federal policy as well as federal investment in disease prevention and health promotion activities.

It is difficult for many health professionals to either follow or understand the processes and activities occurring at the federal level. The purpose of this chapter is to increase your awareness and understanding of federal disease prevention and health promotion program activities and to explain how administrative and fiscal support for these activities can be influenced. To accomplish this task the chapter is divided into five sections: (1) the legislative process, (2) congressional committees, (3) the appropriations process, (4) the regulatory process, and (5) federal departments and agencies.

Legislative Process*

Fig. 6-1 depicts the steps in the legislative process. The first step in the legislative process involves the introduction of a bill into the House or the Senate. A bill is a draft of a law that is introduced into a legislature for approval. Bills are introduced to create new laws, to make changes in existing laws, to establish new programs or extend existing ones, or to provide funds to support programs. The person presenting the bill is referred to as the sponsor of the bill. Frequently, the sponsor is joined by other representatives or senators in introducing the bill; these persons are referred to as cosponsors of the bill. The names of a bill's sponsor and cosponsors appear on the face page of the bill—important information for persons planning to lobby for or against the bill.

Although all bills are introduced into the legislative process by members of the House or Senate, the stimulus for the bill's writing can come from a variety of sources. A representative or senator may have a special interest in an issue and decide to write a bill pertaining to some aspect of the issue. For example, former Senator Richard Schweiker (R-Pa.) had a special interest in diabetes and was responsible for introducing bills pertaining to diabetes research and treatment. However, a minority of the bills introduced in Congress are written as a result of a representative's or senator's special interests.

Important stimulus for writing bills also comes from the executive branch. High-ranking officials and spokespersons within the executive branch can work with members of the House or the Senate to write a bill.

---

*Background information for this section was obtained from *The Legislative Process: How A Bill Becomes a Law* prepared by the National Heart, Lung and Blood Institute.

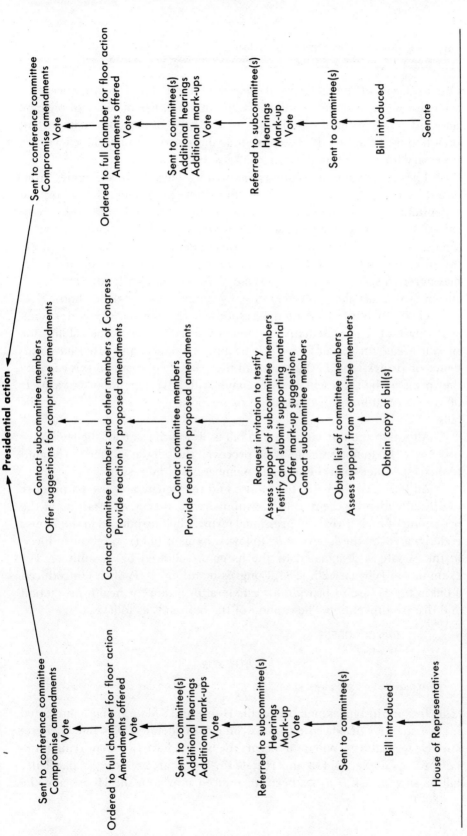

Fig. 6-1. Steps in the legislative process.

Often officials of the executive branch write the bill and then request that a senator or representative introduce it. Although the majority of bills are not written as a result of stimuli from the executive branch, it is an important option in that it allows the executive branch to introduce bills it believes are necessary for the administration's policies to be enacted.

The most common stimulus for writing bills, however, comes from outside the legislative and executive branches. Representatives of private organizations, professional associations, business and industry, and private citizens are the most frequent sources of ideas for bills. A representative or senator or his or her staff is often approached about an idea for a bill. If the proposed bill is of interest to the representative or senator he or she may agree to sponsor the bill. In these cases the bill may be drafted by the citizen or organization representative, by congressional staff, or both.

Finally, bills may be written in response to the interests of congressional staff. Staff of a representative or senator usually have responsibility for specific areas, for example, energy, health, or finance, and often have academic or professional backgrounds in their assigned areas. In this capacity they provide the representative or senator with advice on important aspects of issues, including the desirability of introducing or supporting specific bills.

Although the introduction of a bill is always the start of the legislative process, it also initiates the lobbying process if the bill was written to respond to interests other than those of the members of Congress.

All bills introduced in the House and the Senate are given a number to officially identify them. Bills are numbered consecutively starting at the beginning of each 2-year congressional term. A bill introduced in the House is designated by the letters *H.R.* followed by its number; a bill introduced in the Senate is designated by the letter *S.* followed by its number. For example, on February 26, 1981, Congressman Pursell (R-Mich.) introduced a bill in the House to provide for a federal program for health promotion and disease prevention. The caption of the bill reads as follows:

97th CONGRESS
1st SESSION

H.R. 2212

To provide for a federal program for health promotion and disease prevention.

In some instances members of the House and Senate are both interested in an issue and decide to introduce similar or identical bills into their respective legislatures. When this occurs the bill will have two identifying numbers, for example, S.1413 and H.R.4715. If you are following a particular bill be sure to ask if it has been introduced into both the House and the

Senate. If so, request both versions; this allows you to identify the bills' sponsors and cosponsors and to compare the House and Senate versions of the bill.

However, it is not necessary that bills be introduced into both chambers. If a bill is passed in one chamber and a similar bill does not exist in the other chamber, it can be referred to the other chamber for action. If similar but not identical bills are passed by both chambers they are referred to a conference committee for action, which often results in a compromise version of the bills that is then sent to both chambers for action.

The next steps in the legislative process involve congressional committees and subcommittees. Following introduction of a bill into the House or Senate it is referred to the committee that has legislative jurisdiction in that area. A bill may be assigned to more than one committee if its contents involve multiple legislative areas, for example, research grants, tax incentives, and surveillance activities. The committee chairperson(s) then assigns the bill to the appropriate subcommittee(s), which analyzes the specifics of the bill in considerable detail.

At this stage you should contact the committee chairperson to determine the subcommittee(s) to which the bill was referred. You should also secure a list of the members of the committees and subcommittees that have jurisdiction over the bill. If you want to provide input on the contents of the bill or influence the committees' actions, it is the members of the assigned committees and subcommittees that you must contact. Collect as much information as possible on the committee members' anticipated reactions to the bill. You can, for example, check their voting records to determine how they voted on bills similar to the one pending. If similar bills have not been introduced previously, it may be possible to anticipate their reaction on the basis on their past voting record on issues within the same general area, for example, health education, safety legislation, or education research grants. More direct and detailed reaction to the bill may be received by writing, telephoning, or visiting the committee member's office (be sure to make an appointment). In most instances you will not be able to talk to or meet with the committee member; you will be referred to the staff person assigned responsibility for following the bill (this staff person will also respond to your letter). Do not be disappointed by your inability to contact committee members directly because their staff ultimately provide them with a synthesis of public input on the bill and recommend whether the bill should be supported in its current form. In essence, congressional staff are responsible for most of the work related to the analysis and modification of a bill, so close contact with them should be maintained throughout the legislative process.

Public hearings on the bill are scheduled at the subcommittee level. The purpose of the public hearings is to provide a forum for individual citizens and representatives of various organizations to comment on the bill or any of its parts. The length of a hearing can vary from 1 day to several months, depending on the complexity and significance of the bill and the public's interest in it.

The format of hearings is similar—invited witnesses present a brief statement outlining their reactions to the bill, followed by a series of questions directed at them by subcommittee members. However, the question and answer segment often develops into open dialogue involving several sub-committee members and the witness(es). It is important to note that the participation of subcommittee members at hearings varies. During some hearings all subcommittee members attend and actively participate; other hearings may not be of particular interest to some subcommittee members and only a few may attend and participate in the hearings.

At the end of the hearings a transcript of the proceedings is produced. The transcript includes a verbatim account of dialogue during the hearings as well as copies of materials submitted "for the record." Often witnesses submit many materials for the record; thus the hearing's proceedings can be quite lengthy.

The lobbying process intensifies before and during subcommittee hearings. If you want to influence a bill's outcome, numerous opportunities exist during this step of the legislative process. As soon as the bill is referred to a subcommittee, contact the chairperson or his or her staff and request an invitation to appear before the subcommittee as a witness. Subcommittee chairpersons have the authority to select witnesses from a variety of groups, including representatives of federal agencies that are likely to be affected by the bill, members of Congress, experts on the subject matter of the bill, representatives of organizations or businesses potentially affected by the bill, and private citizens. When requesting an invitation be prepared to indicate (1) the organization(s) that you represent, if any, (2) the reason for your interest in the bill, and (3) the general nature of your testimony. If your request is rejected or not acted on by the subcommittee chairperson or his or her staff, contact your representative or senator and ask him or her to approach the chairperson with your request.

If invited to appear before the subcommittee as a witness, you have an excellent opportunity to affect the outcome of the bill, especially if you follow four basic rules. First, keep your testimony short and simple and make only two or three major points related to the bill's content. Second, conclude your testimony with specific, realistic recommendations. If your recommendations are not consistent with the prevailing political atmosphere of Congress they may be ignored or, worse yet, may be detrimental to your cause. Third, provide detailed material for the record in support of your testimony. This material is placed in the proceedings and may affect the subcommittee's members or their staffs, especially if the material is related to the major points of your testimony and is not too voluminous. Finally, be certain to maintain contact with the subcommittee staff and the staff of the subcommittee members. Express a willingness to provide them with additional materials or assist them in whatever capacity they deem appropriate.

The legislative process continues with the "mark-up" subcommittee meetings. During these meetings the bill is reviewed sentence by sentence and provisions of the bill are crossed out and changed to reflect information and analyses developed during the hearing phase. In fact, the subcommittee may refer to the transcripts from the hearings when making changes. Alternative language and amendments to the bill are offered during the mark-up sessions. Staff of both the subcommittee and its members are very involved in this step of the process. When the major points have been resolved the subcommittee votes to send the bill back to the full committee. In some instances the bill sent back to the full committee is similar to the original bill. In other instances, however, the bill sent from the committee is significantly different from the original and is referred to as a "clean bill." When this occurs it is given a new number as it often has few similarities with the original bill.

When the bill is back in the full committee it may be accepted as is or reviewed and revised by the full committee. The chairperson may call for additional hearings or mark-up sessions. Following consideration of all amendments and changes, the committee takes a final vote. The committee may vote to (1) table the bill, thereby leaving it in the committee, (2) send the bill back to the subcommittee for revisions (if sent back to the subcommittee the bill can be stalled), or (3) order the bill reported to the full chamber.

When following a bill through the legislative process, continuous attention should be directed to the voting stage in the subcommittee and the committee. Once the bill is referred to a committee you should begin identifying probable support for the bill at the committee and subcommittee levels. The committee and subcommittee members should be grouped into three categories: those supporting the bill, those opposing the bill, and those undecided. Direct your attention first to those members supporting the bill— never take their continued support for granted. Next, direct your attention to those members who you consider to be undecided. If you cannot reach the members directly, contact their staff. If there are sufficient votes for your position in the committee and the subcommittee, your efforts should be spent trying to maintain that support throughout the entire legislative process. If there are not sufficient votes for your position, direct your attention to those committee and subcommittee members who you believe are not entrenched in their position to opposing the bill. In some instances, however, you may not be able to generate majority support for the bill regardless of the scope and intensity of your lobbying effort.

If the committee orders the bill reported to the full chamber, the committee's report is filed with the administrative office of the chamber. Each report is given a number based on when it was reported to the administrative office; for example, Senate Report No. 97-233 would be the 233rd Senate report in the Ninety-seventh Congress.

If you are following the bill, always obtain a copy of the committee report because it reflects "congressional intent" on the bill, that is, what the committee intended as the objectives and impact of the bill. The report usually includes the background and need for legislation, an explanation of proposed changes if the bill consists of amendments to existing legislation, a detailed analysis of the bill's provisions, reprints of actual changes in the law, and dissenting views of committee members who did not concur with all or part of the bill.

As the bill proceeds through the legislative process, the committee report increases in importance. First, it provides a summary and analysis of the bill and surrounding issues for those members of Congress who were not on the subcommittee or committee but must vote on the legislation. Second, federal agencies use the reports as guidance for promulgating the regulations guiding the implementation of the legislation. Third, if regulations or points of law related to the legislation are disputed in the judicial system, the courts may use the committee report in deciding on the dispute.

Once the legislation is reported to the full chamber it can be debated on the floor of the House or the Senate. However, bills reported to the House are sent to the Rules Committee before reaching the floor for debate. The Rules Committee establishes rules for debate, including the number of minutes that each party is allocated for debating the bill and its amendments.

During floor debate a number of actions are possible. The legislation may be relatively straightforward and noncontroversial and receive little attention, or it may be complex and controversial and generate lengthy and heated debate. In either instance amendments may be offered, debated, and voted on. Once debate is completed, including debate on floor amendments, the House or Senate votes on the entire bill. Three voting options are available: (1) they may vote to pass the bill, (2) they may vote to defeat the bill, or (3) they may vote to recommit the bill to committee.

The lobbying effort continues during the floor debate. Contact should be maintained with committee members supporting the legislation to ensure their continued support. Members of Congress who are believed to support or favorably view the legislation should be contacted and provided with whatever information they request about the legislation. Finally, undecided members should be contacted to secure their commitment to support the legislation. However, it is important to remember that the lobbying process does not begin when the bill reaches the floor for debate, rather; this is the point at which prior lobbying efforts yield a "pay-off."

When both the Senate and House have passed bills on a topic, such as to create a federal health promotion program, the two versions are examined for differences. If few differences exist between the House and Senate versions, one chamber can agree to the other's amendments and the bill will be sent directly to the president. If there are significant differences between the two versions, a conference committee will be formed. Conference committees consist of approximately 12 to 15 representatives from the House and Senate subcommittees that considered the original bills.

The conference committee members, called conferees, consider only those points that differ between the two versions of the bill. Conferees cannot add new material to the bill. In instances in which the bills have differing provisions for levels of funding or the effective period of the legislation, the conferees must reach a compromise that falls within the limits set by the highest and lowest figures of such provisions. If conferees cannot reach a compromise they report back to the House and the Senate for instructions regarding the position they should take. In a few instances, new conferees are appointed.

If the bill is sent to a conference committee, the lobbying effort should continue. Members of the House and Senate subcommittees assigned to the committee should be contacted to discuss how the differing points of the bill can be resolved without compromising the basic intent of the legislation. Specific recommendations may be helpful, especially if they reflect a true compromise between the two versions.

Once agreement has been reached the conference committee prepares a report explaining the recommendations and presenting the conference version of the bill. The conference bill is voted on by both chambers. If either chamber rejects the bill it is returned to the conference committee. If, however, both chambers accept the bill, it is sent to the president.

On receipt of the bill the president has three options. First, he can sign the bill, making it law. Second, he can veto the bill and return it to Congress (without his signature) along with a statement outlining his objections. Congress can override a presidential veto with a two thirds vote of both chambers—always a difficult task. Third, the president can choose to take no action. If he takes no action for 10 days (Sunday excepted), the bill automatically becomes law. However, if Congress adjourns within that 10-day period without the president taking any action, the bill does not become law—an action referred to as a pocket veto.

After the president signs a bill it is assigned a number and subsequently published (see example below). For example, the number 95-626 indicates the Congress (Ninety-fifth) and the sequence in which it was passed (626th bill).

Public Law 95-626
95th Congress

An Act

To amend the Public Health Service Act and related health laws to revise and extend the programs of financial assistance for the delivery of health services, the provision of preventive health services, and for other purposes.

Congressional Committees

In both the House and the Senate a number of committees and subcommittees have jurisdiction over particular health areas. In some instances a bill will have parts that fall within the jurisdiction of two or more committees, thereby resulting in the bill being referred to more than one committee. When this occurs the bill's progress is slower than usual and the effort required to follow and influence the bill's outcome is substantial.

House of Representatives. The House committees and subcommittees that most frequently deal with legislation of interest to health educators are identified and described below.

House Committee on Agriculture. The Committee on Agriculture, with 43 members, has jurisdiction over the following areas: (1) adulteration of seeds, insect pests, and protection of birds and animals in forest reserves, (2) agriculture generally, (3) agricultural and industrial chemistry, (4) agricultural colleges and experiment stations, (5) agricultural economics and research, (6) agricultural education extension services, (7) agricultural production and marketing and stabilization of prices of agricultural products and commoditites, (8) animal industry and diseases of animals, (9) crop insurance and soil conservation, (10) dairy industry, (11) entomology and plant quarantine, (12) extension of farm credit and farm security, (13) forestry in general, and forest reserves other than those created from the public domain, (14) human nutrition and home economics, (15) inspection of livestock and meat products, (16) plant industry, soils, and agricultural engineering, (17) rural electrification, (18) commodities exchanges, and (19) rural development. One important subcommittee is the Subcommittee on Domestic Marketing, Consumer Relations and Nutrition.

House Committee on Appropriations. The Committee on Appropriations, consisting of 55 members, is responsible for appropriation of the revenue for the support of the government. This is one of the most important committees because it determines the amount of funds allocated to support programs within the authorization levels. The most important subcommittee of interest of health educators is the Subcommittee on Labor, Health and Human Services, and Education.

House Committee on Education and Labor. The Committee on Education and Labor, with 34 members, has jurisdiction over the following areas: (1) *measures relating to education and labor generally,* (2) child labor, (3) Columbia Institution for the Deaf, Dumb, and Blind, Howard University, and Freedmen's Hospital, (4) convict labor and the entry of goods made by convicts into interstate commerce, (5) labor standards, (6) labor statistics, (7) mediation and arbitration of labor disputes, (8) regulation or prevention of importation of foreign laborers under contract, (9) *food programs for children in schools,* (10) United States Employees' Compensation Commission, (11) vocational rehabilitation, (12) wages and hours of labor, (13) welfare of minors, and (14) work incentive programs. In addition to its legislative jurisdiction under the preceding provisions, the committee has the special oversight function provided for in clause 3(c) of the Rules on House Committees with respect to *domestic education programs and institutions, and programs of student assistance,* which are within the jurisdiction of other committees. Important subcommittees include the Subcommittee on Elementary, Secondary, and Vocational Education; Subcommittee on Health and Safety; Subcommittee on Human Resources; and Subcommittee on Post Secondary Education.

House Committee on Ways and Means. The Committee on Ways and Means, with 35 members, has jurisdiction over the following areas: (1) customs, collection districts, and ports of entry and delivery, (2) reciprocal trade agreements, (3) revenue measures generally, (4) revenue measures relating to the insular possessions, (5) the bonded debt of the United States, (6) deposit of public moneys, (7) transportation of dutiable goods, (8) tax-exempt foundations and charitable trusts, and (9) *national social security, except for health care and facilities programs that are supported from general revenues as opposed to payroll deductions* and work incentive programs.

House Select Committee on Aging. This committee has as its most important subcommittee the Subcommittee on Health and Long-Term Care. This committee has been especially active in Social Security issues. Its chairman, Rep. Claude D. Pepper (D-Fla.), has become a national spokesman for the elderly in the United States.

House Select Committee on Narcotics Abuse and Control. This House committee deals with narcotics trafficking and attempts to limit the importation and sale of narcotics.

Senate. The committees and subcommittees in the Senate that have jurisdiction over issues of most interest to health educators are identified and described below.

Senate Committee on Agriculture, Nutrition, and Forestry. The Committee on Agriculture, Nutrition, and Forestry comprises 17 senators. This committee receives all proposed legislation, messages, petitions, memorials, and other matters relating primarily to (1) agricultural economics and research, (2) agricultural extension services and experiment stations, (3) agricultural production, marketing, and stabilization of prices, (4) agriculture and agricultural commodities, (5) animal industry and diseases, (6) crop insurance and soil conservation, (7) farm credit and farm security, (8) food from fresh waters, (9) *food stamp programs,* (10) forestry, forest reserves, and wilderness areas other than those created from the public domain, (11) *home economics,* (12) *human nutrition,* (13) inspection of livestock, meat, and agricultural products, (14) pests and pesticides, (15) plant industry, soils, and agricultural engineering, (16) rural development, rural electrification, and watersheds, and (17) *school nutrition programs.*

Senate Committee on Appropriations. The Committee on Appropriations, consisting of 29 senators, receives all proposed legislation, messages, petitions, memorials, and other matters relating to (1) *appropriation of the revenue for the support of the government,* (2) recision of appropriations contained in appropriation acts, and (3) *spending authority.*

Senate Committee on Labor and Human Resources. The Committee on Labor and Human Resources comprises 16 senators. This committee receives all proposed legislation, messages, petitions, memorials, and other matters relating to (1) *measures relating to education, labor, health, and public welfare,* (2) *aging,* (3) agricultural colleges, (4) arts and humanities, (5) *biomedical research and development,* (6) child labor, (7) convict labor and the entry of goods made by convicts into interstate commerce, (8) *domestic activities of the American National Red Cross,* (9) equal employment opportunity, (10) Gallaudet College, Howard University, and Saint Elizabeth's Hospital, (11) *handicapped individuals,* (12) labor standards and labor statistics, (13) mediation and arbitration of labor disputes, (14) *occupational safety and health, including the welfare of miners,* (15) private pension plans, (16) public health, (17) railway labor and retirement, (18) regulation of foreign laborers, (19) student loans, (20) wages and hours of labor, and (21) matters relating to health, education and training, and public welfare, which the committee reviews and reports on periodically.

Senate Special Committee on Aging. The Special Committee on Aging, consisting of 15 senators, has the following responsibilities. First, *to conduct a continuing study of any and all matters pertaining to problems and opportunities of older people,* including but not limited to problems and opportunities of maintaining health, of assuring adequate income, of finding employment, of engaging in productive and rewarding activity, of securing proper housing, and when necessary, of obtaining care of assistance. No proposed legislation is referred to this committee, and the committee does not have power to report by bill or otherwise have legislative jurisdiction. Second, from time to time (but not less often than once each year), the committee must report to the Senate the results of the study conducted along with recommendations the committee considers appropriate.

The Appropriations Process

The process of providing operating funds for federal programs is referred to as the appropriations process. The process lasts between 18 and 24 months and involves the House, the Senate, and the executive branch. It culminates in the passage of an appropriations bill providing the various federal departments and agencies with funds to operate their programs for the specified fiscal year (a fiscal year begins October 1 and ends September 30).

Fig. 6-2 outlines the steps in the appropriations process in terms of the passage of an appropriations bill for Fiscal Year (FY) 1985 (October 1, 1984, to September 30, 1985). To add clarity to the explanation, the process is described in terms of its effects on one program unit, in this case the Office of Disease Prevention and Health Promotion (OHPHP), for FY 1985.

The ODPHP lies within the Office of the Assistant Secretary for Health (OASH) and provides leadership for the DHHS disease prevention and health promotion initiatives. OASH has two operating units: the Office of Health Information, Health Promotion, and Physical Fitness and Sports Medicine (OHP) and the Nutrition Coordinating Office (NCO). Fig. 6-3 depicts the position of the ODPHP within the DHHS.

The FY 1985 appropriations process for the ODPHP starts in November 1982. During November the director of the ODPHP meets with his or her staff to discuss the office's program priorities. The discussion includes an examination, on a line-by-line basis, of the office's budget. From these discussions a preliminary plan of program activities for FY 1985 emerges.

Concurrent with this process are discussions within OASH. Program priorities that are established at this level are used by the program units, such as the ODPHP, to narrow their program focus. The program plans are revised and shared with selected persons throughout the Public Health Service (PHS). This phase of the planning process usually lasts through the end of December and is characterized by proposing program options, seeking and receiving feedback, and revising the program plan. By January 1983

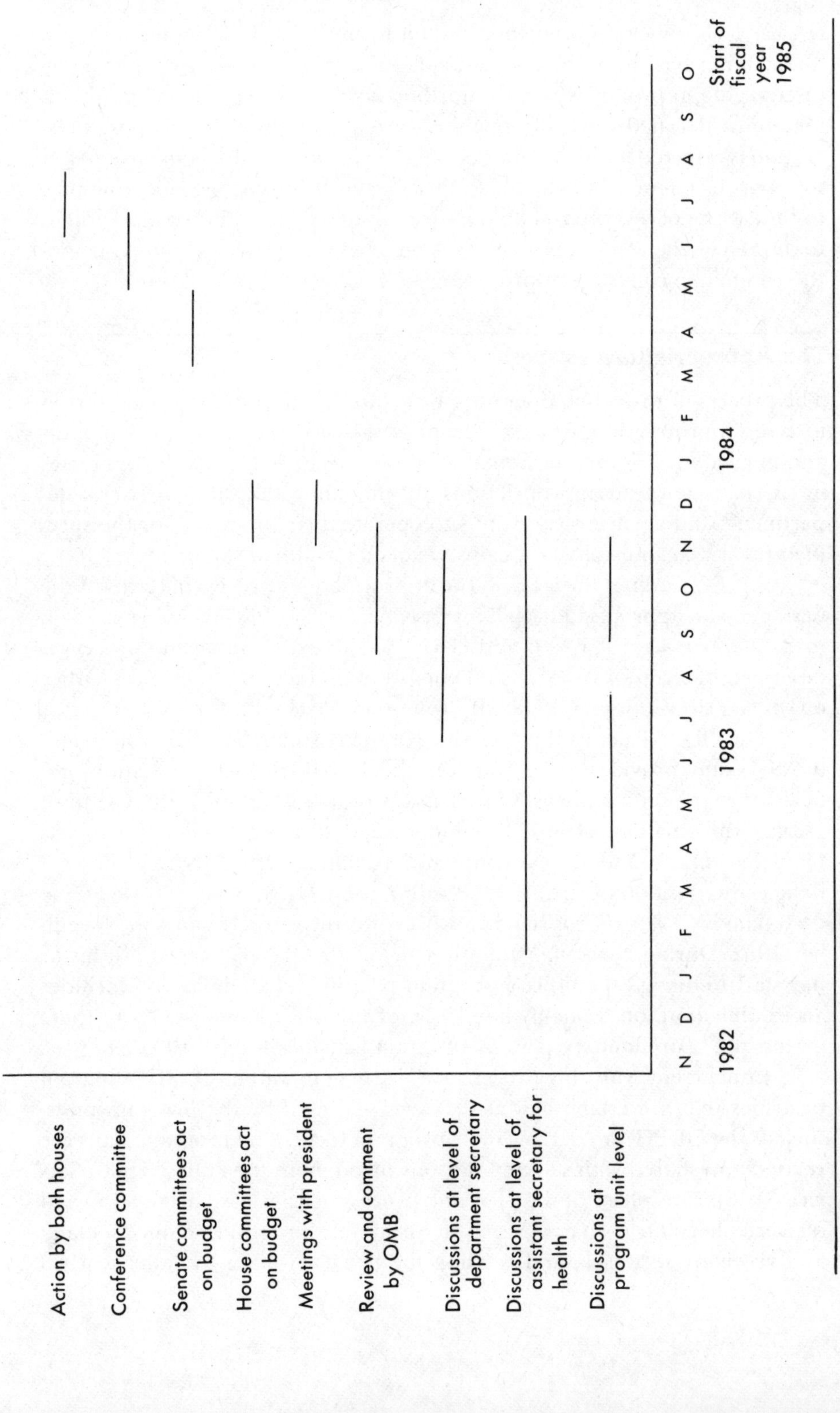

Fig. 6-2. Steps in the appropriations process for passage of the Fiscal Year 1985 budget.

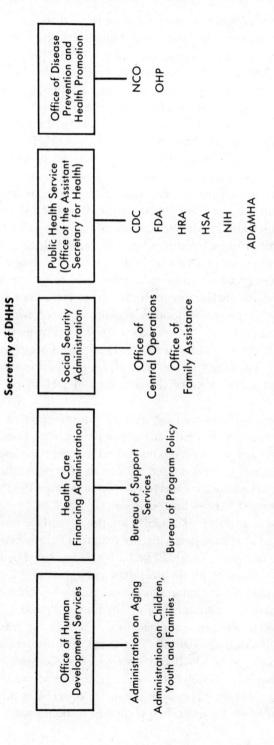

Fig. 6-3. Simplified organization table of the Department of Health and Human Services. *CDC,* Centers for Disease Control; *FDA,* Food and Drug Administration; *HRA,* Health Resources Administration, *HSA,* Health Services Administration; *NIH,* National Institutes of Health; *ADAMHA,* Alcohol, Drug Abuse and Mental Health Administration; *NCO,* Nutrition Coordinating Office; *OHP,* Office of Health Information, Health Promotion, and Physical Fitness and Sports Medicine.

the priorities of the assistant secretary for health are more specific and ordered. Using the assistant secretary for health's program priorities and feedback on the preliminary program plan, the ODPHP program plan for FY 1985 is revised. The program activities are listed in order of priority and estimates of the funds necessary for each activity are made. This phase of the process ends with the delivery of an ODPHP program budget to the Office of the Assistant Secretary for Health by mid-April 1983.

The next phase of the process primarily involves OASH. The proposed program unit budgets, including ODPHP, are reviewed by OASH staff to determine the extent of congruency with the assistant secretary's priorities. In addition, the budget estimates are examined on an activity-by-activity basis. The reviews are usually completed by the end of May, and in June the Assistant Secretary and his or her staff meet individually with directors of the program units to resolve differences identified during the review process. The differences in program or budget focus are resolved through a negotiating process in which there is a great deal of compromise. The program unit review usually lasts through the end of December and is characterized by proposing program options, seeking and receiving feedback, and revising the program plan. By January 1983 the priorities of the Assistant Secretary for Health are more specific and ordered. Using OASH plans, budgets are revised, assembled by OASH staff, and submitted in the form of the PHS budget to the office of the secretary of DHHS no later than August 1.

The PHS budget is reviewed by staff of the secretary of DHHS to determine its consistency with the department's program and budget priorities. Budget changes are noted on the budget tables and these are returned to OASH. A negotiation process is used to resolve differences between the proposed and the marked budgets and by the end of August 1983 the DHHS department's proposed FY 1985 budget is sent to OMB.

The budget sent to OMB is actually a large bound book containing hundreds of pages of narrative justifying the program priorities and dozens of tables containing budget estimates. The budget is reviewed by OMB staff to determine its congruency with the president's program and fiscal intents. This review also includes an examination of all previous alterations in the budget (this information is contained within the budget tables). Changes are noted on the budget tables and returned to the DHHS for transmittal to the program units, including ODPHP. The program units can appeal the budget changes proposed by OMB if a strong justification can be written. The appeal sequence is as follows: from program unit, to OASH, to the DHHS, and finally to OMB. The appeal can be rejected at any of these levels. The usual process, however, is for appeals to be decided within the department, with only the strongest appeals being forwarded to OMB. OMB considers the appeals and returns to the department a final, marked version of the budget tables. This process is usually completed by the end of October.

During November the department has another opportunity to influence the budget. The president meets individually with department secretaries to review their budgets, often on a line-by-line basis. The secretaries are selective in their appeals, only arguing for changes in areas that are of highest personal concern. On completion of this phase of the budget process OMB assembles the president's budget and sends it to the Government Printing Office. To meet congressional time schedules this must occur by the third week of December.

To date, the appropriations process has taken 13 months. During these months the discussions have been within the executive branch (within the DHHS and with OMB), with no opportunities provided for input from the public.

Sometime around the third week of January (1984) the president's FY 1985 budget is delivered to Congress (in the form of a book). Protocol dictates that the budget be delivered to the Speaker of the House and the president of the Senate (who is the vice-president of the United States). The budget is referred to the committees that have legislative jurisdiction in specific budget areas and to the appropriations committees. The committees refer individual sections of the budget to the appropriate subcommittees, where the detailed budget analysis occurs.

Although both the House and the Senate receive the president's budget, it is the House that takes the lead in analyzing the budget's components. Subcommittees of the House Appropriations Committee schedule hearings, starting in mid-Febuary (1984). The hearings are opened by the secretary of the DHHS, who presents and testifies on the DHHS budget. Following this review of the entire budget, the subcommittee initiates a detailed examination of the budget's components, for example, the Health Care Financing Administration and the PHS. The subcommittees often request that DHHS officials with responsibility in specific areas, such as disease prevention and health promotion, appear before the subcommittees to testify.

At this point the appropriations process the public has an opportunity for input. The methods of public input are similar to those described in the preceding section of this chapter, that is, testifying before subcommittees or providing written material for the record. After testimony by department officials and the public, the subcommittees hold mark-up sessions, during which the DHHS budget is reviewed and changes noted on a line-by-line basis. The marked-up version of the budget is then sent back to the DHHS and OMB (however, OMB is not usually directly involved in this phase of the appropriations process).

On receiving the subcommittees' marked-up versions of the budget, the department reviews them to ascertain probable effects on its programs. This analysis is conducted at the program unit level (ODPHP) and at the level of OASH. Staff in the office of the secretary of the DHHS synthesize responses from the various program units and send a department response to the appropriations subcommittees (a copy is also sent to OMB). This document is referred to as the "effects statement" because it contains the department's description of probable program effects if the proposed budget cuts are maintained. A low-key, semiformal negotiation process now ensues between representatives from the subcommittees and the department, culminating in the drafting of subcommittee reports outlining the House actions that are recommended. The subcommittee reports are submitted to the Appropriations Committee and are usually accepted as written. However, the Appropriations Committee may decide to go into a mark-up session to make additional budget changes. If the department is dissatisfied with a subcommittee report it can appeal directly to the Appropriations Committee. When this occurs the appeal is usually based on the department's belief that the subcommittee did not pay sufficient attention to the effects statement or to a portion therein. Ultimately, the Appropriations Committee issues a formal report for consideration of the report by the full House. Substantive changes are seldom made when the report is on the floor for debate. After acting on amendments initiated during floor debate, the Appropriations Committee's report is accepted by the House and issued as a House report around mid-May (1984).

Although the Senate receives the President's budget in late January, it seldom takes action on it before March. There are two primary reasons for the delay in Senate action. First, the House is the legislative body that historically has assumed responsibility for conducting a detailed review of the president's budget. This review is time-consuming and therefore is initiated at the earliest possible date. Second, the Senate's review of the president's budget is more limited than the review by the House. Senators tend to focus on those aspects of the budget that are of personal interest to them. For example, Senator Mark Hatfield (R-Ore.) is personally interested in school health programs; thus a significant portion of his participation at the Appropriations hearings has focused on DHHS involvement with school health programs. The illustration of differences between the review processes of the House and the Senate are not intended to be a criticism of either process. Rather, the differences in budget review reflect the differences in the overall working styles of the two bodies; that is, the House tends to focus on the specifics of an issue and the Senate tends to focus on the issue as an entirety, including its interaction with other federal issues.

From early March through mid-August (1984) the Senate Appropriations Committee and its subcommittees hold hearings on the president's FY 1985 budget. DHHS officials have an opportunity to testify during the hearings and this opportunity becomes especially important if the House has made budget cuts that department officials believe will have an adverse effect on their programs. In cases in which the House has made significant budget cuts, the department often tries to convince the Senate of the need to fund the programs at the DHHS-proposed levels. The basis of this debate is the effects statement document prepared during the House hearings that describes the specific effects on the department's programs if the House budget cuts are maintained. Representatives of various professional organizations and associations and other interested parties may also be invited to testify or submit material for the record. On completion of the hearings the Appropriations Committee submits a report to the full Senate for consideration and action. Sometime around mid-May (1984) the Senate passes its version of the Appropriations bill.

Because the House and Senate versions of the budget seldom agree, the two versions are sent to a conference committee, which resolves differences. The conference committee's report is then sent back to the House and Senate for action. If the report is accepted by both the House and the Senate it becomes the Appropriations Bill for Fiscal Year 1985. Ideally, this process is completed before the end of June (1984). However, because the 1985 fiscal year starts on October 1, 1984, the bill must be passed on or before September 30, 1984. If it is not passed by that date a continuing resolution is passed, allowing the federal government to continue to operate pending passage of an appropriations bill.

Assuming the steps in the appropriations process have been completed within the time frame depicted in Fig. 6-2, a total of 22 months have passed (November 1982 to June 1984) since work on the FY 1985 budget was initiated. During the first steps of the process (November 1982 to January 1983) the preparation of the budget has been within the federal government, with virtually no opportunity for participation by the public. However, once the president's budget has been delivered to the House and the Senate the opportunities for public input as they were described in the legislative process section of this chapter apply. Specifically, you can influence the appropriations process by (1) contacting representatives and senators (or their staff) who serve on appropriations-related committees and subcommittees, and (2) testifying before those committees and subcommittees or providing them with written material for placement in the record.

Finally, it is important to note that the appropriations process is affected by two other concurrent processes. First, the House and Senate committees review existing legislation or introduce new legislation as the appropriations process is taking place. These committees, such as the Senate Committee on Labor and Human Resources, set funding limits for the various programs; that is, they authorize the amount of money that can be appropriated to a program. The appropriations bill cannot designate more funds for a program than are authorized. Second, Congress engages in a process known as the reconciliation process, which is designed to control spending by the federal government. Twice a year, May 15 and September 15, Congress determines the total amount of money that can be appropriated for federal programs. In addition to the total amount of money that can be appropriated, spending ceilings are established for 14 subject areas, such as defense. Managing the reconciliation process is the responsibility of the budget committees in the House and the Senate.

The legislative and appropriations processes provide the authorization and funding for federally sponsored programs. If you want to influence the program sponsored by the federal government or the distribution of funds between and within the various federal departments, it is these two processes with which you must become involved.

EDITORS' NOTE: Proposal writing is a skill that is required of many health educators. A detailed description of grantsmanship can be found in the special edition of *Health Education*, 1978. Also see Jerry Lafferty, Suggestions and Guidelines For Effective Proposal Writing in Health Education, *Eta Sigma Gamman* 13(1), 1981.

The Regulatory Process

The regulatory process differs from the legislative and appropriations processes because it is almost totally within the domain of the executive branch of government. In rare cases, Congress specifically directs the executive branch to develop regulations; usually, however, the initiative to develop regulations is taken by the executive branch. Further, although Congress has the authority to veto regulations proposed by the executive branch, they rarely consider taking such action.

The executive branch is given responsibility for implementing legislation after it has been passed by Congress. In some instances the implementation is rather straightforward and regulations are not required. However, when legislation is complex, regulations are often necessary to ensure proper and complete implementation. In a general sense regulations define the parameters of legislation but subjectively are involved in the interpretation of congressional intent of the legislation, that is, what Congress hoped the legislation would accomplish. Differences in interpretation of congressional intent often slow the process of developing regulations.

Although the specific procedures of developing regulations may differ between federal departments, the general steps taken to develop regulations are similar. To help you understand the process of developing regulations a hypothetical example will be used. Let us assume that legislation has been passed that directs the DHHS, and specifically the OHP, to provide technical and financial assistance to local school districts to develop school health service programs. The legislation also includes language specifying that provision of health services for preschool and elementary school children from low-income families be a priority.

The first step in the regulations development process is a review of the legislation by the OHP staff. Following their review a plan is written, describing how the legislation is to be implemented. If the OHP staff believe regulations are necessary, they state so in the plan and set a timetable for their development. The implementation plan is sent to OASH for review and comment. The plan is then returned, with comments, to the OHP, where program specifications are developed. During this phase of the process the OHP staff try to ensure that the program specifications are consistent with the legislative intent as well as with the priorities and policies of the Administration.

The draft version of the program specifications is then sent to the Regulations Office (within the PHS). Staff of this office review and revise the program specifications and return them to the OHP. Later, staff of the OHP and the Regulations Office rewrite the program specifications into a regulatory format, using regulatory language. This document is now referred to as a *Notice of Proposed Rule Making* and is reviewed by interested parties within PHS. The review comments are assembled and the *Final Notice of Proposed Rule Making* is written.

The next step in the regulatory process involves informing the public of the proposed regulations and soliciting reactions from them. The proposed regulations are published in the *Federal Register,* along with instructions concerning where comments are to be sent and by what date they are to be recieved. The usual practice is to allow 60 days for the review and comment period. At the end of this period the OHP staff review the public's comments and make whatever changes they believe are appropriate. Final regulations are then drafted, along with a preamble to the regulations that includes a synthesis of the public's comments and the resolution of the comments. The final draft is reviewed by interested persons within the PHS before its publication and distribution.

While the final review process is occurring, staff of the OHP prepare a second document that provides clarity to the most complex regulations. This is often referred to as a program guideline document and is designed to assist persons in interpreting the regulations. The program guideline document is not reviewed by staff outside the OHP and is not a legal document. In situations in which the two documents appear to differ, always consider the *Final Regulations* as the document of authority.

Federal Departments and Agencies

The myriad disease prevention and health promotion activities directly or indirectly supported by the federal government virtually defy identification and description. Yet the products of these activities—education materials, research reports, program activity reports, and bibliographies—are probably useful to health educators and others working in the health promotion field. The difficulty facing professionals in disease prevention and health promotion activities is twofold: How does one find out what the various federal departments and agencies are supporting, and how does one get the products from the various federally sponsored activities?

Before outlining the steps necessary to secure information or products, two points are worthy of mention. First, all products produced from federally sponsored activities are within the public domain (unless the products have been classified for national security reasons). Simply, this means that you have a legal right to them. Certain products may be distributed free of charge (such as brochures); some may be sold through the Superintendent of Documents, the National Technical Information Service, or some other outlet (as in the case of research reports and data tapes); and some may have been produced in such limited quantity that none are available for distribution (in this instance you may ask that the document be copied or make arrangements to have it copied). In a few instances, the office or agency may refuse to send you a requested product. If this occurs you can request it through the Freedom of Information Act (the request should go to the Public Affairs Office of the specific department with a copy sent to your senator's or representative's office).

Second, always be specific in your request for a product. Tens of thousands of documents and other products are produced each year as a result of federally sponsored activities. Therefore if your request is not specific there is a good possibility that you will not receive the document you want. Whenever possible your request should include the title of the document (or other product), the office or agency that provided support for the activity, the year the document was completed, and the publication number (if one exists). Although it is not always possible to be this specific in your request, you should make every attempt to provide as much of the above information as you possibly can.

Although the two questions posed are interrelated, for clarity they will be addressed separately. The first question is How does one find out what disease prevention and health promotion program activities the various federal offices and agencies are supporting? The following steps will assist you in securing the information that you desire.

- Write to the offices and agencies identified in this section and others that are of particular interest to you and request (1) a copy of the office's annual report (this report may go to Congress or the office of the Secretary of the department), (2) a list of the office's staff and their areas of responsibility (this is not always available), and (3) copies of office publications that describe current activities. To get the offices' addresses you have four options (listed in priority order): (1) ask the government documents librarian at your local university or college for directories or other documents that contain listings of federal departments, agencies and offices, (2) write the Public Information Office of each of the federal departments and ask for the addresses and telephone numbers of the offices and agencies identified in your letter, (3) contact your representative (at his or her office) and solicit their assistance in securing the addresses and telephone numbers of the federal offices and agencies that you have identified, or (4) write the office or agency using the most complete address that you have (for example, Center for Health Promotion and Education, Centers for Disease Control, Atlanta, Ga.).
- Go to the government documents section of your local university or college library and ask for copies of the appropriations (House and Senate) hearings from the previous year. Be certain to get the relevant subcommittee reports identified in the major report. If your library does not have copies of these reports they can probably be secured through your representative or senator or through the House and Senate Appropriations Committees.*
- Identify the agency or office that appears to be most involved in your particular area of interest (for example, community health education and risk reduction programs would involve the Center for Health Promotion and Education at the Centers for Disease Control). Contact the office (by telephone or letter) and request the specific information you need. In most instances your letter will be answered by staff of the office within 2 to 3 weeks. On receipt of the letter, assess

---

*Their addresses are House Committee on Appropriations, Capitol, Room H-218, Washington, D.C., 20515; Senate Committee on Appropriations, Capitol, Room S-130, Washington, D.C., 20510.

the completeness and appropriateness of the information contained within the letter. If you need or want additional information make a list of the specific questions you want answered. Then telephone the person who answered the letter, thank him or her for the response, and request assistance with the additional questions. In most instances the agency representative will try to be helpful. If they refer you to other persons be sure to get their full names, office affiliations, addresses, and telephone numbers. Once you have made direct contact with persons who have access to the type of information you need make every attempt to retain the contacts (by means of telephone calls or letters). Also, if you are visiting the Washington, D.C., area, contact these persons and arrange for appointments to discuss specific questions or your general information needs. If your requests remain reasonable and intermittent these contacts will probably develop into your best single source for information.

The second question posed was How does one get the products from the various federally sponsored activities? The following steps will assist you in securing these products.

- Write the office or agency that sponsored the activity and request a copy of the product (for example, a document) or information on how it can be secured. Be as specific as possible in your request. Your request should include (1) the name of the product (for example, Guidelines for Health Promotion Activities at the Worksite), (2) the name(s) of the author(s), (3) the publication number (if appropriate), and (4) the year in which it was produced.
- If your request is general (for example, information on diabetes), start by contacting the National Health Information Clearinghouse (1-800-336-4797). This clearinghouse serves as a switchboard for other federal information centers, so your request will be relayed to the most appropriate federal agencies. In addition, the National Health Information Clearinghouse will send you whatever relevant and available material it has.

The federal departments and agencies sponsoring disease prevention and health promotion activities are identified below, along with the offices responsible for directing these activities.

Department of Health and Human Services (DHHS)

The vast majority of disease prevention and health promotion activites of the DHHS are sponsored by the PHS. The PHS, which is directed by the assistant secretary for health, has seven functional units (listed below). Numerous prevention-related research, health services, and health education activities are directed or funded by offices and agencies within these seven units. These units and their offices and agencies that are most involved in disease prevention and health promotion activities are listed, along with selected program units located within OASH.

Office of the Assistant Secretary for Health (OASH)
National Center for Health Statistics (NCHS)
Office of Adolescent Pregnancy Programs (OAPP)
Office of Disease Prevention and Health Promotion (ODPHP)
Office of Health Information, Health Promotion, and Physical Fitness
    and Sports Medicine (OHP)
Office of Health Maintenance Organizations (OHMO)
Office on Smoking and Health (OSH)
President's Council on Physical Fitness and Sports (PCPFS)
Centers for Disease Control (CDC)
Center for Health Promotion and Education (CHPE)
Center for Infectious Diseases (CID)
Center for Prevention Services (CPS)
National Institute for Occupational Safety and Health (NIOSH)
Food and Drug Administration (FDA)
Bureau of Drugs (BD)
Bureau of Foods (BF
Bureau of Radiologic Health (BRH)
Health Resources Administration (HRA)
Bureau of Health Planning (BHP)
Bureau of Health Professions (BHPr)
Health Services Administration (HSA)
Bureau of Community Health Services (BCHS)
Bureau of Health Personnel Development and Service (BHPDS)
Indian Health Service (IHS)
Alcohol, Drug Abuse and Mental Health Administration (ADAMHA)
Division of Prevention
National Institute of Alcohol Abuse and Alcoholism (NIAAA)
National Institute of Drug Abuse (NIDA)
National Institute on Mental Health (NIMH)
National Institutes of Health (NIH)
National Cancer Institute (NCI)*
National Heart, Lung and Blood Institute (NHLBI)*
National Library of Medicine (NLM)

---

*Legislative mandate to conduct education activities.

National Institute of Allergy and Infectious Diseases (NIAID)

National Institute of Child Health and Human Development (NICHHD)

National Institute of Dental Research (NIDR)

Department of Education (ED)

The Department of Education is in a state of transition; thus it is difficult to assess its future involvement in disease prevention and health promotion activities. The Alcohol and Drug Education Program is the office most directly involved in health promotion activities. However, the Department of Education is also involved in health-related activities in such areas as adolescent pregnancy, parent education, diffusion of exemplary education programs, education for the handicapped, consumer and homemaking education, and migrant education.

Department of Agriculture (USDA)

The prevention-related programs administered by the USDA include food and nutrition programs directed to needy infants, children, pregnant women, mothers, elderly persons, and other low-income persons; nutrition education programs, nutrition research, food quality and safety programs; pollution control and abatement; and other environmental protection programs.

The majority of the prevention-related programs are administered by the Extension Service and the Food and Nutrition Service. The Extension Service is the chief educational arm of the USDA and sponsors programs on such areas as nutrition education, meal planning and food selection, prevention of illness, use of available health services and facilities, and safety education. The Food and Nutrition Service administers the following food assistance programs to the needy in cooperation with state and local governments: food stamp programs, child nutrition programs (such as the National School Lunch Program, School Breakfast Program and Special Milk Program), and the special supplement food program for women, infants, and children (WIC).

Department of Commerce (DoC)

The major prevention-related activities of the DoC focus on the monitoring, prediction, control, and abatement of marine and atmospheric pollution.

Department of Defense (DoD)

The Office of the Assistant Secretary of Defense for Health Affairs is responsible for planning and administering the health activities of the DoD, including care and treatment of patients, nutrition programs, drug and alcohol abuse programs, and health personnel education and training.

Department of Labor (DoL)

The Occupational Safety and Health Administration (OSHA) and the Mine Safety and Health Administration (MSHA) within the DoL administer a variety of prevention-related programs, including the development, promulgation, and enforcement of health and safety standards and education and training programs.

Department of Transportation (DoT)

The DoT plays a lead role in highway safety and motor carrier safety by means of its research, demonstration, and education programs. The National Highway Traffic Safety Administration (NHTSA) administers the motor vehicle standards program, the motor vehicle consumer information program, traffic safety programs, drinking driver programs, and emergency medical service programs.

Consumer Product Safety Commission (CPSC)

The CPSC functions as a regulatory agency to (1) protect the public against unreasonable risk of injury associated with consumer products, (2) assist consumers in evaluating the comparative safety of consumer products, (3) develop uniform safety standards for consumer products, and (4) promote research and investigation into the cause and prevention of product-related deaths, illnesses, and injuries. It also sponsors education and information activities designed to reduce injuries by raising public awareness about product safety.

Environmental Protection Agency (EPA)

The EPA's primary responsibilities are in pollution abatement and control and enforcement of antipollution laws and regulations. The EPA also conducts research and development programs to provide a strong scientific basis for the development of standards and effective control measures.

Federal Trade Commission (FTC)

The FTC's major prevention-related functions include (1) prevention of the dissemination of false or deceptive advertisements of consumer products, (2) regulation of packaging and labeling of certain consumer commodities used in the home as well as certain foods, and (3) regulation of cigarette advertising.

National Academy of Sciences (NAS)

The NAS serves in the capacity of an official adviser, on request, to the federal government. No federal funds are appropriated directly to the academy; the principal funding mechanism is the negotiation of contracts with federal agencies. The NAS comprises the National Research Council, the National Academy of Engineering, and the Institute of Medicine. A variety of prevention-related activities are sponsored by the NAS in such areas as child development, substance abuse, habitual behavior, radiation effects, and nutrition.

The American National Red Cross

The Red Cross is the official disaster relief agency of the United States. However, it also offers a variety of prevention-related services to the public, including nursing and health programs that sponsor classes in home nursing, mother's aide, and mother and baby care; safety programs that sponsor courses in first aid, small craft operation, swimming, and water safety; and Red Cross Youth Service Programs in health and safety.

Editors' Remarks

Dr. Iverson has explained and delineated the role of the federal government in the legislative, appropriations, and regulatory processes. As you might imagine, influencing that level of government is not an easy task. It would seem that we would be able to exert more influence closer to home, that is, at the state and local levels. We will attempt to describe some specific ways health educators can influence funding of health education at both the local and state levels.

Community Health Education and Block Grants

After President Reagan took office in January 1981 he announced that he intended to shift administrative and decision-making authority regarding health programs from the federal to state governments. Although federal aid to cities, counties, and other jurisdictions has in the past been transmitted through specific categoric funds and block grants, the new proposal included many human service programs that were consolidated into grants for social service, community development, education, and health through the Federal Omnibus Reconciliation Act of 1981. Block grants have five features that distinguish them from other forms of federal assistance:

1. They authorize funds for a wide range of activities within a broadly defined functional area.
2. They give recipients substantial discretion in identifying problems, designing programs, and allocating resources.
3. They minimize administrative, fiscal reporting, planning, and other federally imposed requirements.
4. They distribute aid by statutory formula, narrowing federal discretion, and offering a sense of fiscal certainty to recipients.
5. They favor general purpose governments as recipients and elected officials as decision makers.

Nine block grants were created from 57 categoric health programs. Although state and local jurisdictions will have authority for these block grants, the funding level has been drastically reduced; therefore all proponents of these human service programs are finding that they must oppose each other to maintain their funding levels. Of these nine block grants, prevention (preventive services) will receive the smallest amount of funding. The prevention block grant consolidated seven categoric programs: hypertension, fluoridation, rat control, health education, risk reduction, comprehensive public health services, and emergency medical services. In addition, a new program for rape prevention was established.

There are several strategies for health educators to initiate concerning the block grant process, funding, and jurisdiction, at both the state and the local levels:

1. Monitor very closely where the funding is going.
2. Let your congressional representatives know where you stand on that funding.
3. Write or call your local health authorities to inform them of the necessity and importance of preventive activities.

4. Apply for funding if you are in a position to do so.
5. Attend the public hearings that are held regarding preventive services and make your views known.
6. Organize a consortium of concerned health educators to act as a local and state lobbying body.

School Health Education and Comprehensive Programs

School health educators would appear to have an advantage over other health workers because they have a captive audience: children 16 years of age and younger must attend school. Although school attendance is compulsory, the teaching of health education is not in most schools throughout the United States.

ASHA completed a survey to determine the status of state-level school health programs in 1978. They found that five states (Florida, Illinois, New York, South Carolina, and Virginia) had legislation requiring comprehensive school health education programs. These states specified content areas and indicated the grade levels at which specific content should be taught. Thirteen additional states had general laws requiring health education but did not specify grade level or content area. Furthermore, five states either had no requirements for health education or had no program in existence.

Health educators would agree that a comprehensive school health education program would be the most beneficial for students, parents, and society. If this is an accepted truth, then why does the present situation exist? A review of an attempt to install a comprehensive health education program in Illinois schools (Creswell and Janeway, 1974) should serve as a model for state and local action to create and implement public policy.

The Illinois Joint Committee on School Health decided in March 1969 to press for legislation that would mandate comprehensive health education in all of the public and secondary schools in Illinois. The committee's officers began a series of meetings with state officials to draft the new legislation. The two chief officers, the state superintendent of public instruction and the director of the Department of Public Health, gave their support to the proposed legislation.

The bill was passed by the state legislature with changes concerning appropriations and teacher certification. In essence, the act was made a law; however, there was no funding to implement the comprehensive health education program. An undaunted Health Education Advisory Committee was appointed as provided for in the act. This committee of 11 was authorized to promulgate rules and regulations in order to implement the provisions of the act. The committee secured a legal interpretation of the new law to determine the relationship of the Comprehensive Health Education Act to older sections of the code specifically related to health, physical education, and training. Furthermore, the committee developed guideline statements that served as the basis for the rules and regulation of the act.

A major and important focus on the Illinois act was that it provided for the establishment of "the minimum amount of instruction time to be devoted to health education," and to establish guidelines for implementation for local school districts. These guidelines were eventually distributed to all schools in Illinois, with the request that each school respond and submit their implementation plans for health education instruction by January 1974. In addition, the Illinois teacher certification board established the Standard High School Certificate for all secondary school teachers, which required a 32-hour major in health education.

These developmental, legislative, and implementation steps for a comprehensive school health education program could only be accomplished through a coordinated effort of professionals, school personnel and administrators, public health officials, and the lay public. The Illinois Comprehensive Health Education Act was several years in the planning and developing stages and became a model for local and state constituencies to emulate. Professionals can be influential!

Summary

Chapter 3, on health promotion, demonstrated the fact that the federal government can have a tremendous influence on health education. It provides funding for manpower training, demonstration projects, and research. It also represents a potential source of employment for hundreds of health educators. In chapter 4, on competencies, we learned that the Role Delineation Project outlines the broad areas of responsibility for health educators regardless of job setting. These skills relate largely to the teaching-learning process, in other words, planning, implementing, and evaluating education programs. Chapter 4 also described the status of health education in relation to its pursuit of professional status and public recognition.

This chapter encourages the reader to consider the potential impact from efforts directed at the federal government. If health education is going to achieve greater public recognition it might begin with the federal government. Current funding for health education represents less than 1¢ of every dollar spent by the government on health. Research and demonstration projects can show the effectiveness of health education, but it seems as though we have always suffered from the "chicken and egg" dilemma. We need money to demonstrate our worth, but the money is not forthcoming until we have demonstrated our worth.

Health education needs to take a more active role in influencing the legislative, appropriations, and regulatory processes. We need to understand how to become advocates for federal programming. There are, of course, advocates for primary prevention who already exist within the Congress and the executive branch of government. But so far we have not used our talents, our time, or our resources in assertive ways to nurture a greater recognition of health education. Perhaps it is possible to mount an effective campaign that exploits our enthusiasm and our commitment to primary prevention. If so, it wll depend on those among us who understand the most productive ways to intervene to be able to gain access to the resources of the federal government.

Questions for Review

1. What legislative bills important to health and education are pending (or have been recently passed) by your state legislature?
2. What is the viewpoint of your congressional representatives toward legislation that affects health education?
3. What is the process for legislation, appropriations, and regulations in your state?
4. Which regulations presented in the *Federal Register* during the past 6 months do you consider to be the most important to health education?
5. How has the most recent presidential election affected the health and social service programs supported by the federal government?
6. What are the major responsibilities of each federal agency listed in the chapter?

Additional Readings

Castill, A., and Jerrick, S.: School health in America, Kent, Ohio, 1979, American School Health Association.

Creswell, W., and Janeway, T.: A comprehensive health education program for Illinois schools, Journal of School Health **14**(6):336-339, 1974.

Davis, K.: Reagan health administration policy, Journal of Public Policy **2**(4):312-332, 1981.

Green, L.: Determining the impact and effectiveness of health education as it relates to federal policy, Health Education Monographs **6**(suppl. 1):28-66, 1978.

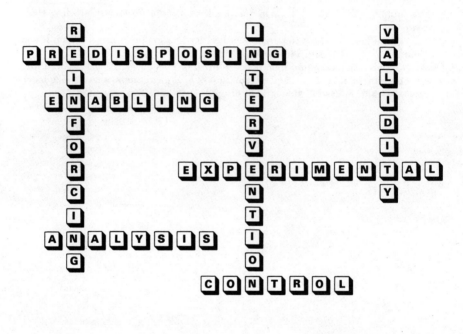

7 Research and Evaluation

Introduction

This chapter introduces some dilemmas, concepts, and approaches to research and evaluation that have particular use in health education. Accountability in the practice of health education should lead the conscientious health educator to approach each program as an experiment. As in a laboratory experiment, the results of an educational program represent the effects or outcomes of an experimental manipulation. If the effect is found, the hypothesis is confirmed and the educational, behavioral, or administrative diagnosis is verified.

Several designs for evaluation are described in simple steps in this chapter, and numerous examples of each are cited in the references. This brief introduction to evaluation and the references cited can serve as springboards for further study of evaluation methods.

The five levels of evaluation begin with the simple record-keeping approach, in which routinely collected data are accumulated and tabulated periodically to show progress toward or achievement of expected goals. In the second level the evaluator does not depend on routinely collected data but instead carries out special surveys periodically. Both of these approaches provide historical comparisons. In the remaining levels of evaluation design one or more comparison groups are added, either in another population receiving a similar program or in the same population (comparing those who receive the health education with those who do not). These last two designs are considered the strongest for scientific purposes, but the "lower-level" designs are adequate and necessary for routine evaluation when the purpose is accountability rather than research.

Dilemmas in Planning and Evaluation of Health Education*

The first part of this chapter will identify some problems peculiar to health education and will emphasize the needs for research and evaluation unique to health education. Because the research methods and evaluation results in related fields of behavioral sciences, marketing, education, epidemiology, and administration are not directly or fully applicable to health education or health promotion, seven dilemmas of this nature will be discussed. The second part of the chapter presents a framework for the documentation of assumptions and decisions in health education plans so that they can be more systematically analyzed in research and evaluation. The third part of this

*Based on Green, L.W.: Evaluation and measurement: some dilemmas for health education, American Journal of Public Health 67:155-161, 1977.

chapter offers a hierarchy of suggested designs, from simple to complex, to account for some of these problems, dilemmas, assumptions, and decisions.

Rigor versus Significance

The implementation of programs in communities and institutions presents organizational, economic, and environmental problems and opportunities to which the creative health educator must adapt his or her strategies and methods. Scientific rigor requires strict adherence to a protocol that specifies the experimental educational treatment in procedural detail. The educational treatment is supposed to be the independent variable, meaning that it should not be subject to or dependent on events that follow or result from the implementation of the program. The attempt to maintain such rigorously defined protocols often results in sterile, perfunctory, or routine educational performance that is not sufficiently adapted to emerging circumstances to be significant in its impact. Thus we end up sometimes with rigorously defined but trivial interventions, and other times with significant interventions that are too vaguely defined to be replicated.

We know that health education works if it is sufficiently adapted to the problem, the population, and the circumstances in which it is implemented. We do not know how to describe those crucial adaptations because they have been restricted or controlled in most experimental evaluations.

How do we resolve this dilemma? There are four ways we can deal with this problem: one requires more complex experimental designs, a second requires more complex statistical analysis, a third requires more detailed documentation and reporting of procedures, and a fourth requires more replication and attention to the cumulative building of the theoretical and research literature in this field. I have described some of these proposals in detail in other places, so will only summarize them here and cite the more detailed references.

Factorial Designs. Most evaluations of health education programs have employed pre-experimental and quasi-experimental designs; those that have used more rigorous experimental designs have usually had only one experimental and one control group with no provision for variations in the experimental treatment.[1] The recognition of the need for adaptations of the educational treatment at different points in the implementation of a program can be accommodated in advance by the sequential assignment of subjects to cells in a randomized factorial design.[2,3] If the size of the available population and the total time available for experimental programming are known in advance, a schedule of programmatic variations can be established at the outset without necessarily knowing exactly what the educational variations will be. Each phase of the program could have its own experimental and control groups, or the control group could be accumulated during one period of the program if there is not systematic bias in the order in which subjects are available for exposure to education.

Analytic Solutions. Even with more simplistic evaluation designs, we could make better use of statistical methods for sorting out the effects of variations in educational treatments during a program.[2-4] Computers are making such methods more accessible.

Documentation and Reporting. Even without factorial designs and adequate data for more detailed analysis of variable program effects, the adaptations and variations in health education interventions could at least be better documented during the program and more explicitly described in published reports. This would allow better understanding of the process of program development as well as the specific elements of health education to which results might be attributed. A framework for documentation of the causal assumptions underlying the design of the program or intervention being evaluated is suggested in the second part of this chapter

Replication and Diffusion. Finally, even with better designs, improved analyses, and more concrete reporting we are left with the dilemma of rigor versus significance unless we can convince practitioners and administrators that our improvements in rigor have indeed made our results more rather than less significant to them. Convincing practitioners will require that results hold up in more than one evaluation, and this will require replication. But even with replicated results we have a persistent "town and gown" problem in this field. Practitioners and administrators are frequently either unequipped or disinclined to consume and use the research literature. The literature itself is partly at fault for having been written often without practitioners as participants or even as the intended audience. It has also lacked cohesiveness as a body of literature, partly because there has been so little replication. The result of this eclectic and noncumulative character of the literature is that the practitioner founders in a sea of print without unifying concepts or theories. Greater efforts at theory building from replicated results, more rigorous training of practitioners in the translation of research and theory, and more continuing education and dissemination of results from evaluation are needed.[5,6]

Internal versus External Validity

A special case of the dilemma of rigor versus significance is the methodologic problem of experimental control in community, classroom, or clinical settings. Internal validity refers to the degree to which we can say with certainty that the results observed after the program are attributable to the program or educational treatment. External validity is the degree to which such results can be expected to recur in other places or at other times. This is sometimes called generalizability. The dilemma is that the harder we strive for internal validity, the more we usually sacrifice external validity; the more we strive for external validity, the harder it is to maintain internal validity or experimental controls.

We know that internal validity is more important when the primary purpose of the evaluation is to determine the efficacy or true effectiveness of a health education method or program design, whereas external validity is more important when the purpose of the evaluation is to demonstrate the feasibility and practical effectiveness of the method or program under actual community or clinical circumstances. What is not known is how and to what degree to sacrifice one type of validity for the other.

The way out of this dilemma would seem to be the development of a set of decision rules for use in striking the right balance between internal and external validity on the one hand, and resources and circumstances on the other. I have proposed a set of hierarchies of optional designs for maximizing either internal or external validity with a minimal sacrifice of the other and with economy and practicability in mind.[7,8] These hierarchies are simplified and translated into a single hierarchy for the practitioner in the third part of this chapter.

Experimental versus Placebo Effects

Medical researchers go to great lengths to remove from their experimental evaluations the element of effect attributable to the faith or confidence the patient has in the treatment. Ironically, this is the very effect that health education attempts to enhance through increased patient participation and informed consent. When we remove the placebo effect from a health education strategy we have a rather sterile and uninteresting intervention. One is tempted, in the face of this dilemma, to regard health education as an organized placebo.

The same dilemma is posed by the behavioral science counterparts of the placebo effect. These are the Hawthorne effect—the change in performance attributable to the attention paid to subjects in an experiment—and the social desirability effect, which is change or response bias attributable to being observed and wanting to do the right thing. These are precisely the effects that participative and normative strategies in health education attempt to mobilize. A well-designed health education program would add to the information (1) an attempt to increase the patient's or consumer's belief in the efficacy of the treatment or preventive measure (placebo effect),[9,10] (2) an attempt to increase the patient's or consumer's perception of having his or her own problems or needs addressed (Hawthorne effect),[11] and (3) an attempt to increase the patient's or consumer's perception that the recommended health practice is socially acceptable and sanctioned (social desirability effect).[12]

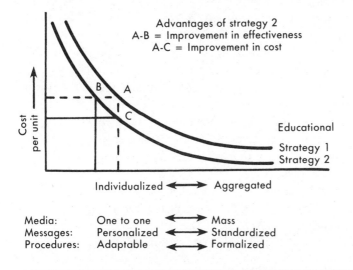

Fig. 7-1. Economy of scale as applied to health education program components. (Modified from Oettinger, A.G., and Zapol, N.: Will information technologies help learning? Teachers College Record 74:5-54, 1972.)

We know that these elements are important components of health education with motivating and reinforcing effects. What is not known is the degree to which and the ways in which health information interacts with these social psychologic forces.[13]

Effectiveness versus Economy of Scale

By aggregating, standardizing, and formalizing health education, we can achieve economies of scale at the expense of some effectiveness at the individual level. The cost per unit of production per patient educated or per message disseminated can be reduced through aggregation. The goal in educational innovation is to design standardized materials, methods, and procedures that can be produced or implemented on a larger scale (therefore at lower unit prices) without sacrificing a proportionate amount of effectiveness inherent in more individualized, personalized, and flexible methods and procedures.

The usual form of the economy of scale curve is illustrated in Fig. 7-1. The vertical axis represents the cost per unit of education. The horizontal axis represents various ways of increasing the scale of educational production, all three of which usually result in reduced effectiveness in terms of behavioral change achieved. Effectiveness is not represented in Fig. 7-1 except as it is negatively correlated with aggregation of educational inputs.

Aggregating Patients. An example of an educational innovation with adults that achieved this kind of economy of scale was group discussion-decision methods, first demonstrated in nutrition education by Lewin,[14] later in breast cancer self-examination by Bond,[15] and more recently in reducing emergency room use and dependency of asthmatics.[16] The beauty of this innovation was that it achieved economy of scale through aggregation while increasing rather than decreasing effectiveness. The group, if properly constituted and guided, proved to be more powerful as an agent of change in health behavior than the individualized exhortations from doctors and nurses. It was also more effective than similarly aggregated education delivered through lectures.

Types of Education Personnel. Another example of an educational innovation that might fit the curve of Fig. 1 for educational strategy 2, relative to the curve for educational strategy 1, is the introduction of indigenous health education aides to carry out health education (strategy 2) in place of health professionals (strategy 1). The cost would be lower at any level of aggregation (A to C), and the effectiveness might be improved at any level of cost (A and B) because the indigenous aide would be able to communicate more personalized messages.[17,18] For example, Cuskey and Premkumar demonstrated that a medium-sized drug treatment center serving about 1000 addicts could save up to $100,000 annually if ex-addict counselors were used in place of professional counselor with graduate level training.[19] Even better than paid indigenous workers for some educational purposes are patients themselves as counselors, recruiters, or reinforcers of other patients. Andrew Fisher has experimentally demonstrated that family planning patients given postcards to pass on to friends achieve recruitment rates at approximately one third the cost per new appointment in comparison with the next most cost-effective method.[20] Another study demonstrated the cost-effectiveness of a clerk in the emergency room assigned to call and remind patients of their return appointments.[21] Any strategy successful in reducing broken appointments must have considerable appeal to hospital administrators and to staff members concerned with continuity of care.

Technology. Other kinds of educational technology that might be expected to meet the criteria of a cost-effective innovation as defined by the difference between the two curves in Fig. 7-1 are programmed instruction and cable television. Teaching machines, or computer-assisted education, as one kind of programmed instruction, can achieve an economy of scale in production and preserve the effectiveness of personalized and adaptable messages and procedures. The marketing problems associated with this technology are beginning to be overcome with microcomputers, which should allow the unit cost to be low enough to achieve the promised economies of scale.[22-24]

The tendency for some hospital administrators to invest in expensive hardware rather than salaries of educational personnel has been based on the sincere but misguided assumption that audiovisual technology is as effective educationally as it is attractive. Campeau concluded from her extensive and scholarly review of experimental studies evaluating audiovisual media in adult education that

> What is most impressive about the formidable body of literature surveyed for this review is that it shows that instructional media are being used extensively, under many diverse conditions, and that enormous amounts of money are being spent for the installation of very expensive equipment. All indications are that decisions as to which audiovisual to purchase, install, and use have been based on administrative and organizational requirements and on considerations of cost, availability, and user preference, not on evidence of instructional effectiveness.[25]

The use of expensive hardware in patient education can be approached on the same purchasing basis as other overpriced medical hardware such as kidney dialysis units, that is, in terms of the regionalization of resources. Health education centers could be established to serve several schools, worksites, hospitals, and clinic through the pooling of their resources. Under these circumstances a total decrease in training time and in provider-patient ratios or teacher-student ratios for all the hospitals, schools, or worksites can be translated into cost savings to the system.[26,27] This situation occurs when computer-assisted instruction or other specialized educational resources can be used for the education and training of professionals as well as patients or students whose special learning needs cannot be met by routine clinical or classroom procedures. Evaluation of computer-assisted instruction and other educational technology in schools has led to essentially the same conclusions.[28,29]

Variety in Approach to Patients. Another aspect of the economy of scale dilemma is that what works for some learners or patients does not work for others. The educational strategy, medium, or message that supports behavior conducive to health in some patients may fail with others. As with prescription drugs, there are differential dose responses and side effects with health education. This poses a specific set of problems for the evaluation of health education programs[2] and calls for a degree of sophistication in educational planning not to be expected of every teacher, doctor, and nurse. It is generally recommended therefore that the person assigned overall responsibility for educational planning be someone with graduate training, preferably in health education or adult education. As with expensive hardware, this often requires the sharing of a specialist on a regional or multihospital basis.

In addition to the principle of "different strokes for different folks," patient education programming also calls for shifting emphasis and technique within a group or population over time. These principles can be seen

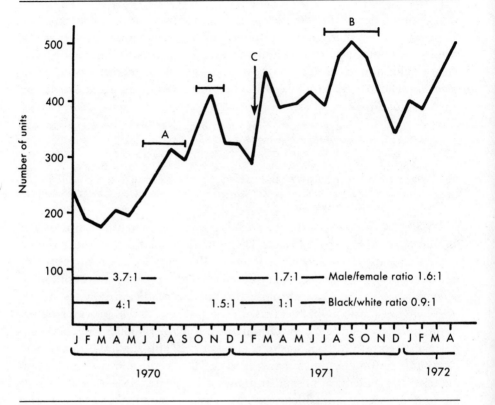

Fig. 7-2. Illustration of design A results: visits to a venereal disease clinic by month.

in terms of benefits in programs requiring sustained behavior over time. An example is illustrated in Fig. 7-2, in which Atwater[30] demonstrated the sequential benefits of different educational approaches during three phases of a venereal disease clinic program over a 2-year period. The benefits of each educational strategy can be noted both in the absolute number of patients appearing at the clinic and in the composition of the patient population. The change in interviewing policy was a change from an investigative approach in which patients were asked for the identification of their sexual contacts to an approach in which patients were encouraged to take the responsibility of getting their contacts under treatment. The change in the male/female ratio of patients as a result of this change in educational approach is most notable.

Risk versus Payoff

Another way of viewing the implications of Figs. 7-1 and 7-2 is to consider that there may be optimal times in the life history of a given health problem or program when spending for specific kinds of educational inputs will minimize risk and maximize payoff. Referring back to Fig. 7-1, as educational methods become more aggregated they tend to minimize risks while usually also minimizing payoff. More individualized methods increase the risks of loss because they are more expensive but they also increase the possibility of benefits because they are usually more effective. The timing of investments in one educational method versus another should follow two decision rules governing the setting of priorities.

The first decision rule is based on diffusion theory. During the early phases of a new program, the people most likely to respond are those who are already motivated to adopt the recommended health practice. During this phase, low unit-cost measures such as written materials (pamphlets, etc.) are effective enough. As the program moves through the at-risk population to increasingly hard to reach and high-risk groups, more expensive educational methods, such as counseling sessions and home visits, may be justified.

The second decision rule is based on setting priorities according to the level of risk or need. The extra cost to reach one high-risk patient will be offset in most cost-benefit computations by the greater benefits accruing from behavioral change in a high-risk as contrasted with a low-risk person or population. In economic terms, the marginal utility of behavioral change is greater in high-risk than in low-risk populations.*

Long-term versus Short-term Evaluation

Most of the benefits of health education are time-dependent.[34] These raise problems of behavioral change that must be taken into account in assessing program effectiveness and benefits. Most of these have to do with the timing of the measurement of outcomes following the educational inputs. Some effects of health education are immediate and temporary; others are slower in developing but are longer lasting. These variations and others are illustrated in Fig. 7-3.

Delay of Impact. Fig. 7-3, *A*, illustrates the error that would be made in underestimating the impact of an educational program if the effect were measured as the difference between observation 1 before the program and observation 2 after the program $(O_2 - O_1)$. The so-called sleeper effect in much behavior change occurs when the audience must go through a process of attitude change between the educational exposure and the actual change in behavior that yields the health benefits. This effect might also be found in cases in which an immediate behavioral change requires additional time before its benefits can be detected in health or administrative terms.

---

*References 4, 17, 18, 31-33.

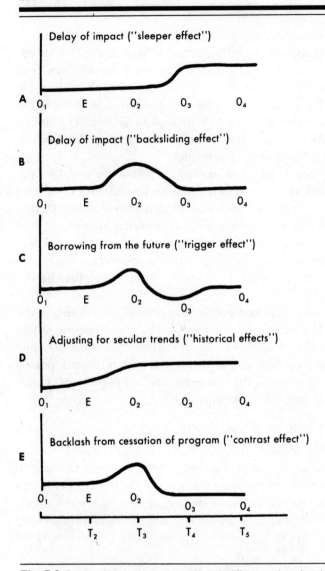

Fig. 7-3. Points of observation in relation to different educational inputs.

Decay of Impact. Fig. 7-3, *B,* illustrates the error in underestimating benefits that might be made if comparative measures were taken only at time *4* or time *5* or in overestimating impact if observations at time *3* were taken as permanent. The backsliding effect is not uncommon with behavioral changes that are complex, such as smoking cessation, diet change, and complicated drug regimens.

Borrowing from the Future. Some educational effects are really only triggers to behavior that would have changed eventually anyway. In such cases the educational program can be regarded as hastening the inevitable. There may be real benefits to be realized from getting earlier action, as with early diagnosis of cancer symptoms, earlier treatment of infections or injuries, earlier prenatal care, and so forth. But it might be an error of overestimation of benefits from some health actions if the observations are taken only at O_1 and O_2. The gains at O_2 may be offset at O_3, so that the net long-term gain is zero. This phenomenon is most notable in some mass communication media campaigns designed to recruit new patients to a screening clinic or a family planning clinic.* The gains immediately after the broadcasts turn out to be patients who would have appeared within a few months anyway. This effect can be seen following the radio broadcasts in Atwater's data on the venereal disease clinic (Fig. 7-2).

Adjusting for Secular Trends. One of the most important purposes served by having a control group in the evaluation of program impact is that the apparent gains following the program can be partitioned into gains resulting from the program and gains that were occurring as part of general trends or extraneous events. The curve in Fig. 7-3, *D,* applies to an experimental group of patients exposed to an educational intervention of some kind. If there were another curve for a control group of patients not exposed to the education, it would probably be parallel to the curve in Fig. 7-4, *D,* because the gains were actually developing and heading toward the O_2 level before the educational intervention. In this case the error without adjustment for secular trends would be one of overestimating the benefits of the program.[31-33]

The secular trend, however, could be negative (downward sloping curve before or during the health education program). In this case, the error would be a false-negative underestimation of the program's impact. In every case a careful plotting of trend lines or the use of a control group not exposed to the program is essential to the accurate estimation of the true benefits of a program.

Contrast Effect. Another dilemma posed by short-term evaluation is illustrated by Fig. 7-3, *E.* Premature termination of the educational treatment may induce a contrast that demoralizes or embitters the experimental group, causing a backlash, a defiant reduction, or a reversal of the behavior advocated. Self-care programs,[16] smoking and diet programs,[17-18] and family planning programs[34] have experienced contrast effects when the educational activities were insufficiently developed, creating expectations that were not met.

---

*This effect may also be obtained when the clinic has difficulty handling and providing adequate service to the new influx of patients. Dissatisfied patients may give negative impressions of the clinic to other potential patients.

How Much to Spend?

Evaluation should lead eventually to knowing how much money to budget for health education. In the meantime, the decision tends to be made in a variety of ways, but the most common way is probably the least rational: budgeting from leftover funds. The alternatives to residual funding for health education require either assumptions or research data. Until we accumulate more specific data, assumptions based on theory and experience must suffice. The alternative criteria for deciding how much to spend on health education are as follows.

Cost-Benefit Analysis. When cost-benefit ratios can be computed comparably for health education and alternative intervention or control mechanisms such as surgery, long-term medication, and hospitalization we will be compelled to budget accordingly. We are so far from having adequate data to compute comparable ratios that there will be few applications of this criterion as an administrative decision tool in the near future.[4] Even then it will apply primarily to public programs and institutions rather than to proprietary hospitals[35] or voluntary health agencies, except when benefits are narrowly defined to refer to the limited goals and survival of that institution or agency.

Cost-Effectiveness Analysis. Unlike cost-benefit data, the prospects for generating comparable cost-effectiveness ratios for different combinations or amounts of health education and other program components are very real. The difference is that specific results can be predetermined for cost-effectiveness analyses, whereas the results of cost-benefit analyses are largely conjectural. Cost-effectiveness data will be equally applicable to public and private programs or institutions. Care must be taken, however, in applying cost-effectiveness estimates from one situation to another or from one population to another.

Threshold Spending. The minimum that should be spent on health education for a specific purpose is the amount required to achieve that purpose. Although this may seem tautologic, it is a tragic fact of much health education funding that the budget is below the minimum required to obtain the desired effect. Parrish notes a similar phenomenon in marketing, in which "massive amounts of advertising dollars are wasted on budgets that are well below minimum effective levels of spending."[36] With health education, as with advertising, a threshold level of input is required before a difference in behavior is perceptible. It is not necessarily true that anything is better than nothing. If the "anything" is insufficient to achieve a desired effect, it may be wasted and, worse, may place health education in disrepute. A "critical mass" is required before a reaction can be expected.

From the first three criteria, decisions about the minimum amount to spend can be made. Cost-benefit estimates can tell you whether anything should be spent on a given educational program. If the ratio of potential benefits to costs is not greater than one, then nothing should be spent, strictly speaking. Cost-effectiveness estimates enable you to compare the costs of two or more methods in achieving the same outcome. Then, depending on how much of that outcome is needed, the threshold level of spending might be obtained directly from the cost-effectiveness measurement by multiplication.

Saturation Spending and the Point of Diminishing Returns. The maximum to be budgeted for a specific health education purpose should be based on data concerning the point of diminishing returns for further input. We are beginning to get an understanding of the point of diminishing returns in some program areas.[37] It has always been clear that quality in educational programming was more important than quantity, but we have seldom tried to determine how much of a good thing was too much, probably because we have seldom had resources enough even to reach threshold levels. The range within which decisions on variable amounts of spending should be made is the range between the threshold level and the point of diminishing returns.

Booster Spending. We are sometimes guilty of claiming too much for health education, as we do when we give the impression that educational effects are usually permanent. In fact, we know a great deal about learning curves and memory curves and the process of forgetting and backsliding. We know that reinforcement is as important to education as booster shots are to sustained immunization. Thus after reaching the saturation level of spending we should allow a period of time to elapse before introducing an additional expenditure on education for the same population. At the point when the behavioral changes achieved begin to deteriorate, booster spending on reinforcement or new educational methods may be necessary.[38] It is a mistake also to assume that educational effects are generally applicable to related but distinct health behaviors. The evidence appears to indicate the need for highly targeted health messages addressed to very specific behaviors rather than more general classes of health behavior.[39]

•   •   •

This survey of the state of evaluation and measurement in health education has attempted to summarize what we know and do not know in relation to the major decisions facing administrators and practitioners today. First, there are some fundamental dilemmas to be reconciled. These dilemmas are posed by the peculiar characteristics of health education that make it resistant to some of the standard applications of research procedures.

Second, there are some problems in measuring the outcomes of health education that require policy decisions on whether benefits are to be expected to accrue rapidly or slowly, temporarily or permanently, in the general population or in high-risk groups, and in what relationship to the economy. Finally, there are questions to which administrators and practitioners must address themselves in the absence of an adequate data base. These particularly concern the decisions that must be made on how much money to spend for various health education efforts. Health education need not be regarded as a bottomless pit, but neither can it be expected to accomplish much without adequate, timely, and well-directed support. Further evaluation is needed specifically to determine the threshold level, the point of diminishing returns, and the saturation level for various programs.

Some of the dilemmas facing health education today cannot be resolved simply by trying harder to measure and evaluate. Some will not yield to quantitative and deductive solutions until they undergo a more thorough conceptual and inductive analysis to clarify the theoretical and experiential basis for much of what passes as health education practice. And all of them require for their rational analysis a more systematic approach to planning and documenting program decisions.

In the next part of the chapter the PRECEDE model for planning and documenting the assumptions underlying each health education program is explained and discussed. The framework is founded on the requirements of four disciplines: epidemiology, social and behavioral sciences, administration, and education. The seven basic phases in the procedure using the PRECEDE model are presented.

The last part of the chapter deals with concepts and approaches to evaluation in health education. Several designs that cover the simple to the complex levels of evaluation are described.

An Organized Approach to Documenting Decisions Underlying Health Education Plans*

The following is a product of a period of growth and development in health education that was at times exhilarating but often painful in the recognition that the field has been without a clear articulation of its boundaries, its methods, and its procedures. Only the philosophy and the intellectual roots of health education were sufficiently understood to appear in textbook form. Over several decades many articles have been published in which practical implications for health education have been derived from specific philosophies, theories, experiences, and occasionally studies. Only a few of these

*Based on Green, L.W., Kreuter, M.W., Deeds, S.G., and Partridge, K.B.: Health education planning: a diagnostic approach, Palo Alto, Cal., 1980, Mayfield Publishing Co.

derived practices have survived long-term analysis and evaluation. From a sociologic perspective health education has been more a movement or a series of successive movements than a single profession. Transforming health education principles from philosophic terms to operational ones has been difficult at times. Health education knowledge has been inadequately codified, and the training of health educators has been relatively devoid of uniformity or consistent standards.

Outstanding programs have been emulated, but often with a supporting understanding of their backgrounds, their methods, or their results. The framework for educational diagnosis and planning that follows was designed to give cohesiveness and consistency to the ways in which theory and previous research are brought to bear on the development and evaluation of health education programs. Without such cohesiveness and consistency there can be little continuity in building the scientific base of health education practice.

Concepts and Philosophy Implicit in Planning

Important to this discussion is the idea of intervention. Organized health education activity is based on the desire to intervene in the process of development and change in such a way as to maintain positive health behavior or to interrupt a behavioral pattern that is linked to increased risks for illness, injury, disability, or death. The behavior is usually that of people whose health is in question, but often it may be the behavior of those who control resources or rewards, such as community leaders, parents, employees, peers, teachers, and health professionals. Whether a health education program is operating at the primary (hygiene or health promotion), secondary (early detection), or tertiary (therapeutic) stage of prevention, it may accurately be seen as intervention of one of the four types shown in Fig. 7-4.

Practitioners in various professions have struggled, often without clear guidelines, to systematize their planning, delivery, and evaluation of health or educational programs. In an effort to codify the practice of health education, the following framework strives to minimize the entrapment of method in philosophy. The methods applied are not entirely value free, but they reflect the main traditions of health education practice. The methodology is presented in such a way as to be acceptable to people who approach the practice of health education from various philosophic vantage points. It is unavoidable, of course, that this philosophy would inform the presentation throughout, so the single overriding principle will be stated at the outset. The overriding principle in this approach to health education is that health behavior must be voluntary behavior. Health behavior should be compelled only in those cases in which the health of others is threatened. Health means different things to different people, serves different purposes for different

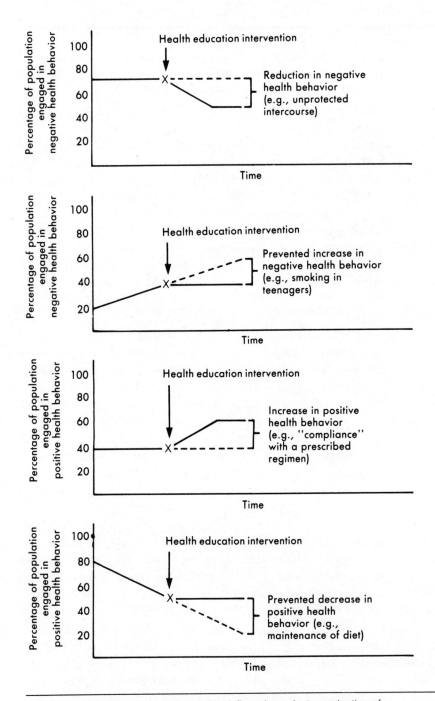

Fig. 7-4. Health education as intervention: influencing voluntary adoption of behavior conducive to health. Reprinted from *Health education planning: a diagnostic approach* by Lawrence W. Green, Marshall W. Kreuter, Sigrid G. Deeds, and Kay B. Partridge, by permission of Mayfield Publishing Company. Copyright © 1980 by Mayfield Publishing Company.

people, and is more or less important than other concerns to different people. Because of this, it is impossible to justify the imposition of rigid criteria of appropriate health behavior unless a behavior has been judged by society as a whole to be a sufficient hazard to the common good to warrant the curtailment of individual choice.

The idea of voluntary behavior has a number of corollaries. First, the reason for a behavior change must be understood by those whose behavior is in question. To accommodate this necessity the model of health education planning to be presented in this chapter has built into it a process to ensure agreement between health practitioners and health education recipients (whether individual or group) on the definition of health-related problems. Indeed, this is the first step in the recommended planning process and is called the social diagnosis or the quality-of-life assessment, it should be taken even before addressing health problems or health behavior.

Second, a recommended behavior must be compatible with the values or value system of the concerned person or community. If it is not, then there must be an opportunity to adjust the value system. These and other corollaries to the definition of health education in terms of voluntary behavior have influenced the form and procedures in the framework for planning proposed in this chapter. Accordingly, health education is defined as any combination of learning experiences designed to predispose, enable, and reinforce voluntary adaptations of behavior conducive to health.

This framework is called PRECEDE (which stands for *p*redisposing, *r*inforcing, and *e*nabling *c*auses in *e*ducational *d*iagnosis and *e*valuation) to draw attention to the necessity of determining what behavior precedes each health benefit and what causes (precedes) each health behavior that must be addressed in a health education plan. The framework, has been built out of a variety of projects in which it has been developed or tested, and has been adjusted in teaching and consultation as it has been applied to an ever-widening range of problems in the health field. Even so, it can be said with confidence that overall the framework and the procedures that substantiate it are serviceable in a variety of populations with a variety of problems. Hundreds of professionals who have used the PRECEDE model in in-service training programs and subsequently in their work have attested to the usefulness of the framework. Additional hundreds of graduate and postgraduate students, including those in the fields of nursing, medicine, health education, health planning, population and family planning, pharmacy, dietetics, and dentistry, have demonstrated their ability to understand the framework and to apply the procedures in the preparation of project proposals. Some of these proposals were taken into the field and subsequently implemented, some of which were funding by government agencies and foundations.

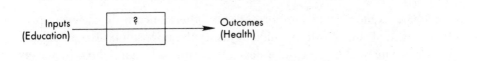

Fig. 7-5. The simplified model of cause-and-effect implicit in the practice of health education.

PRECEDE is not offered as the exclusive road to quality health education. It is, however, a theoretically "robust" model that addresses the acknowledged problem in health education of unsystematic or disjointed planning. It is robust in the sense that it applies to health education in a variety of situations. It has served as a successful model in a number of rigorously evaluated "real world" clinical trials*; as a useful guide to the development of local health department programs that have been adopted by several state health departments[44]; as a guide to the review of maternal and child health projects[45]; as an analytic tool for policy analysis for health education on a national and international scale[46-49]; and as an organizing framework for curriculum development in health education for nurses,[50] pharmacists,[51] and allied health professionals.[52]

Learning to Start from the Other End

Experience suggests that many people responsible for health education programs initiate their programs by considering or even designing the actual intervention to be employed. What's wrong with that? Let us note a presumed cause-effect relationship as shown in Fig. 7-5.

In this scheme *inputs* are interventions (or processes), and *outcomes* are the anticipated results of the interventions in terms of changes in medical or social problems or conditions. Health practitioners, because of their activist orientation, have an understandable tendency to begin with inputs. After a quick glance at the general problem at hand, they immediately begin to design and implement the health education intervention and assume that the outcome will occur automatically.

The PRECEDE framework directs the health educator's initial attention to outcomes rather than to inputs, forcing him or her to begin the health education planning process from the outcome end. It encourages the asking of *why* questions before the asking of *how* questions. Thus, from the standpoint of planning what may seem to be the wrong end to start from is in fact the right one. The health educator begins with the final outcome and determines what must precede that outcome by determining what causes

---

*References, 2, 3, 40-43.

that outcome. The causes of the health outcomes through which health education must achieve its influence are represented by the black box in the middle of Fig. 7-5.

Stated another way, the factors important to an outcome must be diagnosed before the intervention is designed; if they are not, the intervention will be based on guesswork and runs a greater risk of being misdirected and ineffective. The wrong causes of health may be addressed or the wrong processes of change may be set into motion.

Seven Phases of PRECEDE

The PRECEDE model for diagnosis and planning leads the health educator to think deductively, to start with the final consequences and work back to the original causes. There are seven basic phases in this procedure (Fig. 7-6). To provide an overview, they may be superficially described as follows.

Phase One. Ideally, the health educator begins with a consideration of quality of life by assessing some of the general problems of concern to the people in the population of patients, students, workers, or consumers. The demands of social problems a given community experiences are good barometers of the quality of life there.

Phase Two. The task in phase two is to identify those specific health problems that appear to be contributing to the social problems noted in phase one. Using available data and data generated by appropriate investigations, together with epidemiologic and medical findings, the health educator ranks the several health problems and selects the specific health problems most deserving of scarce educational resources.

Many health educators, particularly those working in school health education or patient education, will be given the task of developing a program after someone else has already gone through phases one and two and concluded that educational intervention is needed. We appreciate that situation but advise practitioners to be certain that the first two steps have been done well. Such precautionary action ensures that the existing data are valid and also familiarizes the practitioner with crucial foundation information and assumptions.

Phase Three. Phase three consists of identifying the specific health-related behaviors that appear to be linked to the health problem chosen as deserving of most attention in phase two. As these are the behaviors that the intervention will be tailored to affect, it is essential that they be identified specifically and carefully ranked. Notice in Fig. 7-6 that a category called nonbehavioral factors is linked to the health problems box. Nonbehavioral factors include economic, genetic, and environmental factors. They are acknowledged here because of the power they have, however indirect, to influence health.[53-54] Being cognizant of such forces will enable educators to be more realistic about the limitations of their programs. It will also enable them to recognize that powerful social forces might be affected when the principles of PRECEDE are applied by well-organized health groups and coalitions on the national level. Even at the local level, health-related behaviors influenced by health education can include collective behavior directed at economic or environmental factors.

Phase Four. On the basis of cumulative research on health behavior,[55] we have identified three classes of factors that have potential for affecting health behavior: predisposing factors, enabling factors, and reinforcing factors. Predisposing factors[56] include a person's attitudes, beliefs, values, and perceptions, all of which facilitate or hinder

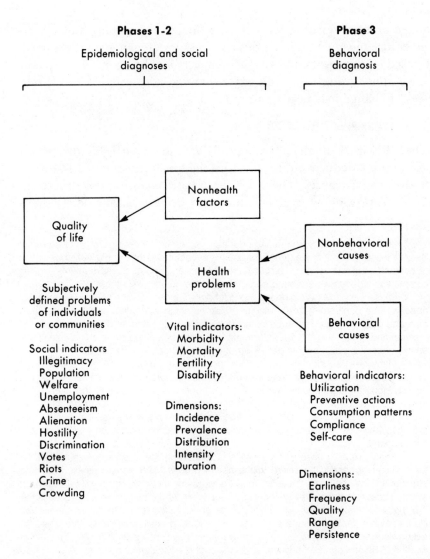

Fig. 7-6. The PRECEDE framework. Reprinted from *Health education planning: a diagnostic approach* by Lawrence W. Green, Marshall W. Kreuter, Sigrid G. Deeds, and Kay B. Partridge, by permission of Mayfield Publishing Company. Copyright © 1980 by Mayfield Publishing Company.

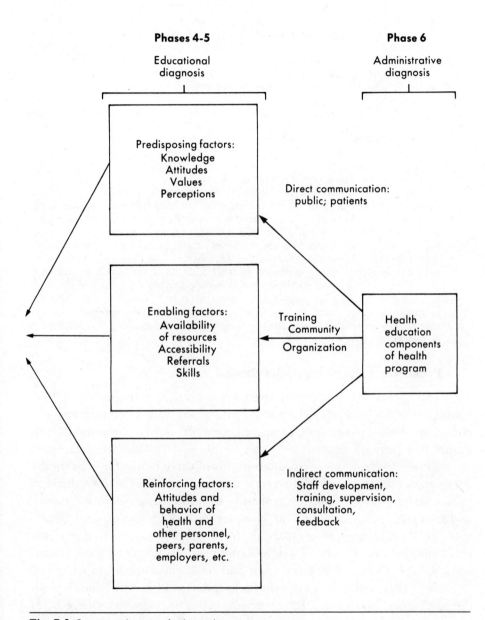

Fig. 7-6. See opposite page for legend.

personal motivation for change. Enabling factors may be considered to be barriers created mainly by societal forces or systems. Limited facilities, inadequate personal or community resources, lack of income or health insurance, and even restrictive laws and statutes are examples of enabling factors. The skills and knowledge required for a desired behavior to occur also qualify as enabling factors. Reinforcing factors are those related to the feedback the learner receives from others, the result of which may be either to encourage or to discourage behavioral change.

The fourth phase therefore is sorting and categorizing, according to the three classes just cited, the factors that seem to have direct impact on the behavior selected in phase two.

Phase Five. Study of the predisposing, enabling, and reinforcing factors automatically takes the educator into the fifth phase of PRECEDE. At this point he or she is called on to decide exactly which of the factors making up the three classes are to be the focus of the intervention. The decision is based on their relative importance and the resources available to influence them.

Phase Six. Armed with pertinent and systematically organized diagnostic information, the health educator is ready for phase six, which is the actual development and implementation of a program. If he or she keeps firmly in mind the limitations of his or her resources, time constraints, and abilities, the appropriate educational interventions will almost be self-evident from the diagnosis of predisposing, enabling, and reinforcing factors. All that remains is the selection of the right combination of interventions and an assessment of administrative problems and resources.

Phase Seven. Listing evaluation as the last phase is misleading. Evaluation is considered an integral and continuous part of working with the entire framework. Criteria for evaluation naturally fall out of the framework during the diagnostic procedure. For example, early on in the framework, clearly stated program and behavioral objectives specify the standards of acceptability before rather than after the program is implemented and evaluated.

Foundations: Staying on Solid Ground

The PRECEDE framework is founded on the requirements of four disciplines: epidemiology, social and behavioral sciences, administration, and education. Although one must necessarily draw on all four throughout, each stands as a primary support to a specific phase of PRECEDE. Successful completion of phases one, two, and portions of three depend heavily on the use of epidemiologic methods and information. Working effectively through phases three and four requires familiarity with social and behavioral theory and concepts. And handling the complex task of designing and implementing a health education program demands knowledge of educational and administrative theory as well as experience. In presenting this framework we are assuming that you have had basic exposure to these several disciplines that constitute the scientific foundation of health education. In the application of PRECEDE, two basic propositions are emphasized: (1) health and health behavior are caused by multiple factors, and (2) because health and health behavior are determined by multiple factors, health education efforts to affect behavior must be multidimensional. It is the multidimensional nature of the health education process that demands the kind

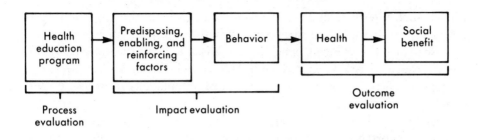

Fig. 7-7. Three levels of evaluation in relation to the PRECEDE framework.
Reprinted from *Health education planning: a diagnostic approach* by Lawrence W.
Green, Marshall W. Kreuter, Sigrid G. Deeds, and Kay B. Partridge, by permission
of Mayfield Publishing Company. Copyright © by Mayfield Publishing Company.

of professional preparation in which several scientific and professional disciplines are integrated. It is not surprising that educators occasionally become discouraged and even disenchanted as they try to synthesize biomedical science, behavioral science, and education. The PRECEDE framework can give direction and focus to such attempts at synthesis. The challenge—to pull together a variety of rapidly developing disciplines as a basis for understanding and in some way contributing to improvements in the quality of life—is what sustains commitment to and hope for health education.

Objects and Designs for Evaluation*
Objects of Interest

We define evaluation as the comparison of an object of interest against a standard of acceptability. There are three levels at which objects of interest in a health education program can be evaluated: in relation to process, in relation to impact, and in relation to outcome (Fig. 7-7). In a process evaluation the object of interest is professional practice and the standard of acceptability is appropriate practice. Quality is monitored by various means, including audit, peer review, accreditation, certification, and government or administrative surveillance of contracts and grants. Standards of acceptability are established both professionally and administratively and are derived chiefly by means of consensus among health education specialists.

The second level is impact evaluation. Evaluation here focuses on the immediate impact the program (or some aspect of it) has on knowledge, attitudes, and behavior. Have the predisposing, enabling, and reinforcing factors that influence the health-related behavior been altered? Have the short-term goals of a program been met? In terms of behavior, the planner

*Based on Green, L.W., Kreuter, M.W., Deeds, S.G., and Partridge, K.B.: Health education planning: a diagnostic approach, Palo Alto, Cal., 1980, Mayfield Publishing Co.

will ask such questions as Does it take as long for members of the target population to seek medical care as it did before the program? Is there an increase in health-enhancing behavior? Are diseases being diagnosed earlier? Has exposure to risk been reduced? Has exercise been increased? Cost-effectiveness is the most succinct standard of acceptability in impact evaluation.

At the third level, the level of outcome evaluation, the objectives of interest are mortality and morbidity. Have the incidence and prevalence of the condition(s) been affected by a program? Have the rate and length of survival following detection and treatment changed? Again, cost-effectiveness in one standard of acceptability; this standard can be expressed more humanely in terms of the number of lives saved or improved. Outcome evaluation is a long-term undertaking requiring large population samples.

When the number of educational booklets distributed is the measure of success, the evaluator is using a process measure of evaluation. The number of patients who made appointments or showed up at cancer screening centers is an impact-evaluation statement. Years later, outcome might be measured in terms of increased survival and reduced mortality and morbidity.

At this point in the history of patient, school, occupational, and community health education, impact evaluation rather than outcome or process evaluation is most needed. Currently, for a number of reasons, it is not efficient to focus exclusively on process. Physicians, nurses, and other health professionals are not uniformly ready for more intensive examination of their skills and effectiveness in such areas as patient education. Even if they were, evaluators are not quite sure what the standards of acceptability for communication with patients should be. It has not yet been possible to translate standards of educational practice in many clinical and community settings into hard criteria for purposes of process evaluation. In addition to the problem of defining criteria, a number of practitioners, including physicians, feel burdened and sometimes threatened by peer review and government surveillance. Process evaluation therefore is not the most fruitful pursuit in community and patient education. In school health education there is a stronger data base for the assessment of communication behavior. Classroom teaching practices have customarily been subjected to intense scrutiny.

It is also premature to expect most programs in their present state of development to have detectable outcomes. Evidence linking specific behaviors to specific medical or health results is still somewhat tenuous. And in some cases health-related behavior is not sufficiently established as medically effective for each individual; they are recommended for populations as good for the average individual. Breast self-examination is one such behavior; restricting cholesterol intake is another. The possible benefits of these practices are established more often on the basis of epidemiologic rather than clinical data. Further, successfully changing some behaviors may have negative consequences. For example, a patient may be encouraged to take a prescribed drug that turns out to have side effects.

Another difficulty with emphasizing outcome evaluation in most community and school programs is that such evaluation cannot be done efficiently. Health outcomes and social benefits often do not appear for long periods of time, and populations rarely remain stable. For example, an evaluation of education and community organization efforts directed toward cancer control in terms of reduced morbidity and mortality would require greater resources, larger populations, and more follow-up time than are likely to be available in those programs.

Designs for Evaluation

At this stage in the development of health education, impact evaluation, the assessment of the changes in knowledge, attitudes, beliefs, and especially behavior that come about as a result of health education programs, is the level of evaluation most likely to produce the greatest improvements in such programs.

Evaluation can be done according to a number of different designs, ranging from the simple but often neglected collection of routine data on an ongoing basis to the collection of data in highly rigorous, highly controlled experimental settings. The historical or record-keeping approach, which is the simplest approach, is applicable to most programs; the controlled experimental approach will usually be impractical. Each approach has its own use. Practitioners will make their selections based on the kinds of data desired and the uses to which the data will be put. All the designs can be implemented in two or three steps.

Design A: Historical or Record-Keeping Approach. Design A, the record-keeping approach, yields charts and graphs that effectively demonstrate what is occurring in a program or community. The procedure is simple. The first step is to construct a dummy graph showing the expected relationship between inputs and outcomes. The second step is to set up a record-keeping procedure to accumulate the data. The last step is to calculate and chart the data periodically, plotting the direction and magnitude to change taking place over time. How often should you tabulate and chart the data? That depends on the number of times the events being tabulated occur.

An example of a design-A graph is given in Fig. 7-2. It demonstrates the sequential benefits of different educational approaches during three phases of a program conducted by a venereal disease clinic over a 28-month period. The impact of each education strategy can be noted in changes in both the absolute number of patients appearing at the clinic and the composition of the patient population. The change in interviewing policy (Fig. 7-2, *C*) was a change from asking patients to identify their sexual contacts to encouraging them to take the responsibility for seeing that their sexual partners received treatment. The behavioral impact in terms of the male/female ratio of patients at this point was most notable.[30] The ratios (looked at in combination with the graph) show increases in females and whites using the clinic until 1972 when the numbers were close to equal.

Design B: Inventory Approach. The inventory approach, which we are labeling design B, requires a special effort to periodically collect data. Sometimes the prevailing record-keeping system does not incorporate the data required, and changing the data system, perhaps expanding it, would be too disruptive to the service program. Rather than accumulating the data on an ongoing basis, as is done with design A, data can be obtained by conducting special surveys.

First the evaluator sets target dates for the assessments. Then he or she identifies the expected target levels. Finally he or she takes the surveys as a way of estimating the levels achieved at the selected points in time.

For some kinds of programs, such as smoking-cessation programs, the critical points for measuring behavior are highly standardized. A review of the literature will reveal the times at which people are likeliest to drop out or backslide in programs dealing with such problems as smoking, antibiotic therapy, oral contraceptive use, and weight control.

Design C: Comparative Approach. Evaluation by means of the comparative approach is an extension of the inventory or the record-keeping approach. The same procedures are followed, except that new data are introduced. You can usually (1) identify similar data on programs in other places; (2) borrow or copy the record forms used in these programs or use a common, standardized format for collecting data or keeping records on the similar programs; and (3) do periodic comparisons between the programs on the same basis as design A or design B.

Various kinds of national data are available for comparison with a local impact or outcome. For example, the National Health Survey provides data derived from standardized questionnaires that can be compared with data collected in local programs. National norms suggest what health educators can expect in relation to breast examination, Pap smears, smoking cessation, and other health behaviors. Comparability is an essential feature of cumulative evaluation. For this reason we recommend using standardized formats for collecting data rather than developing original questionnaires. Examples of the comparative or normative approach can be found in the literature.[57-60]

Design D: Controlled Comparison, Quasi-Experimental Approach. In the controlled comparison approach an evaluator first identifies a community or population similar to the target population but one not receiving the program. He or she then applies design A or B in both the program being evaluated and the comparison program and periodically compares the two communities. The evaluator might want to compare the effects of various kinds of interventions in similar populations in schools or communities. The Stanford three-community study (see Chapter 5) is the most notable contemporary example of the latter application.[61] Three communities were studied, one in which an intensive all-out educational effort had been made, another in which only a mass communication media effort was made, and another in which neither effort was made, although there were comparable resources and facilities. The effectiveness of the strategies used in each of the three experimental communities and their various subpopulations was compared using impact data from surveys. Other examples of this approach can be found in the literature.[62-67]

Design E: Controlled Experimental Approach. The controlled experimental approach is comparable to the clinical trial in medical studies. It requires a formal procedure for random assignments of individuals within the target population to two (and sometimes more) groups. If there are two groups, one will receive the educational treatment and one will not. It should be noted that in this approach it must be possible to deny the treatment to certain people. In some programs in which the treatment being evaluated is known to have some benefit, there may be ethical problems in denying the treatment to a randomized control group; if the treatment is widely *believed* to be beneficial, even if it has not been evaluated, there may be political problems in withholding the treatment from a control group.

Once the groups are set up and the program is under way, the evaluator uses the record keeping (A) approach for the inventory (B) approach for both the experimental and the control groups. Baseline data may be collected on all groups, but this is not essential. Records or survey data over time are then graphed to see how the groups compare at various points in the treatment.[68-73] Smoking cessation and weight control programs are most often evaluated according to this controlled experimental design.

Design F: Evaluative Research Project. The evaluative research project is the most complex of the evaluation designs and is unlikely to be feasible in most community programs. Procedures are similar to those for design E, the controlled experimental approach, with two exceptions: (1) multiple groups rather than only two groups may be randomized to several variations of the experimental treatment in a factorial design, and (2) multiple measures are obtained on intermediate variables such as changes in knowledge, attitudes, and skills as well as on outcomes and impact variables such as behavior and health. Group tendencies are analyzed, as are intragroup variations in impact and outcome. The design can accommodate numerous refinements. Programs consisting of as many as six different treatments applied to various subgroups within randomized groups can be evaluated by means of this design.[74-82]

Somewhere between the simplicity of design A, with its inconclusive but suggestive findings, and the complexity of design F, with its headaches, is a level of evaluation that is feasible and practical as well as rigorous. The problem with the more complicated designs is that they usually have to be carried out under highly controlled conditions, which makes the behavioral circumstances unusual or unnatural.[83] Often it is necessary to remove people from their social milieu, the ordinary context of their behavior. Finding willing participants for controlled, randomized experiments is seldom easy. Further, such designs require informed consent.

In short the gains in internal validity through the more rigorous randomized procedures may be offset by a sacrifice in feasibility and in generalizability of findings. Can data from highly controlled classroom or clinical facilities be generally applicable to private practice and community-based programs?[84-88] The only way to answer this question is to continue to accumulate data in different settings, evaluating programs and methods as they are developed according to careful educational diagnoses.

Editors' Remarks

In this chapter suggestions for improving and conducting research and evaluation of health education were discussed. In order to bring this discussion into focus for the practitioner, we will augment Dr. Green's work with a few examples of research projects that have been conducted by health educators. Projects conducted in schools, in the community, and at the worksite will be used as examples.

School Health Education Research

The PRECEDE model was used in planning a school-based sex education program [89] to (1) explore the effectiveness of a community needs assessment to attempt to reduce negative parental input and facilitate the use of schools as public health resources, (2) identify intervention targets for curriculum development, and (3) develop a method of assessment (a) in which the PRECEDE model would be tested for its usefulness in identifying educational targets in human sexuality, (b) to quantify the model's categories to identify major differences in perceptions between parents and teenagers, and (c) to attempt to explore any underlying constructs in teenage sexuality.

The study was conducted in a small midwestern community in which 600 families reported having at least one teenage child living at home. Three hundred families were surveyed and a total of 204 parents and 210 teenagers responded to the survey. Two questionnaires were developed and tested, both using the seven phases in the PECEDE model. The students completed their questionnaires at a site separate from their school, while their parents were able to complete the surveys at home and mail them to project personnel.

The major results of this study indicated the following: (1) a community needs assessment using the PRECEDE model was effective in reducing negative political input and in facilitating the use of the schools as public health resources, (2) there were major differences between parents and teenagers in perceptions of family life education needs, especially in the identification of important social problems, and (3) the extent of sexual behavior among this group of teenagers.

An intervention program for the population studied was eventually developed and implemented. It should be noted that when developing the curriculum, input from teenagers, parents, school personnel, and project investigators was garnered and used to develop a coherent program that would meet the needs and interests of both the school and community populations.

The preceding example illustrates how a theory related to research and evaluation can actually be applied to real situations. In this particular study, health practitioners as well as university-based personnel were involved in the research effort.

Research in Community Health Education

The long-term effects of a health education program concerning weight control, appointment-keeping behavior, blood pressure control, and mortality were noted for a 5-year period by a group of health professionals at the Johns Hopkins Medical Institutions.[90] A needs assessment was conducted by the research team to identify knowledge and beliefs about hypertension control. This assessment led to the development of a three-part health education program. The first part of the program was an exit interview conducted immediately following the patient's encounter with a medical care provider. The interview was a private session, lasting 5 to 10 minutes, in which instructions for adhering to a medication regimen were reinforced. The family support approach was the second intervention, in which the spouse (usually) of the patient was given an instructional session. In this case the family member was advised how to enable the patient to adhere to the medication regimen. A small group process served as the third health education intervention. This procedure was a series of three 1-hour group sessions that were led by a social worker. All patients were invited to attend the sessions. "The purpose was to provide group support, to strengthen the self-confidence of patients through discussions centering on hypertension management and compliance. The sessions used a broad range of action-related procedures (e.g., role-playing, behavioral rehearsal, problem clarification, cognitive restructuring)."[90]

These interventions were based on behavioral theory and an educational diagnosis of the population, as indicated in the PRECEDE model. The method of a "diagnostic approach to planning and adapting the individual components of such a program to predispose, enable, and reinforce behavior conducive to health would have generalizability to a variety of populations in different organizations of care."[90]

The results of this study were very encouraging for community health educators. The 5-year project and subsequent analyses showed a positive effect on weight control, appointment-keeping, and blood pressure control. In addition, the mortality rates were significantly lower for those patients in the experimental groups than for those in the control group.

Worksite and Research

Until recently, research in health education occurred in community settings or in schools. Presently, as evidenced by several projects, research directed at people in the worksite has taken its rightful place in health education. The American Dental Association received funds to conduct a study in Maine to develop and refine a dental health education program for blue-collar adults in two types of worksites—settings with similar dental prepayment plans and settings without such plans—and to compare the program with an "information only" approach and a no-treatment control group on a variety of variables. These variables included increased access to and use of dental services by workers and their families. In addition, the study team hoped to develop a program that could be implemented in other workplace settings throughout the United States.[91]

As of this writing the results of the proposed project in Maine are not available. However, the important aspect of such an undertaking is that a health education program was developed, implemented, and evaluated for a target group (the blue-collar worker) that had been ignored until this time.

Summary

Some aspiring health educators may believe that research and evaluation are activities reserved for university professors who have a scholarly interest in these areas. Although much of the research in this country is conducted by academicians, this chapter demonstrates that practitioners also need to be involved. Health educators with a professional orientation can establish their own studies in order to determine whether a program is effective or not, whether one program is more effective than another, and whether the benefits of a program justify the expense of the program.

Research and evaluation skills are important to health educators regardless of whether the employer is a public school district, a community agency, or a provider of health care. The school health educator may wonder whether the benefits of programmed instruction materials justify their cost, or whether programmed instruction produces more effective results than traditional classroom activities. In a community setting the health educator may be curious to know whether a planned childhood immunization effort is more successful when a mass communication media campaign is used in place of personal contact, or whether personal contact achieves better results when the facilitator is an expert or an informed member of the target group. Health educators may need to know whether a prescriptive educational program changes long-term behavior when the client receives the education on a one-to-one counseling basis, in groups with others who have the same condition, or with family members.

This chapter encouraged the reader to consider the potential application of research and evaluation techniques. The purpose of having skill in these areas is to be able to answer questions that deal with effectiveness, efficiency of effort, and the allocation of financial resources. Even health educators who do not make the decisions need to understand research and evaluation. Otherwise, their journals have limited value. It would be impossible to translate research findings into a rationale for program implementation. Health educators at all levels, and regardless of job setting, need to be familiar with research and evaluation.

Questions for Review

1. Select an interesting research problem. How would you resolve each of the seven dilemmas raised by Dr. Green?
2. Reviewing recent issues of health journals, how effective were the authors in dealing with the same seven dilemmas?
3. Why is research as important to the practitioner as it is to the scientist?
4. How does a person's philosophy of health education affect his or her program planning? Give some concrete examples.
5. In the PRECEDE model, why does the program planner consider outcomes before inputs?
6. Consider a specific health program, such as community education in cardiopulmonary resuscitation (CPR) procedures. What are some ways that the program could be evaluated in relation to process, to impact, and to outcome?
7. Select an interest in school or community health. Can you identify an evaluation plan using each of the six approaches described in this chapter?

References

1. Green, L.W., and Figa-Talamanca, I.: Suggested designs for the evaluation of patient education programs, Health Education Monographs **2**:54-71, 1974. (Reprinted in Zapka, J., editor: The SOPHE heritage collection of Health Education Monographs, vol. 3, Oakland, 1981, Third Party Publishing Co.
2. Green, L.W., Levine, D.M., and Deeds, S.G.: Clinical trials of health education for hypertensive outpatients: design and baseline data, Preventive Medicine **4**:417-425, 1975.
3. Green, L.W., and others: Two years of randomized patient education experiments with urban poor hypertensives, Patient Counseling and Health Education **1**:106-111, 1979.
4. Green, L.W.: Toward cost-benefit evaluations of health education: some concepts, methods and examples, Health Eucation Monographs **2**(suppl. 1):34-64, 1974. (Reprinted in Zapka, J., editor: The SOPHE heritage collection of Health Education Monographs, vol. 3, Oakland, 1981, Third Party Publishing Co.
5. Green, L.W.: Theory and research vs. practice (editorial), Health Education Monographs **3**:352-358, 1975.
6. Green, L.W., Lewis, F.M., and Levine, D.M.: Balancing statistical data and clinician judgments in the diagnosis of patient educational needs, Journal of Community Health **6**:79-91, 1981.
7. Green, L.W.: Research methods translatable to the practice setting: from rigor to reality and back. In Cohen, S.: New directions in patient compliance, Lexington, Mass., 1979, Lexington Books.
8. Green, L.W.: Research methods for evaluation of health education under adverse scientific conditions. In Bible, B., and Hildreth, R.J., editors: Proceedings of The Extension Seminar on Health Education and Rural Health Care Research Forum, Chicago, 1976, American Medical Association.
9. Becker, M.H., editor: The health belief model and personal health practices. Health Education Monographs **2**:324-473, 1974.
10. Green, L.W.: Health education: Science, placebo, or science of placebo, Century Forum Lecture, Burlington, 1977, University of Vermont Medical School.
11. Windsor, R.A., Green, L.W., and Roseman, J.M.: Health promotion and maintenance for patients with chronic obstructive pulmonary disease: a review, Journal of Chronic Disease **33**:5-12, 1980.
12. Becker, M.H., and Green, L.W.: A family approach to compliance with medical treatment: a selective review of the literature, International Journal of Health Education **18**:173-182, 1975.
13. Green, L.W.: Should health education abandon attitude-change strategies? Perspectives from recent research, Health Education Monographs **1**(30):25-47, 1970. (Reprinted in Mico, P., editor: The SOPHE heritage collection of Health Education Monographs, vol. 1, Oakland, 1981, Third Party Publishing Co.
14. Lewin, K.: Group decision and social change. In Maccoby, E.E., Newcomb, T.H., and Hartley, E.: Readings in social psychology, New York, 1958, Holt, Rinehart & Winston.
15. Bond, B.W.: Group discussion decision: an appraisal of its use in health education, Minneapolis, 1956, Minnesota Department of Health.
16. Green, L.W., and others: Research and demonstration issues in self-care: measuring the decline of medicocentrism. In Consumer self-care in health, National Center for Health Services Research, Research Proceedings Series, DHEW Pub. No. (HRA) 77-3181, Rockville, 1977. (Also in Health Education Monographs **5**:161-189, 1977; reprinted in Mico, P., editor: The SOPHE heritage collection of Health Education Monographs, Oakland, 1981, Third Party Publishing Co.
17. Green, L.W.: Diffusion theory and the adoption of innovations in relation to heart-risk factors by the public. In Enelow, A.J., Henderson, J., and Berkanovich, E.: Applying behavioral science to cardiovascular risk, New York, 1975, American Heart Association.

18. Green, L.W.: Educational strategies to improve compliance with preventive and therapeutic regimes: the recent evidence. In Haynes, R.B., Taylor, D.W., and Sackett, D.M., editors: Compliance in health care, Baltimore, 1974, Johns Hopkins University Press.
19. Cuskey, W.R., and Premkumar, T.: A differential counselor role model for the treatment of drug addicts, Health Services Reports **88:**663-668, 1973.
20. Fisher, A.A.: The characteristics of family planning opinion leaders and their influence on the contraceptive behavior of others, unpublished doctoral dissertation, Baltimore, 1974, Johns Hopkins University School of Hygiene and Public Health.
21. Fletcher, S.R.: A study of effectiveness of a follow-up clerk in an emergency room, unpublished Master of Science thesis, Baltimore, 1974, Johns Hopkins University School of Hygiene and Public Health.
22. Oettinger, A.G.: Run, computer, run: the mythology of education innovation, Cambridge, Mass., 1969, Harvard University Press.
23. Deeds, S.G.: Promises! Promises! Educational technology for health education audiences, Presented at the annual meeting of the American Public Health Association, San Francisco, Nov. 15, 1973.
24. Green, L.W., and others: Health education planning: a diagnostic approach, Palo Alto, 1980, Mayfield Publishing Co.
25. Campeau, P.L.: Selective review of the results of research on the use of audiovisual media to teach adults, AV Communication Review **22:**5-40. 1974.
26. Thompson, J.D.: On reasonable costs of hospital services. In McKinlay, J.B., editor: Economic aspects of medical care, New York, 1973, Prodist.
27. Green, L.W.: The benefits of health education include cost-effectiveness, Hospitals: Journal of the American Hospital Association **50:**51-56, 1978.
28. Butman, R.C.: CAI—There is a way to make it pay (but not in conventional schooling), Education Technology **13:**5-9, 1973.
29. Kreuter, M.W., and Green, L.W.: Evaluation of school health education: identifying purpose, keeping perspective, Journal of School Health **48:**228-235, 1978.
30. Atwater, J.B.: Adapting the venereal disease clinic to today's problem, American Journal of Public Health **64:**433-437, 1974.
31. Bertera, R., and Green, L.W.: Cost-effectiveness of a home-visiting triage program for family planning in Turkey, American Journal of Public Health **69:**950-953, 1979.
32. Campbell, D.T.: Reforms as experiments, American Psychology **24:**409-429, 1969.
33. Morisky, D.E., and others: The relative impact of health education for low- and high-risk patients with hypertension, Preventive Medicine **9:**550-558, 1980.
34. Green, L.W., and others: Paths to the adoption of family planning: a time-lagged correlation analysis of the Dacca experiment in Bangladesh, International Journal of Health Education **18:**85-96, 1975.
35. Knobel, R.J., and Longest, B.B.: Problems associated with the cost-benefit analysis technique in voluntary hospitals, Hospital Administration **19:**42-52, 1974.
36. Parrish, T.K.: How much to spend for advertising, Journal of Advertising Research **14:**9-11, 1974.
37. Wang, V.L., Ephross, P., and Green, L.W.: The point of diminishing returns in home visits to rural homemakers, Health Education Monographs **3:**70-88, 1975. (Reprinted in Zapka, J., editor: The SOPHE heritage collection of Health Education Monographs, vol, 3. Oakland, 1981, Third Party Publishing Co.
38. Green, L.W., and Green, P.F.: Intervening in social systems to make smoking education more effective. In Steinfeld, J., and others, editors: Smoking and health: cessation activities and social action, vol. 2, DHEW Pub. No. (NIH) 77-1413, Washington, D.C., 1977, U.S. Government Printing Office.
39. Green, L.W.: Site- and symptom-related factors in secondary prevention of cancer. In Fox, B.H., Cullen, J.W., and Isom, R.N.: Cancer: the behavioral dimensions, New York, 1976, Raven Press.

40. Levine, D.M., Green, L.W., Deeds, S.G., and others: Health education for hypertensive patients, JAMA **241:**1700-1703, 1979.
41. Maiman, L., Green, L.W., and Gibson, G.: Educational self-treatment by adult asthmatics, JAMA **241:**1919-22, 1979.
42. Roter, D.L.: Patient participation in the patient-provider interaction: the effects of patient question-asking on the quality of interaction, satisfaction and compliance, Health Education Monographs **5:**281-315, 1977.
43. Sayegh, J., and Green, L.W.: Family planning education: program design, training component and cost-effectiveness of a postpartum program in Beirut, International Journal of Health Education **19**(suppl.):1-20, 1976.
44. Health Education Center: Strategies for health education in local health departments, Baltimore, 1977, Maryland State Department of Health and Mental Hygiene. (See also the health education–risk reduction programs in state health departments, sponsored by the Centers for Disease Control, Atlanta, 1980-81.)
45. Green, L.W., and others: Guidelines for health education in maternal and child health, International Journal of Health Education **21**(3, suppl.):1-33, 1978.
46. Green, L.W.: Determining the impact and effectiveness of health education as it relates to federal policy, Health Education Monographs **6**(suppl. 1):28-66, 1978.
47. Green, L.W.: Health promotion policy and the placement of responsibility for personal health care, Family and Community Health: Journal of Health Promotion and Maintenance **2:**51-64, 1979.
48. Green, L.W.: Healthy people: the surgeon general's report and the prospects. In McNerney, W.J., editor: Working for a healthier America. Cambridge, Mass., 1980, Ballinger Publishing Co.
49. Danforth, N., and Swaboda, B.: Agency for International Development Health Education Study, Washington, D.C., 1978, Westinghouse Health Systems.
50. Ackerman, A., and Kalmer, H.: Health education and a baccalaureate nursing curriculum—myth or reality? Paper presented at the 105th annual meeting of the American Public Health Association, Washington, D.C., November 1, 1977.
51. Fedder, D., and Beardsley, R.: Training pharmacists to become patient educators, Paper presented to the section of teachers of pharmacy administration of the annual meeting of the American Association of Colleges of Pharmacy, Orlando, Fla., July 18, 1978).
52. Bennett, B.I.: A model for teaching health education skills to primary care practitioners, International Journal of Health Education **20**(4):232-239, 1977.
53. Milio, N.: A framework for prevention: changing health-damaging to health-generating life patterns, American Journal of Public Health **66:**435-439, 1976.
54. Navarro, V.: Medicine under capitalism, New York, 1976, Prodist.
55. Anderson, R.: A behavioral model of families' use of health services, University of Chicago Center for Health Administration Studies Research Series, No. 25, Chicago, 1968, University of Chicago Press.
56. Becker, M.H., editor: The health belief model and personal health behavior, Health Education Monographs **2:**324-508, 1974.
57. Green, L.W., and Krotki, K.J.: Class and parity biases in family planning programs: the case of Karachi, Eugenics Quarterly (Social Biology) **15:**235-251, 1968.
58. Neill, J.S., and Bond, J.O.: Hillsborough County oral polio vaccine program, Florida State Board of Health Monograph No. 6 (Jacksonville, 1964, Florida State Board of Health.
59. Wang, V.L., Ephross, P., and Green, L.W.: The point of diminishing returns in nutrition education through home visits by aides: an evaluation of EFNEP, Health Education Monographs **3:**70-88, 1975.
60. Ward, G.H.: Changing trends in control of hypertension, Public Health Reports **93:**31-34, 1978.
61. Farquahr, J.W., and others: Community education for cardiovascular health, Lancet **1**(8023):1192-1195, 1977.

62. Green, L.W., and others: The Dacca family planning experiment: a comparative evaluation of programs directed at males and females, Pacific Health Education Reports No. 3, Berkeley, 1972, University of California Press.

63. Maccoby, N., and others: Reducing the risk of cardiovascular disease: effects of a community-based campaign on knowledge and behavior, Journal of Community Health **3:**100-114, 1977.

64. Roberts, B.J., and others: An experimental study of two approaches to communication, American Journal of Public Health **53:**1361-1381, 1963.

65. Stahl, S., and others: Motivational interventions in community hypertension screening, American Journal of Public Health **67:**345-52, 1977.

66. Steinberg, S., and Fitzpatrick, D.: The Paducah Health Education Survey, 1958, American Journal of Public Health **51:**732-745, 1961.

67. Wilkinson G.S., and others: Measuring response to a cancer information telephone facility: Can-Dial, American Journal of Public Health **66:**367-71, 1976.

68. Dershewitz, A., and Williamson, W.: Preventing of childhood household injuries: a controlled clinical trial, American Journal of Public Health **67:**1148-1153, 1977.

69. Phillips, F., and others: An experiment with payment, quota, and clinic affiliation schemes for lay motivators in the Philippines, Studies in Family Planning **6:**326-334, 1975.

70. Robinson, E.: A comparative evaluation of the scrub and brush methods of toothbrushing with flossing as an adjunct (in fifth- and sixthgraders), American Journal of Public Health **66:**1078-1081, 1976.

71. Roter, D.L.: Patient participation in the patient-provider interaction: the effects of patient question-asking on the quality of interaction, satisfaction and compliance, Health Education Monographs **5:**281-315, 1977.

72. Sayegh, J., and Green, L.W.: Family planning education: program design, training component and cost-effectiveness of the postpartum program in Beirut, International Journal of Health Education **19**(suppl.):1-20, 1976.

73. Smith, P.B., and others: The medical impact of an antepartum program for pregnant adolescents: a statistical analysis, American Journal of Public Health **78:**169-172, 1978.

74. Bailey, J., and Zambrano, M.: Contraceptive pamphlets in Columbian drugstores, Studies in Family Planning **5:**178-182, 1974.

75. Dalzell, I.: Evaluation of a prenatal teaching program, Nursing Research **14:**160-163, 1965.

76. Elwood, T.W., Ericson, E., and Lieberman, S.: Comparative educational approaches to screening for colorectal cancer, American Journal of Public Health **68:**135-138, 1978.

77. Fisher, A.A., and others: Training teachers in population education institutes in Baltimore, Journal of School Health **46:**357-360, 1976.

78. Green, L.W., Levine, D.M., and Deeds, S.G.: Clinical trials of health education for hypertensive outpatients: design and baseline data, Preventive Medicine **4:**417-25, 1975.

79. Kupst, M.J., and others: Evaluation of methods to improve communication in the physician-patient relationship, American Journal of Orthopsychiatry **45:**420-429, 1975.

80. Levine, D.M., and others: Health education for hypertensive patients, JAMA **241:**1700-1703, 1979.

81. Maimon, L., and others: Education for self-treatment by adult asthmatics, JAMA **241:**1919-1922, 1979.

82. Peters, R., and others: Daily relaxation response breaks in a working population: effects on blood pressure, American Journal of Public Health **67:**954-959, 1977.

83. Green, L.W.: Evaluation and measurement: some dilemmas for health education, American Journal of Public Health **67:**155-161, 1977.

84. Bertram, D.A., and Brooks-Betram, P.A.: The evaluation of continuing medical education: a literature review, Health Education Monographs **5:**330-362, 1977.

85. Green, L.W.: Change—process models in health education, Public Health Reviews **5:**5-33, 1976.

86. Green, L.W.: Theory and research vs. practice in health education, Health Education Monographs **3:**352-358, 1975.
87. Green, L.W.: Methods available to evaluate the health education components of preventive health programs. In Preventive medicine USA: health promotion and consumer health education, New York, 1976, Prodist.
88. Green, L.W.: What is quality in patient education and how do we assess it? In Squyres, W., editor: Patient education: an inquiry into the state of the art, New York, 1980, Springer Publishing Co., Inc.
89. Rubinson, L., and Baillie, L.: Planning school based sexuality programs utilizing the PRE-CEDE model, Journal of School Health **51:**282-287, 1981.
90. Morisky, D., Levine, D., Green, L., and others: Five year blood pressure control and mortality following health education for hypertensive patients, American Journal of Public Health **73**(2): 153-162, 1983.
91. Ayer, W., Davis, D., and Deatrick, D.: Dental health education in workplace settings, Proposal to National Institute for Dental Research, 1981.

Additional Reading

Green, L., Kreuter, M., Deeds, S., and Partridge, K.: Health education planning: a diagnostic approach, Palo Alto, Cal., 1980, Mayfield Publishing Co. (Appendices B and C).

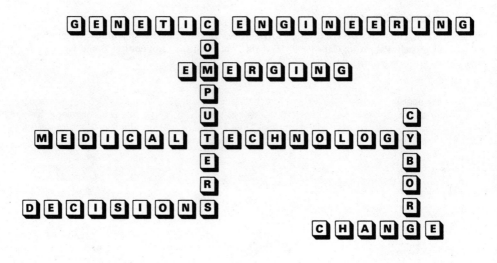

8 Future Issues in Health Education

Introduction

The final chapter of this text offers a window through which you can look into the future and contemplate your role as a health educator. Most of us are busy dealing with day-to-day problems and cast only an occasional glance to the near future. But as Drs. St. Pierre and Shute have observed, many of the significant issues that will affect our world during the last 20 years of this century demand our immediate consideration.

By analyzing current trends and forecasting future ones, the authors encourage you to consider the consequences of decisions related to the environment, medical technology, the family, stress, and the overall quality of life. They recognize that, in addition to the benefits brought about through scientific progress, there may be significant social, legal, political, ethical, moral, and economic trade-offs. The outcomes of these decisions and trade-offs will not only affect our lives as individuals but will also have profound effects on our profession. As you embark on a career in health education you should realize that outside forces that are capable of changing societal values are certainly able to affect the nature of health education. In fact, these future issues may even help to redefine our profession.

Health education has been somewhat analogous to a reed floating in the water, occasionally surrendering to the prevailing current and the arbitrary winds of change. As a result, our efforts have been reactionary and crisis oriented, moving from one concern to the next. Drs. St. Pierre and Shute observe that either we shape the future or we are shaped by it. "Being concerned with the future is not the same as controlling it." During the next several decades, health education has the opportunity and perhaps even the obligation to take a proactive stand on issues related to healthful living. Knowing what the future holds in store, we should be able to prepare ourselves to meet the challenges anticipated in the years ahead.

The Role Delineation Project is seen as an important step in this direction. Chapter 4 on Competencies presented the broad areas of responsibility and the functions of a health educator as listed in the Role Delineation Project. Chapter 8 describes the credentialing process and emphasizes the point that credentialing will have a dramatic effect on the future of health education.

It is quite probable that health education will occur in new and varied settings throughout the next decade. The target populations will be diverse, with a wide range of needs. Content will change as new scientific discoveries are made. The teaching-learning process will appear strange to the "hygiene teacher" of the past as computers, video equipment, and other communication devices become more sophisticated and more available to the general public. Regardless of the nature of the audience, the setting, or the methodology, it is clear that health educators will need to demonstrate their effectiveness and the necessity of having adequate professional preparation to assume their responsibilities. The future is upon us. Will you be ready to accept the challenges that lie ahead?

The Future is Coming!

The future is rushing toward us at alarming speed. Technologic and sociologic advances have often outstripped our ability to understand them. Knowledge is increasing at such a rate that no one expects to be able to master several fields of study. Indeed, many professionals would agree that it is incredibly difficult to stay up-to-date in even one area of specialization. We feel an almost mystical reverence for those individuals in the "near" past, such as Galileo, Isaac Newton, Benjamin Franklin, and Thomas Jefferson, who had a keen grasp of much of the available knowledge of their respective eras. Because of this, they were able to use their brilliant minds to integrate their understandings to bring us many revolutionary scientific, social, and political innovations.

Today our schools and colleges, as well as other professional and technical schools, face the considerable challenge of preparing individuals for careers that in many cases have not yet been fully defined. Our institutions, often slow to react to rapidly changing circumstances, appear to be falling further and further behind. The social, political, moral, and religious customs and practices are being constantly assailed by new discoveries, by the chronic threat of nuclear war, by virtually instantaneous worldwide communications, and by the changing nature of preferred life-styles. For some these changes are so confusing and frightening that they "drop out" or try to turn back to a less demanding existence. Physiologically and psychologically stressful events may cause these people to return with even more vigor to conservative values and practices in a frantic effort to slow progress—at least from their perspective. For some people the pressure of such rapid change will cause stress-related diseases. Others may react to current pressures and the uncertainty of the future by seeking solace in psychoactive drugs or by reaching enthusiastically for every new idea or fad.

Traditionally, however, the future has been endowed with more pleasing qualities. It is a concept of hope, challenge, happiness, and progress. Most of us have grown up with the idea of planning for and looking forward to our future, and we view with considerable disdain those who are not properly concerned with their future.

This concern for the future is typical of people at all ages and in all walks of life. Schoolchildren dream and scheme of many anticipated events—having a career, getting married, taking a final examination in math class. Adults wonder whether they will get promoted at work, be able to buy a new car, or be able to enjoy their retirement years. For most of us our future-directedness is apparently intensely personal and related to our near future. Only rarely do we worry about such philosophic concerns as the future of humanity in general.

Yet being concerned about the future is not the same as studying it with an eye toward shaping and controlling the world's destiny. For much of humanity, preoccupied with day-to-day survival, serious study of the future is idle speculation, something done by science fiction writers, philosophers, and other such "ivory tower sympathizers" (who after all, have little else of importance to do). Futuristic fantasies are certainly curious and interesting exercises for the mind, but who really needs them?

Another difficulty in trying to convince people of the need to consider future issues is that most of us simply fail to recognize the eventual impact of gradual but inexorable change.[1] We expect tomorrow to be pretty much like today—in fact, we count on it! And our expectations are usually fulfilled, lulling us into a false sense of security. Sometimes, of course, we are shocked into looking further forward. Personal involvement in a cataclysmic natural event such as an earthquake, the untimely death of a spouse, or a newly discovered lung tumor can shatter the short-term plans for our lives and force us to actively plan for several years in the future.

But what about other events, those gradual but no less dramatic forces that are working to alter our future in every imaginable way? As an example, Edward Cornish, President of the World Future Society, has noted that "a 2% (yearly) increase in air pollution might attract little attention, yet it means that air pollution would double in 34 years."[2] Another event that may seriously affect all of us is that, in only 20 years, one half million to 2 million plant and animal species now living on earth will be extinct, primarily because of the loss of their habitat through population and industrial expansion and the accompanying pollution.[3] How can we come to grips with the destruction of almost 20% of the earth's living species? Even though we do not notice it, or may choose to ignore it, the future is upon us. The implications of uncontrolled change are enormous. If changes are not planned for effectively or if they occur in an indiscriminate fashion, serious complications could result. It is likely that life as we now know it could cease to exist. Thus change must be approached in a systematic manner in order to ensure a promising future for generations to come.

As a student preparing for a career in health education, you surely have a natural interest in your own personal future. We hope that you will also develop an interest in the *study* of the future so that you will be better prepared to serve your clientele and able to exert some control over the present so that the world of the future will indeed be a bright and healthy place in which to live. This chapter will provide you with some projections of the major health-related issues facing the profession during the next 20 years. We will attempt to describe the health educator of the future and predict the competencies you will need, as well as describe the nature of the settings in which you will ply your trade during the first part of your career.

Please keep in mind that we will present current *projections* for the future. Clearly, depending on the actions we are willing to take today, there are many alternative futures. By looking ahead we are forced to look not only at facts, resources, and educated guesses but also at our needs, desires, values, and goals for humanity and for other life forms on our planet. Will we be able to make responsible decisions that will shape the future rather than allowing events to occur seemingly of their own will? What is the key to a better future? Is it longer life, quality health care, an end to worldwide hunger? Must we return to old ways, basic religious values, and the traditional family values in order to preserve our way of life in America? If so, how will our actions affect the other people of the world? One thing is clear; we must attend to all possibilities and examine available choices rather than just current "facts" and scientific and humanistic principles from the American viewpoint alone.

Future Trends and Issues

The *Global 2000 Report to the President,* presented in 1980 to former President Jimmy Carter, offered rather dismal projections in several key health-related areas. One warning stated that "if present trends continue, the world in the year 2000 will be more crowded, more polluted, less stable ecologically, and more vulnerable to disruption than the world we live in now."[3] We mentioned earlier the expected devastation that will be brought on plant and animal species. Let us examine now, in more detail, some specific forecasts that will deeply affect humans.

Population Pressures. The population of the world in 1950 was about 2.5 billion. By 1970 it had increased to almost 3.7 billion; in 1975 it was over 4 billion. By the year 2000, less than 20 years from now, this planet will support about 6.35 billion people, an increase of nearly 50% from the 1975 figures.[3,4] Ninety percent of the growth in population in the next 20 years will occur in the poorer countries. The U.S. population, by contrast, currently stands at about 220 million. By the year 2000 it will increase to about 250 million, an increase of "only" 16%. Two of the strongest and wealthiest nations in the world, the United States and the Union of Soviet Socialist Republics (U.S.S.R.), account for only 4% and 5% of the total world population, respectively; yet they are the nations most influential on world matters.[3]

Projecting even further, the population of the world could approach 10 billion by the year 2030 and 30 billion by the end of the next century. Thirty billion is a figure that is thought to be close to the maximum capacity of the Earth![3]

Although the developed countries have managed to hold their population growth in check (relatively speaking), the developing countries can look forward to more and more disease and starvation as a result of massive population increases. Compounding this expected increase in population is the fact that the amount of arable land will increase only 4% by the year 2000. The regional water shortages that are becoming more frequent even now are expected to become very severe in the near future, even for the developed countries.

Consider the implications of the above projections in the context of some current hotly debated issues such as family planning and contraception. Some futurists believe that some form of family planning may be forced on us regardless of our religious or moral convictions, customs, or desires. Otherwise, hunger, war, and disease will regulate the population. How does such a concept fit into your value system and professional goals?

Medical Advances and Health Care Problems. The future will bring us many new medical and health-related advances that will revolutionize the way we think about our health status. Some advances may change the way we think about human life itself. Within the next 20 years, experts predict that it may be possible to regenerate severed limbs and replace many internal organs that have succumbed to disease or injury. We may even have a diet supplement that would improve our memory.[4] Also, several projects are under way to test the effectiveness of new drugs that could retard the aging process. And of course new techniques for diagnosis, surgery, and disease management and treatment are on the horizon for all fields of medicine.

Perhaps even more startling is the research into the mysteries of deoxyribonucleic acid (DNA), the chemical that controls heredity. It is already possible to make new chromosomes and entirely new species of simple life forms.[5] Future developments in this area are expected to help medical scientists and physicians in the quest for a cure for heart disease, cancer, and many other chronic diseases.

It must be pointed out, however, that public reaction to the new and prospective advances in medicine has always been mixed. Although some people are truly happy about the possibility for longer, more productive lives, many people view such research with fear and loathing; they raise several questions about the ultimate use and value of such technology. For example:

1. Will a biologic accident release violent organisms on an unsuspecting world?
2. How many organs and other body tissues can be replaced before a human becomes a "cyborg" (humanoid)?

3. Will genetic engineering produce other humanlike species that may replace the basic tasks now performed by humans (for example, will robots perform menial tasks)?

4. Will science be able to produce a super race of human?

Some of these concerns may seem farfetched to you, but some respected thinkers in diverse fields of study believe that the eventual answers to these questions (and others) will revolutionize legal, religious, medical, and ethical views of human life.

Many other issues may be raised in the health care domain that are of more immediate concern to all of us. First, there is a current and worldwide problem of access to quality health care.[6] Even in the United States, we still do not have structure to provide medical help to all those who may need it, regardless of how simple the need may be from a medical standpoint. No matter how advanced our medical technology may become, what use does it serve if most people do not have access to it because of financial or transportation limitations?

Below are some of the health care problems that must be faced in the near future. Perhaps some of them may be solved by the time you read this. We doubt, however, that most of these are amenable to a "quick fix" because of the expense and the political nature of these complex problems.

How can the distribution of physicians be improved?

- In the United States one half of all physicians are in only *seven* states (New York, California, Pennsylvania, Florida, Illinois, Texas, and Ohio). About 135 counties and 5000 towns have *no* physicians at all. Will the training of more nurse-practitioners prove to be an effective way to deal with the poor geographic distribution of physicians?

How will people pay for services rendered?

- In the past decade, rising medical costs have far outstripped the ability of people to pay for care out of their own pockets. Yet millions of Americans have no health insurance, and of course in many catastrophic cases a person's health insurance may be exhausted long before the need for treatment has ended. Do you think a form of national health insurance is the answer?

What can be done to increase the number of general practitioners?

- The tendency of most physicians to limit their practice to one specialty area (such as internal medicine, surgery, or pediatrics) is believed to have been a major factor in the rise of health care costs. Additionally, a patient who sees only specialists may never have a physician who takes time to be concerned with the total health care needs of the patient. What incentives can be devised to encourage a greater number of primary care physicians?

What can be done to improve the standards of quality care?
- As in any field of work, there will always be incompetent, unprofessional, and unethical physicians. Also, there are many others in and around the health field with inadequate skills or abundant greed. So, along with our concerns for eliminating poor physicians, let us not forget to consider standards for other health care professionals, "alternative" practitioners of health care (chiropractors, faith healers, naturopaths, etc.), and the large health quackery industry. Should government take the responsibility for improving the overall quality of care, or do other options exist?

How can health professionals at all levels encourage and assist the public to voluntarily modify their poor health habits?
- It is abundantly clear that many of the diseases that debilitate or kill people are the result of personal behavior selection. It is well established that such voluntary "misbehaviors" as smoking, poor food choices, drug and alcohol abuse, poor safety practices, and too little exercise greatly increase the risk of such health problems as cancer,

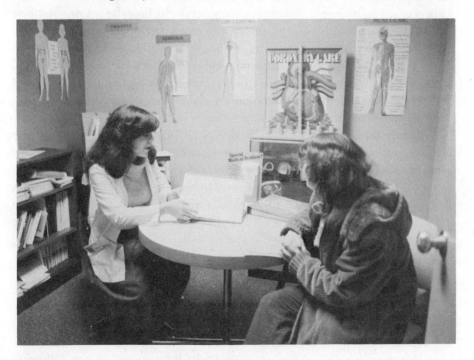

Fig. 8-1. Many health educators are performing the role of health counselor in small group or one-to-one situations. Future health issues may demand more and more of this counseling role by health educators.

emphysema, heart and circulatory diseases, obesity, injuries, drug dependence, and many other debilitating or life-threatening conditions. Is it morally acceptable to encourage a change in behavior when the existing behavior is likely to end in disease?

Without question, new advances in the biomedical field can lead to better, more fulfilling lives for all of us. But perhaps the activity having the greatest potential for future health will be in the area of health promotion rather than in the treatment of disease and injury. The very idea of "wellness" is just beginning to take hold in the public consciousness. It remains to be seen whether the government, health professionals and their organizations, and the social structure will change from an almost mystical belief in medical miracles to a more practical orientation toward developing healthy life-styles.

Two other issues expected to receive greater attention in the near future are acute care and rehabilitation. In spite of the "gee-whiz" technology that exists in some hospital trauma units, many people die because they cannot be kept alive long enough to gain access to this superior technology. Expect more ambulances and other emergency vehicles to be better equipped and staffed with highly trained emergency care personnel and physicians to deal with such acute medical emergencies as heart attacks and physical injuries resulting from burns, accidents, and so on. Because more people will be saved who otherwise would have died, there will be a great need to expand and refine physical and occupational rehabilitation services to help victims resume their lives at maximum potential.

Family Life. Over the past few decades, Americans have altered their life-styles in many significant ways, and perhaps the greatest changes in family life have been attributed to the so-called sexual revolution. Robert T. Francoer[7] has pointed out that the alternative life-styles and flexible attitudes that have emerged over the decades of the 1960s and 1970s have a firm hold on us. Indeed, he believes it is unlikely that we will again experience a return to the values and behavior patterns that followed the Great Depression of the 1930s.[7]

Revolutions imply rapidly changing conditions and accompanying confusion. Although the sexual revolution has brought much personal freedom, it has also been condemned as the destroyer of traditional values, marriage, and family life. Although recent statistics show a drop in the divorce rate, the overall trend indicates that divorce will remain a major social problem. Consider, if you will, the future impact and interactions of the following recent events in the history of sexuality and family living.

1. The women's liberation movement
2. The gay liberation movement
3. The increased number of working women

4. The increased number of unmarried couples living together
5. The increased divorce rate
6. The increased number of "open" marriages
7. The increased number of coed dormitories in colleges and universities
8. The widespread use of contraception and other birth control measures
9. The increased use of sexually explicit language and behavior in the media
10. The increased number of single-parent families
11. The increased publicity given to sex scandals
12. The increase in pornographic materials
13. The increased abortion rate
14. The increased number of "test tube babies" and surrogate mothers
15. The increased number of reported rapes and cases of sexual harassment
16. The increase in child abuse and family violence
17. The increased use of child care centers
18. The increased concern for youthful faces and figures
19. The increased concern about sexual adequacy and sexual performance
20. The increased number of unwanted pregnancies and unmarried mothers, especially adolescents
21. The devaluation of parents and grandparents as mentors and as part of the nuclear or extended family

Certainly there are powerful voices calling for a retrenchment, a return to the basic, conservative values of marriage and family life. But is this a possibility? If so, do we want to move in the direction from which we came? Can we accentuate the positive aspects of these changes and reduce the impact of the negative aspects?

Other factors affect men and women and hence the nature of families. For example, the increased stress placed on working women has led to increases in stress-related diseases such as alcoholism and abuse of other drugs. Men and women are free to adopt androgynous behaviors so that men feel more comfortable about cooking, doing housework, and child-rearing, and women feel more comfortable about being assertive and becoming successful professionals.

Additionally, in tomorrow's world there will be less emphasis on long hours of work and more emphasis on leisure activities.[8] Conventional work routines will be altered significantly to include more on-the-job exercise and other forms of relaxation. The emergence of cooperative versus competitive games will affect the way our children view themselves and their world.

There are, however, opportunities to counteract the forces that have disrupted family living. As new methods of working, playing, learning, and communicating become more widespread, the confusion of the revolution may lead to more satisfying, healthful, but very different family structures.

Other Issues. There are many other concerns to be dealt with in the future that will profoundly affect the health education professional. At a meeting of more than 5000 futurists in Toronto in July 1980, many of these issues were raised and discussed at length.[9] In spite of the dangers of an unguided future, the participants as a whole were cautiously optimistic.

We still have to give more vigorous attention to such critical issues as the disposal of nuclear wastes, poverty, the threat of war, racial unrest, and other social, political, and environmental problems. Yet, in spite of the problems, real advances in communications and computer technology, food production and distribution, and new sources and delivery systems for energy are expected, along with the previously mentioned advances in medicine, population control, and personal and family living structures.

The Challenge for Health Education

When the future of society is viewed from the perspective of the profession of health education several key considerations become apparent. How well the profession adapts to these future needs will dictate the future of health education.

Greater life span, increased leisure time, rapidly changing careers, technologic advances in communications and computers, and other worldwide forces will vastly change our sociologic and psychologic framework. Change and obsolescence demand new educational directions. As June and Harold Shane forecasted:

1. Education of the very young will be a priority.
2. A continuous educational program will emerge in which persons may prepare for a second or third career in their middle years.
3. Life span will increase and individuals will experience more years of good health.
4. Self-instruction and less formal reference and social centers will be developed.
5. A variety of highly advanced electronic listening and viewing devices will become more common.
6. Chemical and electronic means may be used to alter personality and improve learning ability.
7. The physically helpless will have their handicaps reduced or eliminated by means of organ transplants, improved therapy, surgery, and plastic or electronic implants.
8. Genetic controls may be used to eliminate undesirable hereditary factors and birth defects and to allow parents to select the sex of unborn infants.[10]

These and other factors will have an important impact on future educational programs. Whatever your opinions about these changes and issues may be, your future activities as a health educator will have to take into account the relationships between such things as strongly held beliefs about the sanctity of life and facts of the dangers of unchecked population growth. You will have to educate the public about new medical techniques and drugs and you will have to deal with the public's resistance to change their lifestyles in the interest of better health. You will be called on to work within legal, ethical, and social structures to accelerate access to new technologies, systems, and behavior patterns. You will have to serve as an advocate and activist in the interest of public health. You must learn to understand and use new methods of communication to bring the health education message to people of all ages.

Perhaps you will be involved in the development of innovative health education programs for use with home computers and video playback devices. Maybe you will be among the first to expand the new interest in health promotion at the worksite. You may serve as a facilitator of new peer teaching systems so victims of stroke, cancer, and other disabilities can form mutual aid groups for their own education, protection, and progress.

For these things to occur, the health education profession must be amenable to changes in training and practices of the professional. In the following sections of this chapter you will learn of the challenges facing health education professionals and obtain some insight into the nature of health education in the future.

Implications for Professional Preparation of Health Educators

The overall changes anticipated within society in general and within the total health care system specifically have tremendous potential for encouraging creativity in the professional preparation of future health educators. As we enter the final decades of this century the scope and nature of the health education task will undoubtedly be altered. Ethical issues, political activism, concepts of accountability, and the definition of acceptable means of behavioral change will emerge as key concerns.

Ethics. Health educators must be well versed in the ethical and philosophic issues involved in such biomedical considerations as euthanasia, amniocentesis, organ transplants, and a host of related advances. As medical technology continues to create new products and methods, the nature of the educational process related to these advances will be extremely important. In the past, however, health educators have remained on the periphery of involvement in such issues. Perhaps individuals and the professional organizations will find it necessary to take a stand and publicly affirm their values.

Decision Making. The complexity of decision-making tasks facing the health consumer in the future will necessitate a clarification of all facets of each particular health decision, including the ethical aspects. As a result, professional preparation programs will need to design courses that illustrate and clarify the many ethical considerations facing the profession. Most likely

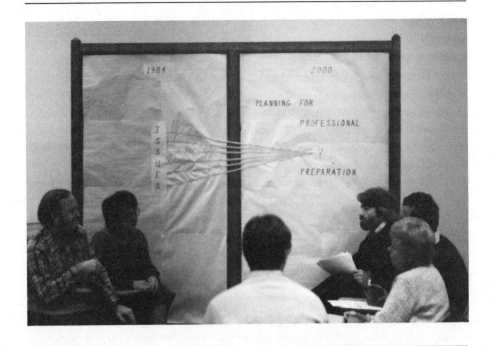

Fig. 8-2. Future issues will help to determine the nature of professional preparation. Faculty planning will enable us to meet the challenges of the future.

these courses will be of an interdisciplinary nature and will broaden the scope of involvement of future health educators by providing an awareness of the role of other health professionals.

A sensitivity to issues such as cloning, for example, will not only facilitate the dissemination of information to consumers but also provide a basis for the health educator to discuss, debate, or interact with other health workers on such topics. Such involvement will begin to enhance both the credibility and acceptance of the health education profession. The profession must anticipate those medical advances requiring ethical decisions and develop effective educational strategies designed to clarify those ethical elements, as well as convey the cognitive components necessary for positive decision making to take place.

Activism. Rarely have health educators been viewed as a politically active professional group. Even though many of the topics and issues covered by health educators have tremendous political implications, health educators have often avoided these political elements. The future, however, appears to indicate a need for greater political awareness and involvement for all health professionals. As more and more health-related programs come under governmental control, either federally or locally, a general understanding of the political process is critical.

Professional preparation programs should direct attention toward the political arena by providing opportunities for students to examine various health-related lobbying interests, to explore the nature and structure of health-related congressional committees, and to understand the complex nature of the total political environment. Innovative practicum experiences and courses specifically designed to examine the politics of health seem particularly appropriate.

Accountability. As health educators and the health education process become more visible in the total health care system, issues of professional accountability are certain to emerge. At no time in the history of health education has this need become more evident. Health educators will be expected to demonstrate program effectiveness regardless of the setting involved. The reduction of federal funds to health-related programs (whether temporary or permanent), coupled with the increased competition for existing dollars, will require sound accountability practices. Health educators must learn the processes for cost-benefit, cost-effectiveness, and behavioral outcome evaluations in addition to the more traditional knowledge and attitude change evaluations.

Understanding expected program outcomes and writing clear, measurable objectives have always been considered important components in health education planning, but now these tasks will need to be refined and made much more explicit. Greater attention to research needs and developing evaluative strategies within all proposed programs will be a necessity for future health education tasks rather than an added frill.

The goal for future health education will be to establish evaluation techniques to determine those outcomes acceptable and desirable to specific target populations and to develop measurement instruments sufficient to monitor program success. Increased public and governmental interest in health promotion, acute care, rehabilitation, and disease prevention (in preference to treatment after the fact) means more sensitive evaluation plans must be initiated.

Behavior Changes. Should health educators be change agents? What limits on the nature of behavioral change strategies should be established? Who decides what behavior should be changed? Which behavioral objectives are reasonable, and measurable, for determining program effectiveness? These ethical concerns related to behavior change are but a few of the questions that future health educators will be expected to answer.

Behavior can be altered in numerous ways: chemically, emotionally, educationally, and legally. And within each category various strategies can be implemented. You may alter moods by drinking alcohol, ingesting drugs, or inhaling fumes. Or you may learn mental and physical techniques to be stimulated or to relax. So it is with education; various teaching strategies can produce desired behavior change. Health educators will need to examine which educational strategies work best and most efficiently, which are acceptable to society, and which border on unethical infringement of individual rights. This concern will become even more critical in the future as technologic advances produce more sophisticated teaching strategies.

The Generalist. Based on our previous discussion of anticipated societal changes and trends it is obvious that a new set of health issues and conditions will emerge in the future. A critical issue confronting professional preparation programs in health education is to prepare professionals who not only understand the various health and science content areas but also have the skills to use their knowledge of sociologic and psychologic forces that shape and control behavior change. Depending on the setting in which the health educators of the future will practice, they must be able to prepare flexible, adaptable materials and methods to help the targeted group, be they school children, hospital patients, employees, the aged, or the physically or mentally impaired.

It may seem illogical to argue that a health educator should be both a specialist and a generalist. However, the process of professional preparation for an entry-level health educator can be quite different from that introduced into graduate education. This generalist-specialist role concept has been addressed by the Role Delineation Project for Health Education, begun in 1978.[11] It is hoped that the outcome of this effort will lead to a more structured and accepted model for developing and maintaining the profession.

So that you may become more aware of the upcoming changes and issues related to the future of health education the chapter on credentialing and role delineation from the final report of the Role Delineation Project for Health Education is reprinted in the following section.

Credentialing and Role Delineation*

As health education developed as a field requiring advanced study, witnessed by the growth of preparatory programs in colleges and universities, practicing and academic health educators have striven to enhance and improve the qualities of the profession. Improvement has come about because of individuals who have continued to professionally grow and develop. New knowledge of health and human behavior has become available, concepts and technology of education have been developed, preparatory programs have sought to improve their curricula, and professional groups have been organized with a goal of establishing an acceptable level of quality while promoting excellence. Indeed, other professions have gone through this process and continue to do so.

Individual professionals promote quality by example, groups of professionals promote quality by establishing standards of preparation and practice of their members. Beyond the associations, a more formal process, credentialing, is used to assure an acceptable standard for those practicing a profession.

---

*Reprinted from Initial Role Delineation for Health Education: Final Report, DHHS Publication No. [HRA] 80-44, Washington, D.C., 1981, U.S. Government Printing Office.

Credentialing, a process of demonstrating evidence of qualification, comprises three related forms:

1. *Accreditation*—The process by which an agency or organization evaluates and recognizes an institution or program of study as meeting certain predetermined criteria or standards.

2. *Licensure*—The process by which an agency or government grants permission to persons to engage in a given profession or occupation by certifying that those licensed have attained the minimal degree of competency necessary to ensure that the public health, safety, and welfare will be reasonably well protected.

3. *Certification or registration*—The process by which a nongovernmental agency or association grants recognition to an individual who has met certain predetermined qualifications specified by that agency or association. Such qualifications may include: (a) graduation from an accredited or approved program; (b) acceptable performance on a qualifying examination or series of examinations; and/or (c) completion of a given amount of work experience.[12]

Briefly, accreditation is a voluntary process which is part of the private sector. Begun by individual professional associations as a way of achieving collective status, accreditation has evolved over the years into an organized, but not necessarily orderly, process. In 1975, the Council on Postsecondary Accreditation (COPA) was developed from two previously existing accrediting umbrella organizations.[13] COPA serves to recognize, review and coordinate accrediting bodies. In turn, the Commissioner of Education, U.S. Office of Education (USOE), recognized accrediting agencies and associations for determining eligibility for federal assistance. Both COPA and USOE publish listings of recognized accrediting bodies. Private accrediting bodies are recognized by COPA. USOE uses COPA recognition, and other criteria, to establish public recognition. This recognition is translated into fiscal and administrative support for educational programs which meet accreditation standards. Due to the burgeoning number of health professions, time and cost of accreditation are placing a burden on institutions considering accreditation either of the institution itself or its programs. Preparatory program personnel in health education must come to grips with these concerns if accreditation is considered to be a viable quality assurance mechanism.

Complicating accreditation concerns for health education is the lack of a currently recognized (COPA and USOE) accrediting body that covers the entire field. Presently there are two accrediting agencies that affect health education: The Council on Education for Public Health (CEPH) and the National Council for Accreditation of Teacher Education (NCATE). CEPH is recognized by COPA and USOE to accredit schools of public health and graduate programs of community health education. (CEPH also has been recognized by USOE in a preaccreditation status for progams of community and preventive medicine.) NCATE accredits college and university programs for the preparation of all teachers and other school personnel at the elementary and secondary levels. CEPH and NCATE primarily focus upon institutional accreditation (e.g., a school of public health or a college of education) rather than emphasizing particular programs (e.g., a department of health education). The concern over programmatic versus institutional accreditation is being debated at the national level. Time and expense now involved in programmatic accreditation for educational institutions is being questioned, as is the utility of accreditation itself.

Licensure of individuals has been among the most rapidly changing of the credentialing mechanisms. As an example, state licensing authorities have had to cope with numerous requests for licensing health professionals. As a result, there is pressure to consolidate individual licensing boards into single state agencies, to eliminate disparities and inequities of licensing practices among the states, and to employ nationally-based examinations as part of the licensing process. Significant attention is being given to assurance of continuing competency of health professionals through means such as continuing education and relicensure.

The conditions existing in the field of licensure coming into and during the 1970's led the Department of Health, Education and Welfare (DHEW) to urge both states and health professions to observe a two year moratorium on legislation that would license a health occupation or role. The first moratorium was recommended in 1971 and was consecutively followed by another one in 1973. In 1977, DHEW recommended that four questions be used by the states to evaluate the need for new licensing requests[14.]

1. How will the unregulated practice of a particular profession clearly endanger the health, safety and welfare of the public?
2. How will the public benefit by assurance of competence?
3. Can the public be effectively protected by means other than licensing?
4. Why is licensure the most appropriate form of regulation?

For health education, answers to these questions and a careful evaluation of the complexities and rapidly changing environment of licensing procedures must be developed to determine the desirability and feasibility of licensing as a credentialing alternative. Also, recognition must be given to the need to approach all of the states to establish licensing legislation.

Certification and registration are processes of a voluntary nature which are more controllable by professional organizations. They can be used to help employers, third party payers, health professionals, preparatory programs, and the public recognize the basic competencies possessed by those certified or registered. Emphasis on the validity of practitioners' competencies is essential to certification, as well as to licensure and accreditation. By establishing certification standards, professional organizations assure that a pool of well-prepared individuals are made available to render needed services to the public. No certification mechanism exists to cover all health educators. This may be due to the fact that no single professional organization concerned with health education speaks for the entire field.

Given the current status of credentialing and the fact that the role delineation process is designed to move the health education profession into these areas, questions of the utility of credentialing of health educators can be raised. While questions regarding the desirability of establishing credentialing mechanisms for health education remain to be answered, the following points should be considered by health educators as immediate professional concerns to be resolved through the development of a credentialing process:

1. Presently the public, as well as other health and education professionals, has difficulty in identifying not only health educators, but those who are capable of delivering services at an acceptable level.
2. Employers of health educators are presented with differing perceptions of health educators, their qualifications, and what they are prepared to do.
3. Functions most often identified as those involving the work of professional health educators are seen as those of other health professionals by employers and other opinion leaders, thus leading to a diffuse or secondary professional identity for health educators.
4. Those paying for health services on an indirect basis (insurance) have not been presented with standards of practice for and qualifications of health educators.
5. Governmental entities who employ and support the preparation of health educators do not have a comprehensive description of the preparation and skills health educators would bring to the federal government. Employment opportunities are unnecessarily restricted. Support for professional preparation is lacking.
6. Other health professions are attempting to establish their professional territory. Those with public contact have educational components within their professional duties. By establishing their own standards, these professions can assume the role performed by health educators on an incremental basis.

The role delineation process and credentialing mechanisms will assist in the resolution of these points. However, the relationship between the Role Delineation Project and credentialing efforts should be understood from the beginning. Fig. 8-3 depicts the relationships between the various aspects of role delineation and credentialing. Following the chart is a brief description of some of the central points which must be considered as the Project is envisioned to progress.

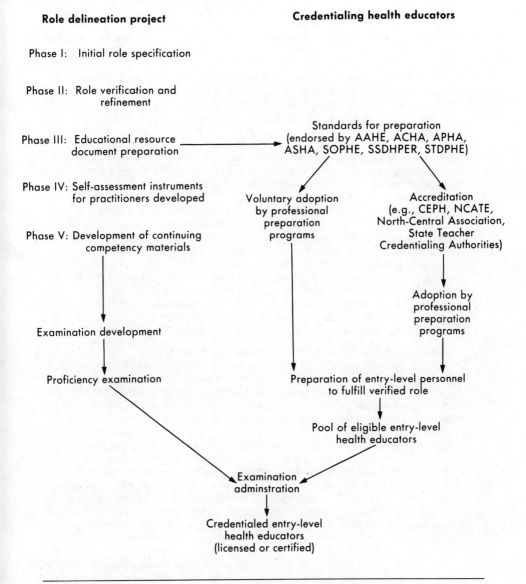

Role delineation project

Phase I: Initial role specification

Phase II: Role verification and
           refinement

Phase III: Educational resource
           document preparation

Phase IV: Self-assessment instruments
          for practitioners developed

Phase V: Development of continuing
         competency materials

Examination development

Proficiency examination

Credentialing health educators

Standards for preparation
(endorsed by AAHE, ACHA, APHA,
ASHA, SOPHE, SSDHPER, STDPHE)

Voluntary adoption
by professional
preparation
programs

Accreditation
(e.g., CEPH, NCATE,
North-Central Association,
State Teacher
Credentialing Authorities)

Adoption by
professional
preparation
programs

Preparation of entry-level personnel
to fulfill verified role

Pool of eligible entry-level
health educators

Examination
adminstration

Credentialed entry-level
health educators
(licensed or certified)

Fig. 8-3. Relationship between the role delineation and credentialing processes.

Critical Points in the Role Delineation and Credentialing Processes
Practitioner Involvement
The entire role delineation process and its relationship to credentialing is based upon a valid description of the responsibilities, functions and skills and knowledge of entry-level practitioners. Such a description must be anchored in the experiences of practitioners.

Academician Involvement
In order for outcomes of the role delineation process to be implemented in the preparation of entry-level health educators, those responsible for such preparation need to be involved so that they are able to evaluate the verified role specification, to participate in development of an educational resource document, to articulate needed changes to their respective administrative units, and to adapt the standards to their respective programs.

Decision Points
At the conclusion of each phase of the role delineation process, health educators, through their organizations, have the opportunity to evaluate and decide upon the need for each subsequent phase. Among the decision points most critical to the entire process is the voluntary adoption or adoption through accreditation of preparation standards embodied in the educational resources document produced in Phase III. Another is the decision on the part of health educators to develop proficiency examinations for entry-level personnel and equivalency examinations for those who wish to become credentialed as health educators. Such decisions will of necessity be made based upon the advantages and disadvantages credentialing offers to the health education profession.

Examination Administration
Following a decision to develop proficiency/equivalency examinations, it will be necessary to create a method for administering such exams. As the process of developing licensure for one profession within each state becomes involved with other professions' licensing requests, the resulting complexity indicates that future additions to licensing among the states will be difficult, time consuming and costly. Alternatively, a certification mechanism, administered by a voluntary association, could be implemented on a nationwide basis. Demonstration of the relationship between certification and possession of basic skills would enable employers, and others, to evaluate and select certified health educators for health education. However, it remains for health educators to establish a mechanism for certification through examination. No such mechanism presently exists.

Adoption of Preparation Standards by Preparatory Programs
As indicated in the chart, adoption can take the form of a voluntary process or adoption can be effected through accreditation requirements (either programmatic or institutional.) Reasons underlying a voluntary adoption would encompass those cited as advantages for credentialing. Essential to adoption is support for the educational resourse document from the organizations represented on the Project's Advisory Committee. Beyond that support, there is no currently recognized (COPA and USOE) accrediting agency which focuses on the profession of health education. As indicated in the chart, there is time for health educators, practitioners and academicians alike, to consider the merits of voluntary association and formal accreditation adoption utilizing COPA and USOE mechanisms. Alternatively, should the profession decide against certification or licensing, graduation from an "approved" or accredited program may provide another mechanism for credentialing. Without significant adoption of the standards for preparation, reflected in the educational resource document, the remaining steps in the role delineation process will lose significance. Adoption is a crucial step in the evolution of the role delineation for health education.

In summary, credentialing mechanisms offer the profession of health education opportunities to address significant issues facing the field. Because of rapid change in the professions and with new professions emerging, credentialing has become complex.

Because of the actual or potential impact on the public by professionals performing their services, the public, Congress, the executive branch of the federal government, state and local governments, the judiciary, employers, insurance companies, professional associations and individual professionals have entered into attempts to judiciously regulate professional practitioners. For health education, interest and involvement in role delineation and in credentialing matters, in anticipation of future need by interested health educators, will help to assure that the profession of health education will fulfill its role in promoting, protecting and improving the health of the public.

Future Settings for Health Education

Traditionally, health education has been considered to be either school-based or community-based. These rather polarized classifications do not begin to clarify the many levels or settings in which health education activities have been or could be undertaken. In the future many health education tasks in the industrial, clinical, and family settings can be anticipated.

Worksite. It is only recently that the opportunities for health improvement that exist in the worksite have begun to be recognized. The business community has only recently become conscious that it is a significant stockholder in the promotion of the health of its employees. In over a decade of existence of the Occupational Safety and Health Act, the principal focus has been on work-related disease and injury *prevention;* only now is attention being given to beneficial potential or employee health *maintenance* and *improvement.* The escalating cost of disease treatment plans, which are reaching levels measured in the hundreds of millions of dollars annually, has been a major factor in drawing attention to health promotion. As a result of economic pressures, business is overcoming a reluctance to get involved in health promotion and, once having done so, is progressively finding that corporate responsibility in health promotion transcends the original issue of cost containment. Additional potential outcomes include increased attendance and productivity on the job, reduced drug, alcohol, and other stress-related problems among individual employees (both management and nonmanagement), and enhanced functional efficiency of the corporate system as a whole.

The worksite has the potential to provide jobs that have become more difficult for health educators to obtain in the school and community settings. If the worksite health promotion movement grows in substance as anticipated, professional preparation programs for health educators will want to include strategies and issues related to worksite health promotion.

Also, worksite health promotion programs have the potential to supplement and reinforce outcomes of existing school and community health education programs. Contact with these programs occurs over a brief, fixed time and then is terminated, while worksite contact is usually long term. As health needs change throughout an individual's life, worksite health promotion contact could help provide flexible, safe, and acceptable strategies

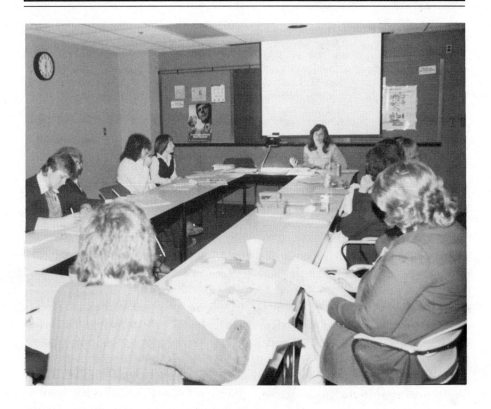

Fig. 8-4. Group counseling at worksite at Carle Wellness Center, Urbana, Illinois. (Photograph by Lyn Lawrance.)

to meet these needs. Thus health education professionals would have greater contact with individuals throughout their life span.

Clinical Settings. Clinical settings for health education (often referred to as patient education) will increase in popularity during the coming years. Health education is a process of modifying or reinforcing knowledge, attitudes, and behavior. It occurs within the clinical setting with or without direction. The process involves not merely experiences but also interpretation of these experiences. Consequently, the movement of a patient (and the patient's family and friends) through a hospital experience cannot help but educate them. Hospital experiences that can be interpreted by the consumer include in-patient care, out-patient care, emergency room care, billing procedures, and community outreach situations. Health educators can provide valuable educational services at each juncture of consumer interaction with clinical personnel.

A hospital is by definition a complex stimulus for knowledge and at-

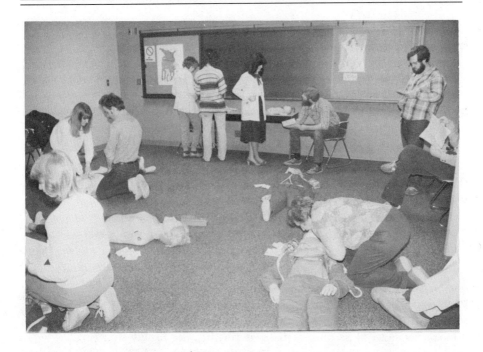

Fig. 8-5. Worksite health education at Carle Clinic, Urbana, Illinois. (Photograph by Lyn Lawrance.)

titudes on health concerns and thus can serve, if used properly, as an advantageous setting for organized consumer health education activities. As health education tasks become more accepted and familiar in the clinical setting, opportunity for growth in innovative educational strategies will emerge.

The health-educated person has the capability of making decisions that have positive health-promotion potential rather than health-limiting consequences. Such decisions are related to personal behavior, the behavior of others, and the environments in which health-promoting decisions are encouraged, facilitated, and reinforced. To arrive and remain at the capability requires an educational process that provides current and relevant information, distinguishes and clarifies the prerogatives and value systems operating within decision tasks, and motivates both action and evaluation of the action. Clinical settings provide an ideal climate for such a process to flourish.

Family Settings. That the family and society are interdependent is a fact widely recognized today. Therefore it is clear that the home cannot be an isolated entity. Public concern for the integrity of the home and family continues to grow, as witnessed by the emergence of new programs on famine and malnutrition, population dynamics, pollution and other environmental hazards and drug dependence. These programs aim to strengthen the family unit so that it can survive the vicissitudes of rapid and complex social change. Concern for health of the family unit is not only limited to the immediate health problems of the pregnant woman and the fetus but also extends to the prevention of problems determined by the social, physical, chemical, and biologic environment of which they are a part.

Health educators will be more and more involved in family intervention strategies. This role has already manifested itself in nutrition and alcohol-related programs with good success. As the importance of the early modification of deleterious life-styles becomes more apparent, the family unit may emerge as the logical setting for the health education process to begin. This may be especially critical if research supports the importance of the early years in the formulation of life-long health habits and life-styles. For example, demonstrating good, sound safety practices within the home may have a greater long-term influence on future safety habits than educational programs offered through the school. Likewise, it is well accepted that parental attitudes toward sexuality have a tremendous influence on the likelihood that sex will be openly discussed within the family structure.

In addition, with the aging of our population, family-oriented health education activities may be the best vehicle with which to reach senior citizens.

Finally, the family setting may prove to be the most likely area for reinforcement of positive life-styles to occur. Thus health education within the family context could be multifaceted—geared toward the parents, child, and related family members in both a content and behavior-oriented fashion.

Because responsibility for good health begins with the individual, it obviously extends to others in the family and even in the community. The role of exemplar is of critical importance for parents who are helping to shape the health practices of their children. Also, by participating in community efforts to ensure the availability of appropriate health services and recreational facilities, and by encouraging the development of sound school health curricula, adults of all ages can enhance their family's health and the quality of life in their community. The family setting therefore holds much promise as the setting for many future health education efforts.

Editors' Remarks

A concept that consistently emerges from the many definitions of health is adaptation. If the profession is to maintain an important role in American society, the profession will have to adapt to changing needs and circumstances. It has been said that with advancing age people become more and more like themselves. That is, they not only maintain their basic values but also exaggerate those values until they become caricatures of themselves. Health education will not be able to maintain its present vitality if it simply evolves into an exaggeration of what it has been. Instead, the profession must explore new horizons, test new ideas, remain alert to opportunities, and be willing to risk adventure into the realm of uncertainty. The ability to adapt will determine our professional niche in the future.

If health implies a quality of life, and if health education is intended to help people achieve quality of life, then the profession must keep abreast of trends and norms. The superstition of yesterday is today's fact, and the fiction of today is tomorrow's reality. We have overcome some of history's most dreaded diseases, such as plague, tuberculosis and polio. They have been replaced by what have become known as the diseases of life-style; cancer, heart disease, and mental illness, to name a few. Health education adapted to meet the challenge. If medical science comes up with a prevention for cancer, what new conditions or diseases will command the attention of the profession, and how will it change health education as we know it today? The educational content will most certainly change as the process of discovery adds new material to the existing body of knowledge. It has been said that all accumulated knowledge doubles every 9 years. One significant challenge will be to keep pace with accurate information. Another challenge will be the search for effective educational strategies that encourage people to seek quality from life.

Just as information is rushing toward us at an alarming speed, so too, are changes within the social environment. It seems that life gets more complicated with each passing year; rules that used to apply now have become exceptions. When divergent points of view fall within narrow parameters it is fairly easy to deal with exceptions to one's own values because the differences will not be all that great. But what happens to a person (health educator) when the range of values are quite divergent? How do we deal with those values furthest from our own positions? Given the complexity of current social issues, it is apparent that the potential for divergence will become more and more pronounced. To illustrate, consider the topic of death and dying. In its early development courses focused on health content and scientific information. Gradually, the social aspects of death and dying—euthanasia, suicide, capital punishment, abortion, and cryogenics—became the focal points. Each of these issues can create a diversity of viewpoints. Will the health educator seek to provide information, to explore the breadth of ideas, to motivate individuals toward a belief that more closely approximates the norm, or will the health educator seek something else from the educational effort?

We believe that the role of the health educator will become increasingly complex as health issues become more social in nature. The role of the medical care provider, the counselor, the social worker, and the educator will blend as the interrelated needs of the individual (and the community) gain greater recognition. In some cases this will cause conflict, just as law and medicine have squared off on issues such as the definition of death, the withholding of treatment, organ transplantation, and abortion. But is is hoped that the interaction between health educators and other professionals working in the human services will be cordial. The extension of knowledge and skills nurtured by cooperation can help to strengthen the individual professionals as well as to benefit the clients whom they serve.

That brings forth another issue—the clients. Probably the variety of clients, and with them the variety of needs, will become more diverse. Will we see the day when health education requires a postgraduate residency similar to the specialty fields of medicine? Will programs of professional preparation train health educators to work specifically with retired people, adolescents, minority populations, pregnant women, patients who have had postcardiac surgery, labor unions, or executives? Will health educators form group practices for consultation, material development, research, and evaluation? Will health education (more broadly defined) become a reimbursable item from third party payers such as insurance companies, Medicaid, and Medicare? Will health educators be trained to work in physicians' and dentists' offices, or will physician assistants and dental assistants be taught to provide health education? Will the school health educator have dual functions as a counselor, or will counselors be trained in the educational content, methods, and materials of health education? These questions raise interesting considerations for discussion. More importantly, they create a need for the development of strategies directed toward resolution of the issues. Effective planning may help to carve a niche for health education that is more attractive than the niche created by chance. A few projections are presented below.

1. Health educators will need to be able to work with computers. No matter how "user-friendly" the design of a computer, it will need someone who speaks the language in order to communicate. Additionally, software packages will become increasingly available as instructional aids. Computer-assisted instruction may become the educational strategy of choice in one or more of the educational settings.

2. Health educators will need to understand the principles of behavioral science in order to deal effectively with individuals and groups of people. As illness concerns shift from a physical orientation to mental and spiritual orientations, the need for psychology and sociology skills will increase.

3. Health educators will need to use communication media in order to attract attention, to inform the public, and to reinforce previous educational messages. Skills such as telecommunications, videotaping, production, and script writing may play an important role as education becomes less institutionalized and more informal. Instead of going to a seminar held at the local church, school, town meeting hall, or hotel conference room, the individual may simply turn the television on to one of the many cable channels and learn at home.

4. Health educators will need marketing skills in order to "sell" health education to new audiences. Too often in the past, marketing people with no expertise in health have capitalized on technology, added some of their own ingenuity, and come up with a high-profit product. Health education marketing would seem to be a career of the future if corporations maintain their current interest in selling health information.

5. Health educators will need to become more active as lobbyists who work to secure healthful legislation and the establishment of agencies that have a positive influence on health education. To cite a few past examples: when the Health Planning and Resources Development Act was passed, a side effect was the employment of health educators as employees of the health systems agencies. The risk reduction grants available through state and federal funding created jobs that involve health education skills. Legislation that funded the development of health maintenance organizations (HMOs) had a "spin-off" effect on health education because HMOs find it cost-effective to educate their clients.

Our challenge to you is to answer these questions: What does the future hold in store for health education? Will the profession be shaped by unfolding events or will we help to shape those events? How will health education in 20 or 30 years from now be similar to or different from health education of today? How do your personal and professional goals fit into the picture of the future? How will you contribute to the profession? How will your skills benefit your clients and society at large? Is health education really the profession to which you want to commit yourself? By answering these questions, and by taking appropriate steps to turn your dreams into realities, you will be formulating your own foundations for the future.

Summary

In this chapter we have presented, albeit briefly, many of the forces that may influence our future as individuals and as a society. Many of these forces have direct and profound implications for those planning careers in health education. Because our health is affected not only by our personal behavior choices but also by inexorable changes in our environment, health educators of the future will need to be more adaptable and better trained than in the past, especially if the profession is to have any measurable impact in improving the health of society. The professional organizations have recognized the need for keeping pace with the changes of the future. It remains to be seen whether we can adapt fast enough to be truly effective proponents and change agents for the health of the human species.

You face a tremendous challenge as you prepare for your career. The issues of the future will certainly be complex. For you to be able to understand the complexity of the issues and to translate the scientific information into relevant learning experiences will be difficult enough; to provide relevant learning experiences that also motivate a diverse population of students will require individuals with extraordinary talent. We hope that your continued study of future trends and issues will help to increase your potential for service and personal fulfillment.

Questions for Review

1. What issues do you think will have the greatest significance during the next 20 years? Why?
2. What are some of the technologic advances that have so challenged existing norms that the ability of society to adapt is in question?
3. Between the time that an issue becomes prominent and the time that school curricula consider the issue, several years have probably passed. What can schools do to become more responsive to current events and even future-oriented curricula?
4. This chapter discussed three major issues: population pressures, medical advances, and family life. How will health education respond to these issues?
5. How will professional preparation programs need to change in order to meet these future issues? How can the dilemma of specialist versus generalist be resolved?
6. How will the unregulated practice of health education endanger the health, safety, and welfare of the public? How will the public benefit by assurance of competence? Can the public be effectively protected by means other than licensing?
7. The section of the chapter that discusses the Role Delineation Project offers six concerns related to the credentialing process. How can the profession respond to these concerns?
8. Can you describe the proposed process for credentialing health educators?

References

1. Cornish, E.: The study of the future: an introduction to the art and science of understanding and shaping tomorrow's world, Washington, D.C., 1977, World Future Society.
2. Cornish, E.: Towards a philosophy of futurism. In Cornish, E., editor: 1999—the world of tomorrow, Washington, D.C., 1978, World Future Society.
3. Barney, G.O., study director: The global 2000 report to the president: a report prepared by the Council on Environmental Quality and the U.S. Department of State, Washington, D.C., 1980, U.S. Government Printing Office.
4. What the next 20 years hold for you, U.S. News and World Report, p. 51-53, December 1, 1980.
5. Genetic engineering: a revolution in medicine, U.S. News and World Report, p. 74, March 16, 1981.
6. Cornacchia, H.J., and Barrett, S.: Consumer health, ed. 2, Saint Louis, 1980, The C.V. Mosby Co.
7. Francoer, R.T.: The sexual revolution, The Futurist **14**(2):3-12, 1980.
8. Jennings, L.: Future fun: tomorrow's sports and games, The Futurist **13**(6):417-431, 1979.
9. Seaborg, R.: The 1980's: a hopeful outlook, The Futurist **14**(5):3-8, 1980.
10. Shane, J., and Shane, H.: Cultural change in the curriculum, 1970-2000 A.D., Educational Technology **10**(4):13-14, 1970.
11. Initial role delineation for health education: final report, DHHS Pub. No. (HRA) 80-44, Washington, D.C., 1980, U.S. Government Printing Office.
12. Report of licensure and related health personnel credentialing, DHEW Pub. No. (HSM) 72-11, Washington, D.C., 1971, U.S. Government Printing Office.
13. The balance wheel for accreditation, Washington, D.C., The Council on Post Secondary Education (pamphlet).
14. Credentialing health manpower, DHEW Pub. No. (OS) 77-50057. Washington, D.C., 1977, U.S. Government Printing Office.

Additional Readings

Feuer, R.: Effective health education in a senior citizen center, The Eta Sigma Gamman, **14**(1):16-19, 1982.

Freudenberg, N.: Shaping the future of health education: from behavior change to social change, Health Education Monographs **6**(4):372-377, 1978.

Institute of Society, Ethics, and the Life Sciences: The Hastings Center report, Hastings-on-Hudson, New York.

Russell, R.D.: Some futures for health education in the 1980's, The Eta Sigma Gamman **12**(2, suppl.):3-7, 1980.

Glossary

accreditation The process by which a review agency evaluates an institution. Individuals representing the agency, normally peers who work outside the institution, determine whether the institution meets specific predetermined criteria of acceptability. If so, the agency endorses the institution. In the case of higher education, students graduating from accredited schools are given the opportunity to become certified.

appropriations process The process of providing operating funds for governmental programs. A legislature determines the amount of money available and the conditions for distribution.

behavioral health An interdisciplinary field dedicated to promoting a philosophy of health that stresses individual responsibility in the application of behavioral and biomedical science knowledge and techniques to the maintenance of health and the prevention of illness and dysfunction by a variety of self-initiated individual or shared activities.

behavior health hazard appraisal A questionnaire that attempts to identify the problems of health and survival based on individual life-style behaviors. Many appraisal forms are computerized and use a data base to make projections about an individual's health status or health potential.

behavioral medicine A field concerned with the development of behavioral science knowledge and techniques relevant to the understanding of physical health and illness and the application of this knowledge and these techniques to prevention, treatment, and rehabilitation.

caduceus The staff and serpent symbol of the physician.

categorical health education approach The process of teaching about health by means of a particular content area. A school curriculum may offer instruction on consumer health, sex education, or environmental health. Each unit or course stands alone as an educational experience.

certification The process by which a quasigovernmental agency or association grants recognition to an individual who has met certain predetermined qualifications specified by that agency or association. In some cases certification is synonymous with licensure. For example, in most states only certified teachers may be employed by public school districts.

cognitive dissonance A conflict between beliefs and behavior. For instance, a cigarette smoker who knows the health consequences of smoking is in a state of cognitive dissonance. Theoretically, this state is uncomfortable and individuals will seek to resolve the dissonance either by altering their perception of the risk or by giving up smoking.

comprehensive health education approach An approach that provides learning experiences based on the best scientific information in an effort to promote the understanding, attitudes, behavioral skills, and practices of students with respect to their health. Although the curriculum may be made up of individual units, there is opportunity to show relationships across units of instruction. Comprehensive health education also implies that the teacher is certified as a health educator. This is in contrast to the categoric approach in which teachers certified in other areas may offer instruction in health.

criterion-referenced A clear description of a set of skills determined to be essential to performance of a role that can be used in a test situation to determine an individual's possession of those skills.

demonstration program An experiment that attempts to demonstrate the viability of a concept or idea. Usually outside funding from private or public sources establishes the program to demonstrate potential benefits.

didactic teaching Teaching that uses the lecture method in an information-giving atmosphere. The focus of instructional activitiy is on the teacher rather than the student.

disease A scientific, medical, and technical territory that encompasses what is known about biologic impairment.

entry level The point at which an individual is capable of meeting the specifications of the role identified. Skills and knowledge necessary to perform the role can be obtained through successful completion of a bachelor's degree program at an accredited university or college with a major emphasis in health education.

ethics A branch of philosophy that attempts to discover whether conduct is good or bad, right or wrong. An ethic is a value, a standard. Professions establish a code of ethics in order to govern conduct among its members.

evaluation The comparison of an object of interest against a standard of acceptability.

external validity The degree to which results of an experiment can be expected to recur in other places at other times.

hawthorne effect A change in performance that is attributable to the attention paid to subjects in an experiment.

health* An elusive term that usually encompasses the notion of individual and collective well-being with physical, social, and psychologic dimensions.

health education* The process of assisting individuals, acting separately and collectively, to make informed decisions about matters affecting individual, family, and community health. Based on scientific foundations, health education is a field of interest, a discipline, and a profession.

health educator* An individual prepared to assist other individuals, acting separately or collectively, to make informed decisions regarding matters affecting their personal health and that of others.

health promotion Activities intended to encourage behavior that leads to good health. Some activities, such as aerobic exercise and nutrition education, are directed at the individual, while other activities, such as immunization and hypertensive screening, are directed at target audiences who are at risk. Health promotion includes all those activities that enable a person to enjoy a more healthful life than otherwise would have been possible.

independent variable That treatment that is not subject to or dependent on events that follow or result from implementation of a program. Hypotheses are stated as if x, then y. In this situation x is the independent variable since it is the causative variable rather than the outcome variable.

interactive teaching A teaching method in which teacher and students interact with each other. Interactive learning demands that students are active participants in the learning situation. Role playing and values clarification activities are examples of interactive learning.

internal validity The degree to which we can say with certainty that the results observed after the program are attributable to the program or educational treatment.

---

*As defined by the Role Delineation Project. Reported in *Focal Points*, U.S. Department of Health and Human Services, July 1980.

issue A matter or question disputed between contending parties. Both issues are neither right nor wrong. Only the evidence used to support the contention is right or wrong. Issues are usually settled on the "weight of evidence."

licensure The process by which an agency or government grants permission for occupation by certifying that those licensed have attained the minimal degree of competency necessary to ensure that the public health, safety, and welfare will be reasonably well protected.

paradigm Provides the context in which research is conducted and knowledge is accumulated.

philosophy A humanistic discipline that attempts to obtain an informed understanding of reality.

PRECEDE A model wherein the predisposing, reinforcing, and enabling factors are considered as part of the program planning process.

preventive medicine A medical approach concerned with general preventive measures aimed at improving the healthfulness of our environment and our relations with it. Preventive medicine rarely means prevention of disease. Instead, it refers to early detection, diagnosis, and treatment as a means of preventing more serious consequences.

primary prevention An attempt to prevent sickness. Examples include life-style intervention strategies such as regular exercise, coping with stress, and balanced diet.

registration Same as licensure.

Role Delineation Project The purpose of this project is to define and verify the role of the health educator and to develop a guide for academic programs preparing health educators, as well as self-assessment tools and continuing education materials for practitioners.

scientific rigor Strict adherence to a protocol that specifies the experimental education treatment in procedural detail.

secondary prevention Preventive measures that consist of those activities that allow for early detection of a disease even before symptoms become apparent. Examples include high blood pressure screening, Pap smears, x-ray examinations and blood tests.

shamans Presently referred to as teachers, doctors, and health professionals.

social desirability effect A change or response bias attributable to being observed and wanting to do the "right" thing.

tertiary prevention Refers to the minimization of consequences caused by a disease in order to prevent further complications or reoccurrence. Tertiary prevention includes activities such as surgery, chemotherapy, and physical therapy.

Appendix A

Promoting Health/ Preventing Disease—Objectives for the Nation

These objectives for the nation are reprinted from *Promoting Health/Preventing Disease— Objectives for the Nation,* U.S. Department of Health and Human Services, U.S. Public Health Service, Washington, D.C., 1980, U.S. Government Printing Office.

High Blood Pressure

By 1990 at least 60 percent of the estimated population having definite high blood pressure (160/95) should have attained successful long term blood pressure control, i.e. a blood pressure at or below 140/90 for 2 or more years.

By 1990, the prevalence of significant overweight (120 percent of desired weight) among the U.S. adult population should be decreased to 10 percent of men and 17 percent of women, without nutritional impairment.

Family Planning

By 1990, there should be virtually no unintended births to girls 14 years of age or under. Fulfilling this objective would probably reduce births in this age group to near zero.

By 1985, oral contraceptives containing more than 50 micrograms of estrogen should not be used for family planning methods, and sales of these preparations should have been reduced to 15 percent. (In 1978, about 27.1 percent of preparations sold were at this level.)

Pregnancy and Infant Health

By 1990, the national infant mortality rate (deaths for all babies up to 1 year of age) should be reduced to no more than 9 deaths per 1,000 live births. (In 1978, the infant mortality rate was 13.8 per 1,000 live births.)

By 1990, no county and no racial or ethnic group of the population (e.g., black, Hispanic, Indian) should have an infant mortality rate in excess of 12 deaths per 1,000 live births. (In 1978, the infant mortality rate for whites was 12.0 per 1,000 live births; for blacks 23.1 per 1,000 live births; for American Indians 13.7 per 1,000 live births; rate for Hispanics is not yet available separately.)

By 1990, the neonatal death rate (deaths for all infants up to 28 days old) should be reduced to no more than 6.5 deaths per 1,000 live births. (In 1978, the neonatal death rate was 9.5 per 1,000 live births.)

By 1990, the perinatal death rate should be reduced to no more than 5.5 per 1,000. (In 1977, the perinatal death rate was 15.4 per 1,000. NOTE: The perinatal death rate is total deaths, late fetal deaths over 28 weeks gestation plus infant deaths up to 7 days old, expressed as a rate per 1,000 live births and late fetal deaths.)

By 1990, the maternal mortality rate should not exceed 5 per 100,000 live births for any county or for any ethnic group (e.g., black, Hispanic, American Indian). (In 1978, the overall rate was 9.6; the rate for blacks was 25.0, the rate for whites 6.4, and for American Indians 12.1; the rate for Hispanics is not yet available separately.)

By 1990, the proportion of women in any county or racial or ethnic group (e.g., black, Hispanic, American Indian) who obtain no prenatal care during the first trimester of pregnancy should not exceed 10 percent. (In 1978, 40 percent of black mothers and 45 percent of American Indian mothers received no prenatal care during the first trimester; percent of Hispanics is unknown.)

By 1990, low birth weight babies (2,500 grams and under) should constitute no more than 5 percent of all live births. (In 1978, the proportion was 7.0 percent of all births.)

By 1990, no county and no racial or ethnic group of the population (e.g., black, Hispanic, American Indian) should have a rate of low birth weight infants (prematurely born and small-for-age infants weighing less than 2,500 grams) that exceed 9 percent of all live births. (In 1978, the rate for whites was about 5.9 percent, for Indians about 6.7 percent, and for blacks about 12.9 percent; rates for Hispanics are not yet separately available; rates for some other Nations are 5 percent and less.)

By 1990, the incidence of neural tube defects should be reduced to 1.0 per 1,000 live births. (In 1979, the rate was 1.7 per 1,000.)

By 1990, Rhesus hemolytic disease of the newborn should be reduced to below a rate of 1.3 per 1,000 live births. (In 1977, the rate was 1.8 per 1,000.)

Toxic Agent Control

By 1990, virtually all communities should experience no more than one day per year when air quality exceeds an individual ambient air quality standard with respect to sulphur dioxide, nitrous dioxide, carbon monoxide, lead hydrocarbon, and particulate matter. (In 1979, the level was estimated to be 50 percent.)

By 1990, at least 95 percent of the population should be served by community water systems that meet Federal and State standards for safe drinking water. (In 1979, the level was 85 to 90 percent for the National Interim Primary Drinking Standards.)

By 1990, a broad scale surveillance and monitoring system should have been planned to discern and measure known environmental hazards of a continuing nature as well as those resulting from isolated incidents. Such activities should be continuously carried out at both Federal and State levels.

By 1990, a central clearinghouse for observations of agent/disease relationships and host susceptibility factors should be fully operational, as well as a national environmental data registry to collect and catalogue information on concentrations of hazardous agents in air, food, and water.

By 1990, every individual residing in an area with a population density greater than 20 per square mile or in an area of high risk should be protected by an early warning system designed to detect the most serious hazards.

By 1990, every populated area of the country should be able to be reached within 6 hours by a toxic agent or chemical emergency team in the event of exposure to a serious environmental hazard.

Occupational Safety and Health

By 1990, workplace accident deaths for firms or employers with 11 or more employees should be reduced to less than 3,750 per year. (In 1978, there were 4,170 work-related fatalities for firms or employers with 11 or more employees.)

By 1990, work-related disabling injuries should be reduced to 8.3 cases per 100 full-time workers. (In 1978, there were approximately 9.2 cases per 100 workers.)

By 1990, lost workdays due to injuries should be reduced to 55 per 100 workers anually. (In 1978, approximately 62.1 days per 100 workers were lost.)

By 1990, among workers newly exposed after 1985, there should be virtually no new cases of four preventable occupational diseases—asbestosis, byssinosis, silicosis, and coal worker's pneumoconiosis. (In 1979, there were an estimated 5,000 cases of asbestosis; in 1977, an estimated 84,000 cases of byssinosis were expected in active workers; in 1979, an estimated 60,000 cases of silicosis were expected among active workers in mining, foundries, stone, clay and glass products, and abrasive blasting; in 1974, there were an estimated 19,400 cases of coal worker's pneumonoconiosis.)

By 1990, at least 25 percent of workers should be able to state the nature of their occupational health and safety risks and their potential consequences prior to employment, as well as be informed of changes in these risks while employed. (In 1979, an estimated 5 percent of workers were fully informed.)

By 1985, an ongoing occupational health hazard/illness/injury coding system, survey, and surveillance capability should be developed, including identification of workplace hazards and related health effects, including cancer, coronary heart disease, and reproductive effects.

Accident Prevention and Injury Control

By 1990, the motor vehicle fatality rate should be reduced to no greater than 18 per 100,000 population. (In 1978, it was 24.0 per 100,000 population.)

By 1990, the motor vehicle fatality rate for children under 15 years of age should be reduced to no greater than 5.5 per 100,000 children. (In 1978, it was 9.2 per 100,000 children under 15.)

By 1990, the home accident fatality rate for children under 15 years of age should be no greater than 5.0 per 100,000 children. (In 1978, it was 6.1 per 100,000 children under 15.)

By 1990, the mortality rate from falls should be reduced to no more than 2 per 100,000 persons. (In 1978, it was 6.3 per 100,000.)

By 1990, the mortality rate from drowning should be reduced to no more than 3.0 per 100,000 person. (In 1978, it was 3.2 per 100,000.)

By 1990, the number of tapwater scald injuries requiring hospital care should be reduced to no more than 2,000 per year. (In 1978, it was 4,000 per year.)

By 1990, the number of accidental fatalities from firearms should be held to no more than 1,700 per year. (In 1978, there were 1,800.)

By 1990, accidental deaths from residential fires should be reduced to no more than 4,500 per year. (In 1978, there were 5,400.)

Dental Health

By 1990, the proportion of children 9 years of age who have experienced dental caries in their permanent teeth should be decreased to 60 percent. (In 1971-74, it was 71 percent.)

By 1990, the prevalence of gingivitis in children 6 to 17 years of age should be decreased to 18 percent. (In 1971-74, the prevalence was about 23 percent.)

By 1990, in adults the prevalence of gingivitis and destructive periodontal disease should be decreased to 20 percent and 21 percent, respectively. (In 1971-74, 25 percent of adults 18 to 74 years of age had gingivitis and 23 percent had destructive periodontal disease.)

By 1990, at least 99 percent of the population on community water systems should be receiving the benefits of optimally fluoridated water. (In 1975, it was 60 percent.)

By 1990, at least 50 percent of school children living in fluoride-deficient areas that do not have community water systems should be served by an optimally fluoridated school water supply. (In 1977, it was about 6 percent.)

Surveillance and Control of Infectious Diseases

By 1990, the (risk-factor-specific) incidence of nosocomial infections in acute-care hospitals will be reduced by 20 percent of what otherwise would pertain in the absence of hospital control programs. A similar percentage reduction should be seen in long-term care and residential care facilities.

By 1990, data reporting systems in all States should be able to monitor trends of common infectious agents not now subject to traditional public health surveillance (respiratory illnesses, gastrointestinal illnesses, otitis media) and to measure the impact of these agents on health care cost and productivity at the local and State levels and, by extension, at the national level.

Smoking and Health

By 1990, the proportion of adults who smoke should be reduced to below 25 percent.

By 1990, the proportion of women who smoke during pregnancy should be no greater than one-half the proportion of all women who smoke. (Baseline data unavailable.)

By 1990, the proportion of children and youths 12 to 18 years of age who smoke should be reduced to below 6 percent.

By 1990, the sales-weighted average "tar" yield of cigarettes should be reduced to below 10 mg. The other components of cigarette smoke known to cause disease should also be reduced proportionately. (In 1978, the sales-weighted average "tar" content was 16.1 mg.)

Misuse of Alcohol and Drugs

By 1990, the cirrhosis mortality rate should be reduced to 12 per 100,000 per year.

By 1990, other drug related mortality should be reduced to 2 per 100,000 per year.

By 1990, fatalities from motor vehicle accidents involving drivers with blood levels of 0.10 percent or more should be reduced to less than 9.5 per 100,000 population per year.

By 1990, fatalities from other (nonmotor vehicle) accidents, indirectly attributable to alcohol use (e.g., falls, fires, drownings, ski-mobile, aircraft), should be reduced to 5 per 100,000 population per year.

By 1990, per capita consumption of alcohol should not exceed current levels.

By 1990, the proportion of adolescents 12 to 17 years of age who are not using alcohol or other drugs should not fall below 1977 levels. (In 1977, it was 46 percent for alcohol and a range for other drugs from 89 percent for marijuana to 99.9 percent for heroin.)

By 1990, the proportion of problem drinkers among all adults 18 years of age and over should be reduced to 8 percent. (In 1979, it was about 10 percent.)

By 1990, the proportion of young adults 18 to 25 years of age reporting frequent use of other drugs should not exceed 1977 levels. (In 1977, it was less than 1 percent for drugs other than marijuana and 19 percent for marijuana.)

By 1990, the proportion of adolescents 12 to 17 years of age reporting frequent use of other drugs should not exceed 1977 levels. (In 1977, it was less than 1 percent of youths for drugs other than marijuana and 9 percent for marijuana.)

By 1990, adverse reactions from medical drug use that are sufficiently severe to require hospital admission should be reduced to 25 percent fewer such admissions per year. (In 1979, estimates ranged from approximately 105,000 to 350,000 admissions per year.)

By 1990, pharmacists filling prescriptions should routinely counsel patients on the proper use of drugs designated as high priority by the Food and Drug Administration, with particular attention to prescriptions for pediatric and geriatric patients and to the problems of drinking alcoholic beverages while taking prescription drugs. (Baseline data unavailable.)

By 1990, standard good medical and pharmaceutical practice will include drug profiles on 90 percent of adults covered under the Medicare program and on 75 percent of other patients with acute and chronic illnesses being cared for in all private and organized medical settings. (Baseline data unavailable.)

Nutrition

By 1990, the mean serum cholesterol level for those 18-74 years of age should be at or below 200 mg/dl.

By 1990, the mean serum cholesterol level for those 1-17 years of age should be at or below 150 mg/dl.

By 1990, the average daily sodium ingestion (as measured by excretion) by adults should be reduced at least to the 3 to 6 gram range. (In 1979, estimates ranged between averages of 4 and 10 grams sodium. NOTE: One gram salt provides approximately .4 grams sodium.)

Physical Fitness and Exercise

By 1990, the proportion of children and adolescents ages 10 to 17 participating in daily school physical education programs should be greater than 60 percent. (In 1974-75, the proportion was 33 percent.)

By 1990, the proportion of adults 18 to 65 participating regularly in vigorous physical exercise should be greater than 60 percent. (In 1978, the proportion who regularly exercised was estimated at over 35 percent.)

By 1990, 50 percent of adults 65 years and over should be engaging in appropriate physical activity, e.g. regular walking, swimming, or other aerobic activity. (In 1975, about 36 percent took regular walks.)

Stress and Violent Behavior

By 1990, the homicide rate among black males 15-24 years of age should be reduced to below 60 per 100,000. (In 1978, it was 72.5 per 100,000.)

By 1990, the suicide rate among people 15-24 years of age should be below 11 per 100,000. (In 1978, it was 12.4 per 100,000.)

Government-Sponsored Health Promotion Programs

These health promotion programs are reprinted from *Prevention '80,* U.S. Department of Health and Human Services, U.S. Public Health Service, Office of Disease Prevention and Health Promotion, Pub. No. 81-50157, Washington, D.C., 1981, U.S. Government Printing Office.

U.S. Department of Health and Human Services
Office of the Assistant Secretary for Health

National Toxicology Program—a program established in 1979 to coordinate the prevention efforts of the scientific institute and regulatory agencies.

Office of Disease Prevention and Health Promotion

Regional Forums on Community Health Promotion—eight regional forums conducted to encourage business, labor, health educators, media, and civic leaders to organize health promotion programs.

National Conference on Health Promotion Programs in Occupational Settings—a conference for the identification of model worksite health promotion programs.

National Conference on School Health—a conference that examined methods of integrating school health services with health instruction.

Health Works—an outdoor health fair in Washington, D.C., to serve as a model for other communities.

Minority Group Health Promotion—a series of five 1-day workshops addressing the health priorities of minority populations.

HEALTHSTYLE Campaign—a self-test developed to help individuals assess the relative risks to their health.

Office of Management—The President's Council on
Physical Fitness and Sports

National Conference on Physical Fitness and Sports for All—reviewed the central physical fitness issues for all age groups.

White House Symposium on Physical Fitness and Sports Medicine—a symposium on the prevention and treatment of injuries caused by sports and exercise.

Office on Smoking and Health

1979 Surgeon General's Report on Smoking and Health.

1980 Surgeon General's Report on Smoking and Health—a report describing the health consequences of smoking for women.

National Poster and Essay Contest—a contest for seventh-grade students designed to increase awareness among youth of the health consequences of smoking.

National Media Campaign: Evaluation—an evaluation of the effectiveness of smoking messages on television, radio, print media, public transit, and point-of-sale displays.

Office of Adolescent Pregnancy Programs
Grant Program—a program that awarded $6.4 million to provide health education and social services to pregnant teenagers and young parents.

Office of Population Affairs
The Office of Population Affairs was set up to promote healthy families and to prevent the physical, emotional, and social ills associated with unplanned or unintended pregnancies and births.
Evaluation of Counseling in Family Planning Programs—a program to determine whether these services provide an effective means of preventing unintended pregnancies.

Office of Health Research, Statistics, and Technology
Health Hazard/Risk Appraisal Research.
Cost Models: Cigarette Smoking—an assessment of the impact of various techniques to reduce smoking.
Health Practices Survey—a series of telephone interviews to determine the prevalence and stability of health practices.
Prevention Profile—a mechanism to formally track the health of the nation.

Office of Health Maintenance Organizations
Preventive Services Demonstrations—demonstrations of the effectiveness of health promotion services delivered in a clinical setting.

Office of International Health
United States–People's Republic of China—a program to share Health Cooperation—new approaches to research and control influenza, cancer, population, and the mental health, food, and drugs.

Alcohol, Drug Abuse and Mental Health Administration
Prevention Division—established to coordinate prevention efforts with National Institute on Alcohol Abuse and Alcoholism, National Institute on Drug Abuse, and National Institute of Mental Health.
National Conference on Prevention.
National Program on Insomnia and Sleep Disorders—an effort to educate physicians and consumers in the use and misuse of sedative-hypnotic drugs and the treatment of sleep disorders.

National Institute on Alcohol Abuse and Alcoholism—supports research, training, and education programs to prevent and treat alcoholism.
Public Education Campaign—a media campaign on alcohol abuse and the effects of alcohol on fetuses.
Symposium on State Drinking Age Laws.
"Here's Looking at You" Curriculum—a K-12 curriculum with a teacher's guide, films, charts, instructional games, and puppets. The curriculum emphasizes coping and decision-making skills.

National Institute on Drug Abuse
The National Institute on Drug Abuse supports research on the misuse of drugs, trains personnel in prevention and rehabilitation, and explores innovative educational approaches. The National Clearinghouse for Drug Abuse is housed within the institute.
State Drug Abuse Prevention Grant Program—a program in each state in which a prevention coordinator supervises program planning, implementation, and evaluation.
The Center for Multi-Cultural Awareness—a program to develop prevention materials to meet the needs of ethnic minority groups.

National Institute of Mental Health
Prevention Research Funds—a program that sponsored 34 grants with emphasis on marital disruption, the impact of severely disturbed parents on children, stress, and minorities.
Prevention Grants for Child Mental Health.

Centers for Disease Control
Reorganization—the name of the center was changed to Centers for Disease Control and six operational units were established: the Center for Environmental Health, the Center for Health Promotion and Education, the Center for Prevention Services, the National Institute for Occupational Safety and Health, the Center for Professional Development and Training, and the Center for Infectious Diseases.
Studies of Radiation Carcinogenics and Nuclear Bomb Testing—assessments of the relationship between radiation and cancer by studying the military personnel who were present at the 1957 atmospheric nuclear bomb detonation in Nevada.
Study on Human Exposure to DDT.
Polio Containment in Amish Communities—a prevention program that limited the 1979 outbreak of polio to only 15 cases by initiating a vaccination program in Amish communities.
Study of Contraception and Risk of Cancer.
Microbiologic Guidelines for Hemodialysis Centers.
Hepatitis B Vaccine—evaluation of a vaccine to control the spread of infection in high-risk health care environments.

Bureau of Health Education
School Health Education Models—a program that developed, tested, and distributed health education models for grades K-7. The School Health Curriculum Project is being used by more than 5000 teachers and is being evaluated against three other programs.
Risk Reduction Grants—grants to help state health agencies conduct health education programs aimed at life-style and health risk behaviors.

Bureau of Laboratories
The Bureau of Laboratories was established to improve laboratory methodology and to standardize clinical laboratory methods and materials.
Legionnaires' Disease—a program that led to the identification of the bacterial cause (*Legionella pneumophila*) of legionnaires' disease.
Botulism Detection—this effort improved the accuracy of diagnosis from 33% to 87%.
Schistosomiasis drug—this program developed a promising new drug for the treatment of schistosomiasis with minimal side effects.

Bureau of State Services
The Bureau of State Services coordinates a national program of state and local health agencies in the prevention and control of serious infectious diseases such as sexually transmitted diseases, rubella, measles, and tuberculosis.
Sexually Transmitted Disease Training Clinics.
Fluo dation Initiative—a series of grants to fluoridate 45 water systems serving nearly a ha million people in small communities.
Childhood Immunizations.
Influenza Immunization.

Bureau of Training
The Bureau of Training assists prevention and control programs in the application of scientific, technical, and operational knowledge.
Training for Immunization Program Managers.

National Institute for Occupational Safety and Health

Criteria Documents and Health Hazard Evaluations—criteria that recommend environmental exposure limits for a given hazard.

Educational Resource Centers—twelve strategically located centers to provide education for degree candidates studying industrial hygiene, occupational safety, occupational health nursing, occupational medicine, toxicology, epidemiology, ergonomics, and biostatistics.

Food and Drug Administration

Patient Package Inserts—a program to ensure that most prescription drugs have inserts to inform consumers about the appropriate use of the drug and its possible side effects, written in nontechnical language.

Prescription Drugs—National Consumer Education Campaign.

Fetal Alcohol Syndrome—National Consumer Education Campaign.

Darvon—National Educational Effort.

Food Additives—National Consumer Education Campaign.

Infant Formula Quality Control Procedures.

Diagnostic X-Rays—Consumer Education.

Dental and Mammography Quality Assurance Programs.

Health Resources Administration

The Health Resources Administration is designed to improve access to health care, improve continuity of health care, assure equal access to health education, and enforce partnerships between private enterprise and all levels of government. This agency provides comprehensive primary health care services by encouraging health professionals to establish their practices in medically underserved areas. Comprehensive primary health care centers now serve more than 4.5 million people.

Curriculum models in occupational, industrial, and environmental medicine.

School Nurse Practitioner grant.

Nutrition Curriculum Development—the development of a curriculum intended for medical students, residents, or other health professionals in training to improve nutrition concepts in patient care.

Curriculum Models in Preventive Dentistry—the development of a curriculum to train dental students in the delivery of community prevention services.

Accident Prevention and Injury Control in Children—three demonstration projects to improve the collection and analysis of demographic, epidemiologic, and operational systems data related to accidents involving children.

Family Planning Media Projects—media campaigns to motivate adolescents to act responsibly about sex.

Maternal and Child Health and Crippled Children's Services Research Grants Program—a program providing funding for 50 research grants focusing on the delivery of health care to mothers and children and adolescents, nutrition, and the manpower for care of mothers and children.

Primary Care Research and Demonstration Projects—projects emphasizing health education and the acquisition of self-care skills to promote health and reduce risks.

Indian Health Service

The Indian Health Service was established to elevate the health of Native Americans by helping them meet their own health needs through a network of 51 hospitals, 86 health centers, and 300 field clinics.

National Institutes of Health

The National Institutes of Health comprise 11 institutes, each with its own medical focus.

National Institute on Aging—conducted Conference on the Risks and Benefits of Estrogen

Therapy, a study of exercise and the aging process, and a study on human adaptation to life cycle changes.

National Institute of Allergy and Infectious Diseases—responsible for gonococcus vaccine development contract and hepatitis B vaccine trials.

National Institute of Arthritis, Metabolism, and Digestive Diseases—established recommended dietary allowances.

National Cancer Institute—studied the use of retinoids in cancer prevention and dietary role in cancer and established a consensus on Pap smears.

National Institute of Child Health and Human Development—developed a new program on behavioral and cultural aspects of nutrition, a study of the relationship between oral contraceptives and heart attacks, and a study of the hormonal effects of vasectomy.

National Institute of Environmental Health Sciences—studied Agent Orange and its contaminant, dioxin, and contaminants in mother's milk.

National Eye Institute—promotes prevention and control of eye diseases related to nutritional deficiencies, investigation of the effects of drugs, light, and environmental substances in retinal and lens disorders; and research aimed at prevention of amblyopia and myopia.

National Institute of Dental Research—sponsored demonstration projects to prevent tooth decay.

National Heart, Lung, and Blood Institute—developed public service announcements about high blood pressure, recommendations on health needs of the black community, and methods of dietary control of lipoproteins.

National Institute of Neurological and Communicative Disorders and Stroke—established new section on neurotoxicology and division of research resources, including support for blacks with hypertension.

Health Care Financing Administration

The Health Care Financing Administration—provides reimbursement for medical care of the elderly and the socioeconomically deprived. It also develops and enforces standards for the quality of health care. Medicare and Medicaid are two of its major programs.

Regulations for family planning—regulations that permit reimbursement for counseling, reversal of sterilization procedures, and education for natural family planning to eligible Medicaid beneficiaries.

National Second Surgical Opinion Program.

Early Periodic Screening, Diagnosis, and Treatment Program—a program that screened more than 2 million eligible medicaid children.

Office of Human Development Service—developed immunization initiative, food programs for the elderly, and child abuse and neglect programs.

Other Federal Agencies

Department of Agriculture

National School Lunch Program: Revised Regulations.

Nutrition Education Demonstration Projects.

U.S. Consumer Product Safety Commission

Chronic chemical hazards identification programs.

Development of child-restraint requirements.

Programs to identify safety hazards in children's toys and outdoor mechanical equipment.

Office of Comprehensive School Health

Established in 1979, the Office of Comprehensive School Health provides advice on school health policy, showcases model school health programs, and provides a focus for school health instruction and services within the Department of Education.

Environmental Protection Agency
Curriculum for Environmental Medicine.

Federal Trade Commission
Proposed Rules for Food and Health Advertising—rules that limit unproven claims in food
    advertising, hearing aids, and over-the-counter drugs.

Department of Housing and Urban Development
Alcoholism Outreach Program in public housing.
Environmental Assessment of Housing Sites for the Elderly.

Department of Interior
Exercise trails—more than 600 throughout the U.S.
Urban recreation/health promotion.

Department of Labor
New Directions Grant Program.
Physician Residency Program—designed to provide physicians with in-service training
    for occupational medicine.

Department of Transportation
Child passenger protection—measures to prevent 1500 deaths and 35,000 hospital re-
    ported injuries.

Department of the Treasury
Fetal alcohol syndrome campaign.

Protection, Prevention, and Health Promotion Activities

Recent progress has enabled us to define the preventive services that ought to be delivered to a healthy population based on age and other risk factors that are known to exist. The surgeon general's report included five preventive services having the ability to significantly reduce death, disease, and disability for people at earlier ages.

Measures to Protect People from Harm

It has been estimated that as much as 20% of the premature deaths in this country could be eliminated by protecting the public from environmental hazards. Much of the disease and disability could also be reduced. Over the past 20 years an extensive network of federal agencies has evolved as a means of protecting the public.* The surgeon general has identified five areas in which protection efforts can significantly improve the health of the nation.

Toxic Agent Control

Chemicals developed for industrial and agricultural purposes pose new threats to our health. In some cases it takes a full generation to recognize the harmful effects of a new compound. Yet each year more than 1000 new chemicals are added to the 60,000 that are already being commercially produced. Food, air, and water supplies are being comtaminated. A difficult challenge to the scientific community and to all levels of government is what to do with the by-products created through the manufacturing process.

Occupational Safety and Health

Every year 100,000 Americans die from occupationally related illnesses and nearly 400,000 new cases of occupational disease are diagnosed. Exposure to toxic chemicals, excessive noise, radiation, vibration, and particulate matter can produce a host of chronic and degenerative diseases as well as genetic alterations that may be transmitted to future generations. Yet 90% of industrial workers are inadequately protected from exposure to hazardous chemicals. It has been estimated that as much as 20% of all cancers may be related to workplace exposure to carcinogenic chemicals.

Based on *Healthy people, the surgeon general's report on health promotion and disease prevention,* U.S. Department of Health, Education, and Welfare, U.S. Public Health Service, Pub. No. 79-55071, Washington, D.C., 1979, U.S. Government Printing Office.

*Health protection responsibilities are presently distributed among several federal regulatory and research organizations: the Environmental Protection Agency; the Department of Labor's Occupational Safety and Health Administration; the Nuclear Regulatory Commission; the Consumer Product Safety Commission; the Department of Transportation's National Highway Traffic Safety Administration; the Department of Treasury's Bureau of Alcohol, Tobacco, and Firearms; the Department of Agriculture's Food Safety and Quality Service; and the Department of Health, Education and Welfare's Food and Drug Administration, Centers for Disease Control, National Institute for Occupational Safety and Health, National Institute of Environmental Health Sciences, and National Cancer Institute.

Accidental Injury Control

Each year more than 100,000 Americans die as the result of accidents and 65 million people (one in four) experience nonfatal injuries that require medical treatment. In 1980 the estimated cost of accidents was $83.2 billion. After the first year of life, and until the age of 44, accidents represent the greatest threat to life. The populations at greatest risk include children, teenage males, problem drinkers, and the elderly. Among drivers involved in fatal crashes about half were found to have blood alcohol levels that indicated the driver was under the influence of alcohol. In just 2 years, more Americans die from alcohol-related crashes than were killed in 10 years of fighting in Vietnam. Although seat and lap belts prevent fatalities, only 20% of the population and 7% of passengers under the age of 10 use them. Similar statistics for firearms, falls, burns, and poisonings demonstrate the fact that much can be done to prevent unnecessary physical trauma, disability, and death.

Fluoridation of Community Water Supplies

Tooth decay affects about 95% of the population, making it the nation's most common health problem. Fluoridation may reduce dental decay by as much as 65% at an extremely low cost. Yet less than half of our citizens drink fluoridated water. Part of the delay for not fluoridating community water systems is caused by public misunderstanding and a lack of knowledge about the effects of fluorine. Research over the past 35 years has produced no evidence that fluoridated water is harmful to health.

Infectious Agent Control

Although infectious diseases are not a leading cause of death, they still remain a significant public health problem, accounting for 156 million work days lost and an annual financial consideration of about $24 billion.

Preventive Services Delivered to Individuals

Family Planning

One million legal abortions are performed every year, terminating one in four pregnancies. Currently, birth control prevents an estimated 750,000 unwanted pregnancies among teenagers each year. Even so, about 1 million teenagers (1 of 10) become pregnant and of these, 30% (300,000) elect to have an abortion. The abortion rate demonstrates a consistent rise among women who have already had one, two, or three children. Unplanned births affect the health and social well-being of the mother as well as the health of the child, yet only 39% of the nation's school districts offer information on human reproduction and sexuality.

Pregnancy and Infant Care

Low birth weight is a risk factor for developmental problems, disease, and death. A small percentage of women receive no prenatal care at all, and approximately one woman in four does not receive care until the fourth month of pregnancy.

Immunizations

Each of the major childhood infections that are preventable by immunization can cause permanent disability and death. Before a recent federal and state campaign in 1977 known as the Childhood Immunization Initiative, more than a third of all children under the age of 15 were not fully protected. Effective use of vaccines, disease surveillance, and containment of outbreak can control these diseases. In fact, the complete elimination of measles has been set as a national goal.

Sexually Transmitted Diseases

In one recent year there were an estimated 10 million cases of sexually transmitted diseases. Vaccines to prevent these diseases do not currently exist. An effective approach to control will require the cooperative efforts of clinics, physicians, public health departments, schools, and employers.

High Blood Pressure Control

Hypertension, affecting one in six Americans, is a primary risk factor associated with the half million strokes and 1 to 2 million heart attacks that occur annually. Generally, hypertension cannot be cured but effective treatment is available to control blood pressure. Because high blood pressure is often asymptomatic many people discontinue their medication, thereby allowing the situation to serve as a risk factor for the cardiovascular diseases that kill nearly as many people in this country as all other causes combined.

Promoting Healthy Life-styles

The final group of activities deal with individual and community efforts to promote healthful life-styles. Reducing even a few of the risk factors can have a tremendous effect on the health of the nation. The factors in question not only promote well-being but also require no outlay of money. In fact, implementation of the following health behaviors often saves the individual from spending money in an attempt to "purchase" good health.

Smoking Cessation

Cigarette smoking is the largest preventable cause of disease and premature death, being associated with cardiovascular diseases; cancers of the lung, larynx, pharynx, mouth, esophagus, pancreas, and bladder; respiratory infections and emphysema; stomach ulcers; and retarded fetal growth among smoking mothers. In all, tobacco is associated with about 320,000 premature deaths a year. If there were no smokers among us, coronary deaths could be reduced by 30%, saving more than 200,000 lives a year. Because smoking is a voluntary behavior, theoretically, all of the consequences are preventable.

Reducing Misuse of Alcohol and Drugs

Alcohol misuse is a factor in more than 10% of all deaths in this country. It is associated with greater risk of traffic accidents; cirrhosis; cancer of the liver, esophagus, and mouth; homicide, suicide, and violence; and birth defects among children born to drinking mothers. It is estimated that there are 10 million adult alcoholics and problem drinkers, affecting another 40 million family members.

Improved Nutrition

Food choices are influenced by a host of complex factors. In this country malnutrition is largely a function of overeating and of poor choices rather than a function of having too little to eat. A substantial portion of men and women are obese, a condition that is clearly related to diabetes and high blood pressure. Americans can achieve better health by reducing caloric intake of saturated fat and cholesterol, salt, and sugar and increasing the intake of whole grains, cereals, fruits, vegetables, fish, poultry, and legumes.

Exercise and Fitness

A decline in physical fitness has been the result of an increasingly sedentary life-style. Over the past several years, however, America has witnessed a resurgence of interest in exercise and fitness. Energetic recreational activities, and especially jogging, have become extremely popular. The physiologic and psychologic benefits are tremendous, not only because they diminish one's risk of becoming ill but also because they enhance the quality of life.

Stress Control

Stress has been shown to be a precipitating factor in dozens of illnesses, and may be a causal factor in all diseases. Factors able to mitigate the effects of stress include strong social support among family, friends and community; a strong and positive self-concept; an ability to solve problems through the careful selection of alternatives; and the use of one of the many available techniques that help the individual to relax.

Federal Health Information Clearinghouses

This information is reprinted from *Focal Points*, U.S. Department of Health and Human Services, U.S.P.H.S., Centers for Disease Control, Bureau of Health Education, Washington, D.C., 1980, U.S. Government Printing Office.

The federal government has established a National Health Information Clearinghouse. A project of the OHP, it was established to help the general public and health professionals find appropriate sources of health information. Services of the clearinghouse include:

- A data base containing entries on health-related organizations and programs throughout the country.
- An inquiry and referral system that allows the clearinghouse staff to refer inquiries to the most appropriate resource and allow the resource to respond directly to the inquirer.
- Access to information through a toll-free telephone number (800) 336-4797 (in Virginia call-(703) 522-2590); through the mail, P.O. Box 1133, Washington, D.C., 20013, or by appointment to visit the clearinghouse at 1555 Wilson Boulevard, Suite 600, Rosslyn Va. 22209.
- Occasional invitational forums to promote the exchange of information and stimulate discussion of key health issues.

Files at the clearinghouse are kept for each organization, with copies of materials about the organization, a fact sheet, a publications list, and copies of annual reports. Subject area files hold publications on specific topics, and a small library, including periodicals, is maintained. The library is open to the public by appointment.

Inquiries by phone or mail are answered with material directly from the clearinghouse or a notice of referral to other organizations. Copies of the response are sent to any agency being referred to so that agencies can respond directly to the inquirer and will know where else the query has been sent.

In addition to responding to inquiries, the clearinghouse staff is preparing several publications. A directory, *Health Information Resources in the Department of Health and Human Services*, was recently published and can be obtained free by writing to the clearinghouse. In the near future a poster giving important health-related telephone numbers will be available free on request. A resource guide on health risk appraisal instruments and a directory of organizations that provide information on fitness activities are in preparation. A listing of selected Federal Health Information Clearinghouses is reproduced below.

Aging

National Clearinghouse on Aging
330 Independence Avenue S.W.
Washington, DC 20201
(212) 245-2158

Provides access to information and referral services that assist the older American in obtaining services. Distributes Administration on Aging publications.

Alcohol

National Clearinghouse for Alcohol Information (NCALI)
P.O. Box 2345
Rockville, MD 20852
(301) 468-2600

Gathers and disseminates current knowledge on alcohol-related subjects.

Arthritis

Arthritis Information Clearinghouse
P.O. Box 34427
Bethesda, MD 20034
(301) 881-9411

Identifies materials concerned with arthritis and related musculoskeletal diseases and serves as an information exchange for individuals and organizations involved in public, professional, and patient education. Refers personal requests from patients to the Arthritis Foundation.

Cancer

Cancer Information Clearinghouse
National Cancer Institute, Office of Cancer Communications
9000 Rockville Pike, Building 31, Room 10A18
Bethesda, MD 20205
(301) 496-4070

Collects and disseminates information on public, patient, and professional cancer education materials to organizations and health care professionals.

Office of Cancer Communications (OCC), Public Inquiries Section
Building 31, Room 10A18
9000 Rockville Pike
Bethesda, MD 20205
(301) 496-5583

Answers requests for cancer information from patients and the general public.

Child Abuse

Clearinghouse on Child Abuse and Neglect Information
P.O. Box 1182
Washington, DC 20013
(202) 755-0590

Collects, processes, and disseminates information on child abuse and neglect.

Consumer Information

Consumer Information Center
Pueblo, CO 81009
(202) 566-1794

Distributes consumer publications on topics such as children, food and nutrition, health, exercise, and weight control. The *Consumer Information Catalog* is available free from the center and must be used to identify publications being requested.

Diabetes

National Diabetes Information Clearinghouse
805 15th Street, N.W., Suite 500
Washington, DC 20005
(202) 842-7630

Collects and disseminates information on patient education materials and coordinates the development of materials and programs for diabetes education.

Digestive Diseases

National Digestive Diseases Education and Information Clearinghouse
1555 Wilson Boulevard, Suite 600
Rosslyn, VA 22209
(703) 522-0870

Provides information of digestive diseases to health professionals and consumers.

Domestic Violence

National Clearinghouse on Domestic Violence
P.O. Box 2309
Rockville, MD 20852
(301) 251-5172

Serves as a central resource for information on the problems and issues of domestic violence. Collects and disseminates information in the areas of sexual abuse in the family, psychological studies on domestic violence, counseling the abused and abuser, program management, prevention, acute medical services, and community networking.

Drug Abuse

National Clearinghouse for Drug Abuse Information
P.O. Box 416
Kensington, MD 20795
(301) 443-6500

Collects and disseminates information on drug abuse. Produces informational materials on drugs, drug abuse, and prevention.

Emergency Medical Services

National Clearinghouse for Emergency Medical Services
P.O. Box 911
Rockville, MD 20852
(301) 436-6267

Gathers and disseminates information on emergency medical services for accidents and other medical emergencies.

Family Plannng

National Clearinghouse for Family Planning Information
P.O. Box 2225
Rockville, MD 20852
(301) 881-9400

Collects family planning materials, makes referrals to other information centers, and produces and distributes materials. Primary audience is federally funded family planning clinics.

Food Drug

Food and Drug Administration (FDA)
Office for Consumer Communications
5600 Fishers Lane,
Room 15B-32, (HFE-88).
Rockville, MD 20857
(301) 443-3170

Answers consumers inquiries for the FDA and serves as a clearinghouse for their consumer publications.

Food Nutrition

Food and Nutrition Information Center (FNIC)
National Agricultural Library Building,
Room 304
Beltsville, MD 20705
(301) 344-3719

Serves the information needs of persons interested in human nutrition, food service management, and food technology. Acquires and lends books, journal articles, and audiovisual materials dealing with these areas of concern.

Genetic Diseases

National Clearinghouse for Human Genetic Diseases
805 15th Street, Suite 500
Washington, DC 20005
(202) 842-7617

Provides information on human genetics and genetic diseases for both patients and health care workers and reviews existing curricular materials on genetic education.

Handicapped

Clearinghouse on the Handicapped
330 "C" Street, S.W.
Washington, DC 20202
(202) 245-0080

Responds to inquiries from handicapped individuals and serves as a resource to organizations that supply information to, and about handicapped individuals.

Health Education

Bureau of Health Education (BHE)
1600 Clifton Road, Building 14
Atlanta, GA 30333
(404) 329-3235

Provides leadership and program direction for the prevention of disease, disability, premature death, and undesirable and unnecessary health problems through health education. Inquiries on health education can be directed to BHE.

Health Indexes

Clearinghouse on Health Indexes National Center for Health Statistics
Division of Analysis
3700 East-West Highway
Hyattsville, MD 20782
(301) 436-7035

Provides informational assistance in the development of health measures to health researchers, administrators and planners.

Health Information

National Health Information Clearinghouse (NHIC)
P.O. Box 1133
Washington, DC 20013
(703) 522-2590 in VA
(800) 336-4797

Helps the public locate health information through identification of health information resources and an inquiry and referral system. Health questions are referred to appropriate health resources that, in turn, respond directly to inquirers.

Health Planning

National Health Planning Information Center (NHPIC)
3700 East-West Highway,
Room 6-50
Hyattsville, MD 20782
(301) 436-6736

Provides information for use in analysis of issues and problems related to health planning and resource development. Limits information services to the Health Systems Agencies and the State Health Planning and Development Agencies.

Health Standards

National Health Standards and Quality Information Clearinghouse (NHSQIC)
11301 Rockville Pike
Kensington, MD 20795
(301) 881-9400

Collects materials concerning standards for health care and health facilities, qualifications of health professionals, and evaluation and certification of health care providers serving federal beneficiaries. While free to federal agency personnel, searches are billed at cost to other requesters.

High Blood Pressure

High Blood Pressure Information Center
120-80 National Institutes of Health
Bethesda, MD 20205
(301) 652-7700

Provides information on the detection, diagnosis, and management of high blood pressure to consumers and health professionals.

Injuries

National Injury Information Clearinghouse
5401 Westbard Avenue,
Room 625
Washington, DC 20207
(301) 492-6424

Collects and disseminates injury data and information relating to the causes and prevention of death, injury, and illness associated with consumer products. Requests of a general nature are referred to the Consumer Product Safety Commission's Communications Office.

Mental Health

National Clearinghouse for Mental Health Information
Public Inquiries Section
5600 Fishers Lane,
Room 11A-21
Rockville, MD 20857
(301) 443-4513

Acquires and abstracts the world's mental health literature, answers inquiries from the public, and provides computer searches for the scientific and academic communities.

Occupational Safety

Clearinghouse for Occupational Safety and Health Information
4676 Columbia Parkway
Cincinnati, OH 45226
(513) 684-8326

Provides technical information support for National Institute for Occupational Safety and Health research programs and supplies information to others on request.

Physical Fitness

President's Council on Physical Fitness and Sports
Washington, DC 20201
(202) 755-7478

Conducts a public service advertising program and cooperates with governmental and private groups to promote the development of physical fitness leadership, facilities, and programs. Produces informational materials on exercise, school physical education programs, sports, and physical fitness for youth, adults, and the elderly.

Poison Control

Division of Poison Control (FDA)
5600 Fishers Lane
Rockville, MD 20857
(301) 443-6260

Works with the national network of 600 poison control centers to reduce the incidence and severity of acute poisoning. Directs toxic emergency calls to a local poison control center.

Additional information about various health promotion and disease prevention activities is available from a number of sources. Both government agencies and private, non-profit groups are listed. These agencies and organizations comprise only a portion of the total possible sources. Many other qualified sources of such information exist, including State and local health agencies which generally provide a comprehensive repository of consumer-oriented health information. Most groups listed offer free or low cost literature.

Preventive Health Services*
Family Planning
Planned Parenthood Federation of America, Inc.
810 Seventh Avenue
New York, New York 10019
(212) 541-7800

---

*This material is reprinted from *Healthy people, the surgeon general's report on health promotion and disease prevention*, U.S. Department of Health, Education, and Welfare, U.S. Public Health Service, Pub. No. 79-55071, Washington, D.C., 1979, U.S. Government Printing Office.

National Family Planning and Reproductive Health Association, Inc.
Suite 350
425 Thirteenth Street, N.W.
Washington, D.C. 20004
(202) 783-1560

American College of Obstetricians and Gynecologists
Resource Center
Suite 2700
1 East Wacker Drive
Chicago, Illinois 60601
(312) 222-1600

National Clearinghouse for Family Planning Information
6110 Executive Blvd., Suite 250
Rockville, Maryland 29852
(301) 881-9400

Pregnancy and Infant Care
Office of Maternal and Child Health
Program Services Branch
Bureau of Community Health Services
Health Services Administration
Room 7A20, Parklawn
5600 Fishers Lane
Rockville, Maryland 20857
(301) 443-4273

National Foundation—March of Dimes
Public Health Education Department
1275 Mamaroneck Avenue
White Plains, New York 10605
(914) 428-7100

American College of Obstetricians and Gynecologists
Resource Center
Suite 2700
1 East Wacker Drive
Chicago, Illinois 60601
(312) 222-1600

American Academy of Pediatrics
1801 Hinman Avenue
Evanston, Illinois 60204
(312) 869-4255

Immunizations
Centers for Disease Control
Bureau of State Services
Technical Information Services
Centers for Disease Control
Atlanta, Georgia 30333
(404) 452-4021

National Institute of Child Health and Human Development
Office of Research Reporting
Room 2A34, Building 31
National Institutes of Health
Bethesda, Maryland 20205
(301) 496-5133

Sexually Transmissible Diseases
Centers for Disease Control
Bureau of State Services
Technical Information Services
Centers for Disease Control
Atlanta, Georgia 30333
(404) 452-4021

American Social Health Association
260 Sheridan Avenue
Palo Alto, California 94306
(415) 321-5134

VD National Hot Line
260 Sheridan Avenue
Palo Alto, California 94306
(800) 227-8922

High Blood Pressure and Heart Disease
National High Blood Pressure Information Center
Suite 1300
7910 Woodmont Avenue
Bethesda, Maryland 20014
(301) 652-7700

National Heart, Lung, and Blood Institute
Public Inquiries Office
Room 4A21, Building 31
National Institutes of Health
Bethesda, Maryland 20205
(301) 496-4236

American Heart Association
7320 Greenville Avenue
Dallas, Texas 75231
(214) 750-5300
(or local chapters)

Consumer Information Center
Consumer Information Center
Pueblo, Colorado 81009
(303) 544-5277, ext. 370

Health Protection

Toxic Agent Control

Centers for Disease Control
Chronic Diseases Division
Bureau of Epidemiology
Building 1, Room 5127
Centers for Disease Control
Atlanta, Georgia 30333
(404) 329-3165

Environmental Protection Agency
Office of Public Awareness
Environmental Protection Agency
401 M Street, S.W.
Mail Code: A-107
Washington, D.C. 20460
(202) 755-0700

National Institute of Environmental Health Sciences
National Institutes of Health
Post Office Box 12233
Research Triangle Park, North Carolina 27709
(919) 541-3345

American Lung Association
1740 Broadway
New York, New York 10019
(212) 245-8000
(or local chapter)

Occupational Safety and Health

Occupational Safety and Health Administration
Office of Public and Consumer Affairs
U.S. Department of Labor (Room N3637)
200 Constitution Avenue, N.W.
Washington, D.C. 20210
(202) 523-8151

Clearinghouse for Occupational Safety and Health
National Institute for Occupational Safety and Health
Centers for Disease Control
Robert A. Taft Laboratory
4676 Columbia Parkway
Cincinnati, Ohio 45226
(513) 684-8326

National Safety Council
444 North Michigan Avenue
Chicago, Illinois 60611
(312) 527-4800

American Industrial Hygiene Association
475 Wolf Ledges Parkway
Akron, Ohio 44311
(216) 762-7294

American Occupational Medical Association
Suite 2240
150 North Wacker Drive
Chicago, Illinois 60606
(312) 782-2166

Accidental Injury Control
Consumer Product Safety Commission
Consumer Education and Awareness Division
5401 Westbard Avenue
Washington, D.C. 20207
(202) 492-6576
(or local Poison Control Centers)

Department of Transportation
General Services Division (NAD-42)
National Highway Traffic Safety Administration
Department of Transportation
400 Seventh Street, S.W. (Room 4423)
Washington, D.C. 20590
(202) 426-0874
ATTN: E. Kitts

National Safety Council
444 North Michigan Avenue
Chicago, Illinois 60611
(312) 527-4800

American Red Cross
National Headquarters
18th and E Streets, N.W.
Washington, D.C. 20006
(202) 857-3555

Community Water Supply Fluoridation
Centers for Disease Control
Dental Disease Prevention Activity (E107)
Centers for Disease Control
Atlanta, Georgia 30333
(404) 262-6631

National Institute of Dental Research
Public Inquiries Office
Room 2C34, Building 31
National Institutes of Health
Bethesda, Maryland 20205
(301) 496-4261

American Dental Association
Bureau of Health Education and Audiovisual Services
American Dental Association
211 East Chicago Avenue
Chicago, Illinois 60611
(312) 440-2593

Infectious Agent Control
Centers for Disease Control
Public Inquiries
Management Analysis and Service Office
Building 4, Room B2
Centers for Disease Control
Atlanta, Georgia 30333
(404) 329-3534

National Institute of Allergy and Infectious Diseases
Office of Research Reporting and Public Response
Room 7A32, Building 31
National Institutes of Health
Bethesda, Maryland 20205
(301) 496-5717

Health Promotion
Smoking Cessation
Technical Information Center for Smoking and Health
Office on Smoking and Health
Department of Health, Education, and Welfare
Room 1-16, Park Building
5600 Fishers Lane
Rockville, Maryland 20857
(301) 443-1690

Office of Cancer Communications
National Cancer Institute
Room 10A18, Building 31
National Institutes of Health
Bethesda, Maryland 20205
(301) 496-5583

American Cancer Society
Public Information Department
777 Third Avenue
New York, New York 10017
(212) 371-2900, ext. 254
(or local chapter)

American Lung Association
1740 Broadway
New York, New York 10019
(212) 245-8000
(or local chapter)

American Heart Association
7320 Greenville Avenue
Dallas, Texas 75231
(214) 750-5300
(or local chapter)

Reducing Misuse of Alcohol and Drugs
National Clearinghouse on Alcohol Information
Post Office Box 2345
Rockville, Maryland 20852
(301) 468-2600

National Clearinghouse on Drug Abuse Information
Room 10A53, Parklawn Building
5600 Fishers Lane
Rockville, Maryland 20857
(301) 443-6500

National Council on Alcoholism
733 Third Avenue
New York, New York 10017
(212) 986-4433

Alcoholics Anonymous
General Services Office (6th Floor)
468 Park Avenue South
New York, New York 10016
(212) 686-1100
ATTN: Public Information Department

Improved Nutrition
Food and Drug Administration
Office of Consumer Communications (HFG-10)
Food and Drug Administration
Room 15B32, Parklawn Building
5600 Fishers Lane
Rockville, Maryland 20857
(301) 443-3170

U.S. Department of Agriculture
Human Nutrition Center SEA
Room 421A
U.S. Department of Agriculture
Washington, D.C. 20250
(202) 447-7854

Consumer Information Center
Consumer Information Center
Pueblo, Colorado 81009
(303) 544-5277, ext. 370

Nutrition Foundation
Suite 300
888 Seventeenth Street, N.W.
Washington, D.C. 20006
(202) 872-0778

National Nutrition Education Clearinghouse
Suite 1110
2140 Shattuck Avenue
Berkeley, California 94704
(415) 548-1363

Exercise and Fitness
President's Council on Physical Fitness and Sports
Department of Health, Education and Welfare
Room 3030 Donohoe Building
400 Sixth Street, S.W.
Washington, D.C. 20201
(202) 755-7947

American Alliance for Health, Physical Education, Recreation, and Dance
Promotions Unit
1201 Sixteenth Street, N.W.
Washington, D.C. 20036
(202) 833-5534

American College of Sports Medicine
1440 Monroe Street
Madison, Wisconsin 53706
(608) 262-3632

Stress Control
National Clearinghouse for Mental Health Information
National Institute of Mental Health
Room 11A33, Parklawn Building
5600 Fishers Lane
Rockville, Maryland 20857
(301) 443-4517

Mental Health Association
1800 North Kent Street
Arlington, Virginia 22209
(or local chapters)
(703) 528-6405

Public Affairs Committee, Inc.
Room 1101
381 Park Avenue South
New York, New York 10016
(212) 683-4331

Blue Cross and Blue Shield Associations
Public Relations Office
840 North Lake Shore Drive
Chicago, Illinois 60611
(312) 440-5955

Public Health Service
Bureau of Health Education
Building 14
Centers for Disease Control
Atlanta, Georgia 30333
(404) 320-3111

Office of Health Information and Health Promotion
Office of the Surgeon General
Department of Health, Education, and Welfare (Room 721B HHH)
200 Independence Avenue, S.W.
Washington, D.C.
(202) 472-5370

National Organizations
National Association of Community Health Centers, Inc.
Suite 420
1625 Eye Street, N.W.
Washington, D.C. 20006
(202) 833-9280

National Center for Health Education
211 Sutter Street (4th Floor)
San Francisco, California 94108
(415) 781-6144

State and Local Levels
Contact your family physician
Contact your local health department
Contact your county's cooperative extension service

Sample Worksite Health Promotion Programs

On March 16 to 18, 1981, representatives of nearly 60 insurance companies met for the first industry-wide conference on health education and promotion. One aspect of the conference invited selected representatives from industry to discuss existing health promotion programs at their respective places of employment. Several program descriptions presented by these representatives are offered in this appendix.

Ford Motor Company
Beverly G. Ware, Dr. P.H., Corporate Coordinator, Health Education Programs
In 1971, at a time when health care costs were already beginning to escalate, the Employee Insurance Department of Ford Motor Company commissioned a study to determine the sources of rising costs. A random sample of eight hundred salaried persons in the world headquarters complex of Ford Motor Company was used to examine the costs and nature of medical incidents over a two-year period. A key finding was that coronary heart disease represented 29% of the total costs, close to 1.5 million dollars each year, but only 1.5% of the total medical incidents.

A recommendation of this study was to urge the development of programs designed to prevent the occurrence of myocardial infarctions, the major cost incident. It was predicted that at least one-half million dollars might be saved by prevention through early identification of persons with risk, and subsequent risk reduction.

The earliest program was in effect from 1972 to 1974, and consisted of a screening protocol and questionnaires designed to assess risk. Subsequent appropriate interventions consisted primarily of personal counseling and group behavior modification. The staff consisted of a health educator and a dietician.

In 1976, the program was revised and reinitiated. The program goal remains to reduce the incidence of heart disease and the ensuing disability. Objectives of the program are: 1) determine the feasibility of a cardiovascular risk intervention program within the workplace; 2) design an educational intervention that is cost effective and reliable, and 3) demonstrate to the company the cost benefit of the program.

The program consists of recruitment followed with screening performed by nurses in early morning hours in the medical department. Screening procedures include blood pressure, skinfold, height, weight, pulse, HDL and cholesterol measurements, as well as a questionnaire which assesses personal/family history and smoking habits. On the basis of these results, individuals are placed into one of five risk categories ranging from lowest risk to high risk. Those at lowest risk receive a personalized letter containing their assessment results and risk reduction advice. Those at highest risk are referred to physicians. Those intermediate between these risk categories are invited to participate in group interventions. One series of five sessions is held once a week

From Kotz, H.J., and Fielding, J.E.: Health Education and promotion, agenda for the eighties. A summary of an Insurance Industry Conference on Health Education and Promotion, Atlanta, Ga., March 16-18, 1980, New York, 1980, American Council of Life Insurance and Health Insurance Association of America.

outside of work hours. These sessions address such issues as the meaning of risk factors, proper diet and weight control, proper exercise, and control of blood pressure and stress. Those who smoke are invited to participate in a four-session smoking cessation program followed by a maintenance program.

As of October, 1979, 1,537 new screens had been performed. Forty-five percent of those persons were classified as either moderate or high risk. Fifty percent of those screened were overweight, thirty percent had elevated cholesterol levels, thirty percent were smokers and ten percent had elevated blood pressure.

Although the program is popular among employees, very little data are available on the cost effectiveness and cost benefits of the program. Much more thorough evaluation is now underway, including a health care cost and benefit study by the systems staff of the Finance Department, and comparison of participants in intervention groups with a matched sample of participants not volunteering for group sessions.

Keys for future health promotion program development include the following: 1) support from top management as well as participants, 2) specific measurable outcomes, 3) creation of interest in participation by focusing on existing needs and program accessibility, and 4) planning for cost containment.

Johnson and Johnson
Gene E. Hollen, Vice-President, Special Products, Corporate Staff

The Johnson and Johnson Health Promotion Program was conceived when James E. Burke, Chairman of the Board of Johnson and Johnson, became concerned about the rising cost of health care to the Corporation. He stated two goals for the program: 1) to provide the means for Johnson and Johnson employees to become the healthiest in the world, and 2) to control and reduce the spiraling illness and accident costs to the Corporation. He also felt that, as one of the world's leading health care products companies, Johnson and Johnson had a responsibility to its consumers, the industry and the nation to pioneer the emerging concepts in health promotion that could have a long-range effect upon the health of our nation.

With projections of the nation's health care costs reaching $1 trillion by the year 2000, and with the fact that corporations pay about 40 percent of this bill, it is difficult to see how health care, as we know it today, will be affordable in the future.

The magnitude of the potential offered by effective lifestyle improvement was another clear stimulus for putting into operation the "Live for Life" program at Johnson and Johnson. The target of the program was primarily cardiovascular disease and the poor lifestyles that contribute to that disease. The program emphasizes pirmary prevention, and was developed under the following guidelines:

First, the program should emphasize health and the benefits of being well. Striving for wellness means that we are alive, vital and challenged.

Second, the program had to be accepted gradually; a slow build up rather than a campaign effort that would peak quickly and then die out.

Third, the program had to be based on sound scientific information. The credibility of the information had to be established and the employees educated as to the possible harm in inaccurate information.

Fourth, the results needed to be measurable in order to determine changes in health and the economic benefit of those changes.

Last is the need for personal employee involvement to actually bring about lifestyle changes.

To implement this philosophy, interested employees were invited to form a leadership group to design and implement the "Live for Life" program. The staff of the Live for Life Institute helped the leadership group organize into task forces to change the work environment so that it was more conducive to individual employee lifestyle change. For example, the nutrition and weight loss task force worked in the company cafeteria to improve the healthfulness of the food. They introduced a salad bar, a breakfast program, and fresh fruit for dessert. They reduced the display of junk foods, and encouraged more fish and fowl to be served and less beef. The exercise task force emphasized aerobic fitness and offered classes in aerobics to music, jazz dancing, volleyball, badminton, and other special programs. The substance abuse task force developed smoking and alcohol policies. The stress task force provided a "quiet" room and stress reduction tapes for employees. The publicity task force published a newspaper on the program and also coordinated the annual banquet for the leadership group.

Once the leadership group has changed the work environment to support lifestyle changes, they invited their fellow employees to participate in the program, which consists of the following steps:

First, employees are asked to complete a 93-item lifestyle questionnaire.

Next, they undergo a health screen which measures height, weight, blood pressure, cholesterol and HDL.

One month later, employees attend a lifestyle seminar in which the results of their health screens are distributed in the form of a lifestyle profile. This instrument describes their current health status, and defines those changes that should be made to improve their health status.

Employees are then asked to join action groups which concentrate on a specific change, such as smoking, weight reduction, exercise, nutrition or stress reduction. Action groups of approximately ten participants are led by a professional through a course that meets once a week for eight to ten weeks. As employees complete one action group, they may sign up for another.

To date, the results of the action groups have been excellent. The weight loss has averaged about 13 pounds per participant; some smoking groups have had as high as 100% success; and the stress groups have successfully taught more than 70% of their participants to relax effectively.

The initial enthusiasm of the employees suggests that the program is considered to be a highly desirable benefit. The "Live for Life" program has enhanced employee morale and improved communications. Research to determine cost benefit and cost effectiveness is in progress.

Kimberly-Clark Corporation
Robert E. Dedmon, M.D., F.A.C.P., Staff Vice-President, Medical Affairs

The goal of Kimberly-Clark's Health Management Program is to achieve a higher level of wellness among employees and thereby improve productivity and reduce absenteeism and health care costs. Longer term objectives are to reduce the prevalence of cardiovascular disease risk factors and ultimately the incidence of coronary heart disease.

Principal program components include, first, a computerized medical history and health hazard appraisal, multiphasic screening (including hemoglobin, fasting blood sugar, triglycerides, HDL and total cholesterol, liver function and urinalysis) and physical examination (including blood pressure and skinfold thickness measurements, spirometry, chest x-ray, electrocardiogram, audiometry, visual testing, homoccult tests, and proctoscopic examinations on all employees over 40 years of age), and an exercise test using either the Bruce treadmill protocol or the YMCA bicycle ergometer protocol. These procedures are followed with a personal health review by a physician or nurse practitioner. At this review, the employee receives a health prescription addressing the particular health problems that he/she manifests.

Prescribed interventions include an aerobic exercise program carried out in the Kimberly-Clark exercise facility, which provides a swimming pool, 100-meter jogging track, exercise equipment, sauna, whirlpool and shower/locker facilities. Participants may engage in jogging, swimming, stationary cycling, cardiac rehabilitation, aerobic dancing, rope jumping, or a water exercise class, as their needs and interests dictate.

Health education classes are offered in the areas of diet management, the meaning of risk factors, smoking control, cancer, breast self-examination, high blood pressure, low back pain, basic life support and stress reduction. Employees with an alcohol or chemical dependency are referred to an Employee Assistance Program that addresses these problems specifically.

To date, over 90% of salaried employees have had multiphasic screening and exercise tests, about 50% have attended exercise orientations, and 25% currently use the exercise facility.

Hypertension was found in 9.6% of male and 3.7% of female employees. Elevated serum cholesterol was found in 45% of male and 35% of female employees. About 15% of employees had abnormal ST segment response to treadmill exercise, 22.6% of male and 14.4% of female employees had at least two risk factors for coronary heart disease, and 4.6% of males and 1.8% of females had at least three risk factors.

Significant reductions in blood pressure and triglycerides have occurred along with a significant increase in treadmill time, but no significant change has yet occurred in weight, percent body fat, total or HDL cholesterol in the first small group of employees re-tested. About 65% of referred employees have been successfully rehabilitated through the Employee Assistance Program. No definite impact on health care costs or absenteeism has been observed thus far. A ten year study of these two work related variables is in progress.

Kimberly-Clark's experience has identified several key points to be considered in planning an employee health promotion:

1. The crucial role of the chief executive officer and other senior management, the corporate medical director, and occupational health nurses in making health promotion programs effective.
2. The importance of persuasive, medically valid, well-designed, clearly presented and attractive communications in motivating employees to participate in the program.
3. The application of educational diagnosis and evaluation with specific, practical and achievable behavioral objectives for the program.
4. The development of simple user run and managed information and data systems which provide clear and meaningful information to be used for program evaluation and management decision making.
5. Cooperation in sharing data, experience and ideas among companies.
6. Training programs for health educators, occupational physicians, nurses, and managers in effective health education strategies and survey and outcome evaluation techniques.
7. Mini-screening and maxi-intervention and the need to constantly re-evaluate yield and cost effectiveness of various screening tests.
8. Achieving involvement and support of local employees' personal physicians as reinforcement for implementation and maintenance of behavior change.

Kimberly-Clark's Health Management Program experience to date is consistent with the above points. It is also important to view a health promotion program as part of a company's total health care cost containment efforts. Such programs also support and give credibility to senior management objectives of showing real concern and respect for the health needs of employees. Effectively helping people to achieve their normal life expectancy as healthy, motivated and productive citizens is the real bottom line.

SAFECO Life Insurance Company
Roger Butz, M.D., Vice-President, Individual Department and Medical Director

SAFECO's motivation for starting a health promotion program is clear: As a life insurance company it is vitally interested in effective measures that promote health and prolong life. The program is based upon four main principles:

1. The program must be universally applicable to all employees.
2. The data compiled as a result of the program must be kept strictly confidential.
3. The program must be non-medical.
4. The results of the program must be measurable, which involves defining goals and taking baseline measurements at the beginning of the program.

SAFECO's health promotion program, called SHAPE, begins with a voluntary questionnaire that is quick, simple and assesses certain health habits, attitudes and behaviors. It includes a 24-hour dietary recall, as well as specific questions on height, weight, pulse rate and exercise and smoking habits. From the results of this questionnaire, a Health Quality Profile is prepared for each participant which rates him or her on a scale from 1 to 100 according to smoking habits, weight, exercise habits, pulse rate and percentage of fat in food. With this profile, the participant is given a health notebook with educational information regarding the above parameters as well as information on stress reduction. It is a goal clarifying kit, with a written exercise that involves the participant in setting his or her own health goals, and helps the individual make specific plans that will facilitate reaching these goals. The notebook makes use of already available materials on health promotion and education, including a copy of Kenneth Cooper's book on aerobic exercise. It includes a pocket calorie counter to permit calculation of total caloric intake and percentage of fat in food. Colorful calendars and charts enable the participants to measure progress toward stated goals.

In addition, the SHAPE program publishes a monthly newsletter that provides professional comment of such topics as smoking, diet and exercise. One of the most attractive features of the SHAPE program is its low cost, which is approximately $25 per participant, including a one-year subscription to the Newsletter.

The SHAPE program has enjoyed enthusiastic acceptance and participation. Results of the effect of the program on outcomes such as absenteeism and productivity are pending.

SAFECO's experience suggests four basic principles which should be considered when developing an employee health promotion program:

1. The program must suit the particular goals and constraints represented by personnel policy, geographic limitation, etc.
2. The program must have clear objectives.
3. The program must be carefully planned and budgeted.
4. The program managers must exercise strict objectivity in establishing benchmarks for measuring results.

In summary, similarities and differences can be observed in program components and implementation strategies in each of the four model programs. Each worksite setting presents various needs, interests and resources that must be considered when developing a work-site health promotion program. Because of these situation specific differences, it would be unrealistic to expect that any two work-site health promotion programs be identical in content and process. As previously stated, work-site health promotion programming requires careful and thorough assessment and planning in the very initial stages of program development. This step will serve to identify employee interest in participation and management expectations as well as give indication of attainable and measurable program goals and objectives.

Appendix F

Employee Health Promotion Resource List

This resource list* is presented to serve as a starting place for individuals interested in identifying information concerning work-site health promotion.

Publications

Goldbeck, W.B., Egdahl, R.H., and Walsh, D.C., editors: Mental wellness programs for employees, New York, 1980, Springer-Verlag New York, Inc.

Egdhal, R.H., and Walsh, D.C., editors: Health services and health hazards: the employee's need to know, New York, 1978, Springer-Verlag New York, Inc.

The Egdahl/Walsh publications are available through the Boston University Center for Industry and Health Care, Boston University Health Policy Institute, 53 Bay State Road, Boston, MA 02215.

Employee Health–Fitness (monthly), 67 Peachtree Park Drive, N.E., Atlanta, GA 30309.

Erfurt, John C., and Foote, Andrea: Blood pressure control at the worksite. Manual of procedures for blood pressure control programs in industrial settings. Copies may be obtained from Worker Health Program, 401 Fourth Street, Ann Arbor, MI 48103.

Hospitals, October 1, 1979 (Health Promotion: A Special Issue).

Kotz, Heather J., M.D., M.P.H., and Fielding, Jonathan E., M.D., M.P.H., editors: Health education and promotion, Agenda for the Eighties. A Summary of an Insurance Industry Conference on Health Education and Promotion 1980. Available through the American Council of Life Insurance and Health Insurance Association of America, 1850 K Street, N.W., Washington, DC, 20006.

McGill, Alice M., Ph.D., editor: Proceedings of the National Conference on Health Promotion Programs in Occupational Settings, January 17-19, 1979. U.S. Department of Health, Education and Welfare. For sale by the Superintendent of Documents, U.S. Government Printing Office, Washington, DC, 20402.

Parkinson, R.S., and associates: Managing health promotion in the work place: guidelines for implementation and evaluation, Palo Alto, CA, 1982, Mayfield Publishing Co.

Public Health Reports 95(2), March-April, 1980. (Special Section 1, Health Promotion at the Work Site.)

Sehnert, Keith W., M.D., and Tillotson, John K., M.D.: A national health care strategy: how business can promote good health for employees and their families, The National Chamber Foundation, 1615 M Street, N.W., Washington, DC 20062.

USDHHS, *Toward a Healthy Community,* Center Building, 3200 East-West Highway, Hyattsville, MD 20782.

Walsh, D.C., and Egdahl, R.H.: Payer, provider, consumer: industry confronts health care costs, New York, 1977, Springer-Verlag New York, Inc.

---

*Compiled by the Washington Business Group on Health, 922 Pennsylvania Avenue, S.E., Washington, DC 20003.

Corporations and Organizations

The American Association of Fitness Directors in Business and Industry (AAFDBI), Dennis L. Colacino, Ph.D. (1980-81, President), Pepsico Inc., Anderson Hill Road, Purchase, NY 10577.

The American Health Foundation, Richard Osborn, 320 East 43rd Street, New York, NY 10017.

The American Hospital Association, Center for Health Promotion, Ruth Behrens, Director, Lynn Dickey Jones, M.S., 840 North Lake Shore Drive, Chicago, IL 60611.

AT&T, Rebecca Parkinson, M.P.H., Basking Ridge, NJ 07920.

Armco, Inc., David Klaiber, Supervising Corporate Safety Engineer, 703 Curtis Street, Middletown, OH 45043. (The Armco Off-the-Job Safety Program is available for sale to other corporations and organizations.)

Association of Labor-Management, Administrators and Consultants on Alcoholism, 1800 North Kent Street, Suite 907, Arlington, VA 22209.

Bureau of Health Education Center for Disease Control, Horace G. Ogden, Director, 1600 Clifton Road, N.E., Atlanta, GA 30333.

Campbell Soup Corporation, Roland Wear, M.D., Medical Director, Campbell Place, Camden, NJ 08101.

Center for Health Enhancement Education and Research, Jonathan E. Fielding, M.D., M.P.H., Director, 924 Westwood Boulevard, University of California at Los Angeles, Los Angeles, CA 90024.

Citibank, Irvine H. Dearnley, Vice-President, 399 Park Avenue, New York, NY 10022.

Control Data Corporation, Barbara Merrill, P.O. Box 0, Minneapolis, MN 55440.

Ford Motor Company, Beverly G. Ware, Dr., P.H., Corporate Coordinator, Health Education Programs, 900 Parklane Towers West, 1 Parklane Boulevard, Dearborn, MI 48126.

HELP (Health Evaluation and Longevity Planning) Foundation, Glenn M. Friedman, M.D., Suite 203, 7300 Fourth Street, Scottsdale, AZ 85251.

Henroten Hospital, Tom Sanberg, Vice President, Marketing, 111 West Oak Street, Chicago, IL

Hospital Corporation of America, Holly Caldwell, One Park Place, Nashville, TN 37203.

IBM Corporation, Bob Beck, Director of Benefits and Personnel, 15 Old Orchard Road, Armonk, NY 10504.

The Johns-Manville Corporation, Paul Kotin, M.D., Senior Vice-President for Health, Safety, and the Environment, Kenlaryl Ranch, Denver, CO 80217.

The Pennsylvania State University, Health Education Department/Worksite Health Promotion Program, Richard St. Pierre, Chairman, 19 White Building, University Park, PA 16802.

Johnson & Johnson, John Rassweiller, M.D., 317 George Street, New Brunswick, NJ 08903.

Kansas Department of Health and Environment, Virginia Lockhart, Bureau of Health Education, Building 321, Forbes Field, Topeka, KS 66620.

Kimberly-Clark Corporation, Robert E. Dedmon, M.D., FACP, Staff Vice-President, Medical Affairs, 21100 Winchester Road, P.O. Box 999, Neenah, WI 54956.

Metropolitan Life Insurance Company, Clarence Pearson, Vice-President of Health and Safety, Andrew J.J. Brennan, Ph.D., Director, Center for Health Help, One Madison Avenue, New York, NY 10010.

Mobil Oil Corporation, Jack Bleuler, 150 East 42nd Street, Room 837, New York, NY 10017.

National Chemsearch, Inc., Janie Stowers, Fitness Director, P.O. Box 2170, Irving, TX 75060.

National Executive Services Corp., Frank Pace, President, 622 3rd Avenue, New York, NY 10017.

National Federation of Independent Business, James D. McKevitt, Legislative Office, 490 L'Enfant Plaza East, S.W., Washington, DC.

National Health Screening Council, 5161 River Road, Building #20, Washington, DC 20016.

Office of Health Information and Health Promotion, Department of Health and Human Services, Alice McGill, Ph.D., 200 Independence Avenue, S.W., Washington, DC 20201.

Professional Research, Inc., Rosalind C. Hawley, 441 Lexington Avenue, New York, NY 10017. (For information on Health Fairs.)

Prudential, Keith Fogle, Prudential Plaza 2-W, Newark, NJ 07101.

San Francisco Department of Public Health, Teri Dowling, Room 204, 101 Grove Street, San Francisco, CA 94102.

Sun Company, Harry Smith, 100 Matsonford Road, Radnor, PA 19087.

Washington Business Group on Health, Anne Kiefhaber, 922 Pennsylvania Avenue, S.E., Washington, DC 20003.

Xerox Corporation, Craig Wright, M.D., Director of Health Services, High Ridge Park 5-1, Stamford, CT 06904.

U.S. Chamber of Commerce, Jan Peter Ozga, H Street, N.W., Washington, DC.

Educational Materials Available from Three Voluntary Health Agencies

March of Dimes Birth Defects Foundation

Starting a Healthy Family

This is an interdisciplinary program that draws on the fields of medicine, community health, social science, and biology. Composed of four units for study at the junior and senior high school level, the program is intended to present the responsibilities of parenthood. The units explore the life changes that people face when becoming parents, adolescent sexuality, special needs of children, and health promotion during pregnancy to provide a healthy and safe environment for the fetus.

Parenthood Education Program

This program focuses on health care and nutrition during pregnancy. It is effective in serving the needs of school-age parents. The program can be used in junior and senior high schools, prenatal care clinics, hospitals, WIC sites and public health departments. A Spanish language version is also available.

The Curriculum Guide for Health Education: Nutrition

This project was prepared through a March of Dimes grant to the National Catholic Educational Association. The curriculum encourages students to design a personalized, balanced diet based on their own preferences for food. The four units include nutrition, consumer education, community resources, and the handicapped.

Healthy Mothers, Healthy Babies

This project is being carried out by a coalition of representatives from more than 50 agencies. Government, professional, and voluntary health organizations with a common interest in prenatal and infant health are working together to provide public education. Some of the activities are (1) publication of a newsletter to disseminate information, (2) development of a directory of educational materials, (3) posters, and (4) public service announcements narrated by the surgeon general and produced jointly by the March of Dimes and the U.S. Public Health Service.

American Heart Association

Putting Your Heart Into the Curriculum

This guide for teachers is actually a K-12 curriculum. It includes a detailed section on teaching methodology. Another 102-page section suggests creative learning activities, many of them designed to be used with American Heart Association educational materials. A third section of the guide offers suggested teacher resources, presented by topical area.

Heart Health Curriculum

This heart attack prevention program incorporates affective education as well as the traditional cognitive approach. The four modules include (1) body systems and functions, (2) diet and weight control, (3) fitness, and (4) prevention. Filmstrips, activity sheets, personal health logs, and supplementary materials are used to reinforce the objectives for each module.

School Health Packet

The Schools and Colleges Task Force of the Texas Affiliate developed materials for teacher use in cardiovascular health. The curriculum guide for elementary teachers and another one for secondary teachers includes concepts, subconcepts, suggested learning opportunities, and resources. A teacher's guide provides classroom games appropriate for grades K-12. Overhead transparencies explain the benefits of exercise. The children's cookbook offers healthy recipes that can be prepared by children.

American Cancer Society

Take Joy

This program is intended for elementary age students. The film portrays experiences familiar to most children while evoking positive feelings toward the systems of the body. The teacher's guide includes an overview of each system and a series of duplicating masters.

An Early Start to Good Health

This is a four-unit, multimedia package that promotes good health habits for children in grades K-3. Progressively, the units are entitled, "My Body," "My Self," "My Health," and "My Choice." Cartoon characters are used to encourage healthy attitudes. Each unit contains a musical sound filmstrip, a teaching guide with suggested lesson plans, a wall poster, and duplicating masters.

Health Network

This is a multimedia package for grades 4 to 6. The primary focus is on understanding one's responsibilities for good health. Each unit contains a sound filmstrip, teaching guide, wall poster or game, and several duplicating masters to be used with activities suggested in the teacher's guide.

Cancer Challenge to Youth

This teaching kit is designed to acquaint adolescents with factual information about cancer. It emphasizes personal responsibility for health. The kit includes a filmstrip, discussion questions and activities, student study sheets, a list of resources available from the American Cancer Society, a glossary, and pre- and post-tests.

Who's in Charge Here

A film for high school students that examines the immediate and long-term physical effects of smoking. A booklet encourages follow-up activities and offers related American Cancer Society resource materials. Correlated health content includes topics such as blood pressure, air pollution, stress, prenatal health, physiologic dependence, and peer pressure.

Voluntary agencies promote health through many of their own activities. Using a small paid staff and volunteer help they have undoubtedly contributed a great deal to the nation's health. A few examples will demonstrate this fact.

March of Dimes Birth Defect Foundation
• Financial support for neonatal intensive care units
• Development of hotlines between community hospitals and a major care facility
• Creation of genetic service units for diagnosis and counseling
• Establishment of an annual birth defects conference for medical personnel
• Sponsorship of an Institute on Education for responsible childbearing and a program for school administrators on the topic of adolescent pregnancy
• Publication of a birth defects compendium that is the most complete compilation available to physicians

- Development of the Birth Defects Information System, a 24-hour computerized system for physicians at 60 medical centers

American Heart Association

- Educational programs on hypertension published for the elderly, blacks, health care personnel and patients
- Development of guidelines for advanced cardiac life-support in high-density population areas such as stadiums and terminals
- Taking the initiative to develop programming about health on Saturday morning television
- Certification of individuals in cardiopulmonary resuscitation
- Production of the AHA Heart Book as a recording for the blind

American Cancer Society

- Financial support for comprehensive cancer centers that form a network for research, diagnosis, treatment, and rehabilitation
- Publication of *CA–A Journal for Clinicians*, which has a circulation of more than 380,000.
- Maintenance of the world's largest reference center for the collection and dissemination of unproven methods of cancer management
- Encouragment of support groups such as "Reach to Recovery" and the International Association of Laryngectomies
- Series of Cancer Prevention Studies to identify risk factors associated with cancer.

Index

A